Cardiac Pacing
and Defibrillation
in Pediatric and
Congenital Heart
Disease

Cardiac Pacing and Defibrillation in Paediatric and Congenital Heart Disease

EDITED BY

Maully Shah, MBBS, FACC, FHRS, CCDS, CEPS

The Children's Hospital of Philadelphia
Philadelphia, PA

Larry Rhodes, MD

West Virginia Univ. of Health Sciences
Morgantown, WV

Jonathan Kaltman, MD

National Heart, Lung, and Blood Institute
Bethesda, MD

WILEY Blackwell

This book is dedicated to my family, especially my parents who taught me that nothing is impossible, my husband Shaun for making everything possible, and my son Neil who reminds me every day of the endless possibilities that lie ahead.

I am deeply grateful to Dr. Larry Rhodes for his mentorship, Dr. K.M Cherian for believing in me when I emerged fresh out of fellowship, Dr. Frank Cecchin for imparting his exemplary technical skills, Dr. Paul M. Weinberg for his rigorous teachings of cardiac anatomy, and Dr. Victoria Vetter for her support in creating a Device Implantation & Lead Extraction program at The Children's Hospital of Philadelphia. I am also very grateful to my Division of Cardiology Chief, Dr. Robert Shaddy and Department of Pediatrics Chair, Dr. Joseph St. Geme for their support of a sabbatical which allowed me to complete this project. Last but not the least, this book is dedicated to the Cardiology and Electrophysiology fellows who motivate me every day to learn more and become a better teacher.

–Maully Shah

Thanks to Dr. Ed Walsh for teaching me Electrophysiology, Dr. Vickie Vetter for letting me practice Electrophysiology, my fellows for making Electrophysiology fun, and my family for putting up with me.

–Larry Rhodes

I would like to thank my mentors, Larry Rhodes and Gail Pearson, my EP colleagues and friends and most importantly, Becca, Maddie and Jacob.

–Jonathan Kaltman

Contents

Foreword, ix

List of Contributors, xi

Preface, xv

About the Companion Website, xvii

Part 1: Introduction

1 History of Cardiac Pacing and
   Defibrillation in the Young, 3
   Larry Rhodes and Robert Campbell

2 Clinically Relevant Basics of Pacing and
   Defibrillation, 12
   Maully Shah and Erick Cuvillier

Part 2: Clinical Concepts

3 Indications for Permanent Pacing,
   Device, and Lead Selection, 37
   *Philip M. Chang, Christopher Carter, and
   Yaniv Bar-Cohen*

4 Indications for Implantable
   Cardioverter Defibrillator Therapy,
   Device, and Lead Selection, 62
   Mitchell I. Cohen and Susan P. Etheridge

5 Hemodynamics of Pacing and Cardiac
   Resynchronization Therapy (CRT) for
   the Failing Left and Right Ventricle, 91
   Kara S. Motonaga and Anne M. Dubin

6 Sensor Driven Pacing: Ideal
   Characteristics in Pediatrics, 118
   David Bradley and Peter S. Fischbach

7 Implantable Cardioverter-Defibrillator
   Testing in Pediatric and Congenital
   Heart Disease, 123
   Elizabeth A. Stephenson and Charles I. Berul

Part 3: Implantation Techniques

8 Permanent Transvenous Pacemaker,
   CRT, and ICD Implantation in the
   Structurally Normal Heart, 133
   Akash R. Patel and Steven Fishberger

9 Permanent Pacemaker, CRT, and ICD
   Implantation in Congenital Heart Disease, 147
   Ian Law and Nicholas H. Von Bergen

10 Permanent Epicardial Pacing: When,
   How, and Why? 163
   Larry Rhodes and Maully Shah

11 Managing Device Related
   Complications and Lead Extraction, 172
   Avi Fischer and Barry Love

12 Temporary Pacing in Children, 195
   Anjan S. Batra and Ilana Zeltser

Part 4: Device Programming and Follow-Up

13 Pacemaker and ICD Programming in
   Congenital Heart Disease, 211
   Jonathan Kaltman and Jeffrey Moak

14 Pacemaker Troubleshooting and
   Follow-Up, 231
   Ronn E. Tanel and Frank Zimmerman

15 ICD Troubleshooting and Follow-Up, 252
   Steven Fishberger and Maully Shah

16 CRT device Programming and
   Optimization, 271
   Anoop Singh and Seshadri Balaji

17 Implantable Syncope and Arrhythmia
   Monitors, and Automated External
   Defibrillators, 280
   John R. Phillips and Pamela S. Ro

18 Electromagnetic Interference and
    Implantable Devices, 294
    Karen Smoots and R. Lee Vogel

19 Quality of Life, Sports, and Implantable
    Devices in the Young, 302
    Elizabeth Saarel

20 Device Innovations and the Future of
    Device Therapy for Arrhythmia and
    Heart Failure Management, 308
    Michael P. Carboni and Ronald J. Kanter

Glossary, 322

Index, 325

Foreword

Children represent only about 5% of the market for implantable cardiac rhythm management devices and adults with congenital heart diease certainly form an even smaller segment. It is easy to forget, therefore, that much of the impetus for the development of pacemakers in the early days was to answer a major problem: namely the occurrence of a complete atrioventricular block as a complication of open heart surgery to close septal defects. Unique clinical needs often drive innovation in medicine, and those developmemnts are then noticed and put to use by the larger community of practitioners. The endless variation in heart size and anatomy seen in children with congenital heart disease, along with the rapid development of new approaches to surgical repair, mean that we will continue to have a need for innovation in this field.

The field of pediatric electrophysiology has matured from a small group of practitioners trying to fit a square peg into a round hole into a true international professional body called PACES (Pediatric and Congenital Electrophysiology Society) that is innovating and advocating for pediatric and congenital heart disease specific device therapy. The editors have put together a group of authors that are leaders in this field, providing in this book their knowledge and experience, which is the round peg.

Doctors Shah, Rhodes, and Kaltman have edited and provided us with a textbook that fills a major gap and a pressing need focused on device management in children given the absence of specific leads or device features that meet the challenges of implantation and extraction of devices in children as a result of their smaller size, anticipation of growth, unique activity spectrum, and the relative overrepresentation of anatomic variants and congenital heart disease in the pediatric group. These challenges have been addressed by experienced implanters with idiosyncratic technical modifications at implant or device programming, and until now, there has been no targeted work that summarizes the approaches best suited for pediatric device practice.

Due to the comprehensive nature of this textbook it will find its home in a broad range of readers. For the trainee it will be a syllabus, for the the general practitioner it will provide the background and detail needed to comanage these patients and for the practicing electrophysiologist it will be a daily reader.

This textbook importantly explains the technical approaches in the normal pediatric heart as well as devoted sections for device management in congenital heart disease. Innovative and useful features that enhance the value of this textbook include a pacemaker and ICD glossary and a dedicated companion website that helps test the readers' knowledge and understanding as well as videos that help implanters in picturing the special needs in children. I have no doubt that *Cardiac Pacing and Defibrillation in Pediatric and Congenital Heart Disease* will be a must-have on the shelves of all of us who help manage rhythm disturbances in children and the adult congenital heart disease population.

Samuel Asirvatham, MD
Frank Cecchin, MD
George F. Van Hare, MD

List of Contributors

Seshadri Balaji, M.B.B.S, F.R.C.S (U.K.), Ph.D
Director, Arrhythmias Pacing and Electrophysiology
Doernbecher Children's Hospital
Professor of Pediatrics
Oregon Health & Science University
Portland, Oregon, USA

Yaniv Bar-Cohen, M.D.
Director of Cardiac Rhythm Devices
Children's Hospital Los Angeles
Associate Professor of Clinical Pediatrics and Medicine
University of Southern California
Los Angeles, California, USA

Anjan S. Batra, M.D., M.B.A, F.H.R.S
Director of Electrophysiology
Children's Hospital of Orange County
Division Chief and Vice Chair of Pediatrics
University of California, Irvine
Orange, California, USA

Nicholas H. Von Bergen, M.D.
Pediatric Electrophysiologist
The University of Wisconsin – Madison
Pediatric Cardiology.
Associate Professor of Pediatrics
The University of Wisconsin – Madison
Madison, Wisconsin, USA

Charles I. Berul, M.D.
Co-Director, Heart Institute
Children's National Health System
Professor of Pediatrics
George Washington University School of Medicine
Washington, DC, USA

David Bradley, M.D.
Director Pediatric Electrophysiology
C.S. Mott Children's Hospital
Professor of Pediatrics
University of Michigan School of Medicine
Ann Arbor, Michigan, USA

Robert Campbell, M.D.
Pediatric Cardiologist
Children's Healthcare of Atlanta
Sibley Heart Center Cardiology
Professor of Pediatrics
Emory University School of Medicine
Atlanta, Georgia, USA

Michael P. Carboni, M.D.
Pediatric Electrophysiologist
Duke Children's Hospital and Health Center
Assistant Professor of Pediatrics
Duke University School of Medicine
Durham, North Carolina, USA

Christopher Carter, M.D.
Pediatric Electrophysiologist
Children's Heart Clinic of Minnesota
Minneapolis, Minnesota, USA

Philip M. Chang, M.D.
Pediatric Electrophysiologist
Medical Director, Adult Congenital Heart Disease
Care Program
Keck Medical Center of University of Southern California
Assistant Professor of Clinical Medicine, Keck School of
Medicine of University of Southern California
Los Angeles, California, USA

Mitchell I. Cohen, M.D., F.A.C.C., F.H.R.S
Co-Director of the Heart Center and Chief
Pediatric Cardiology
Phoenix Children's Hospital
Clinical Professor of Child Health
University of Arizona College of Medicine-Phoenix
Phoenix, Arizona, USA

Erick Cuvillier, MSc
Director, Clinical Research and Education
Medtronic s, Inc. Puerto Rico
Minneapolis, Minnesota, USA

Anne M. Dubin, M.D.
Professor of Pediatrics
Stanford University School of Medicine
Director, Pediatric Electrophysiology
Lucile Salter Packard Children's Hospital Heart Center
Palo Alto, CA, USA

Susan P. Etheridge, M.D.
Pediatric Electrophysiologist
Primary Children's Hospital
Professor of Pediatrics
University of Utah
Salt Lake City, Utah, USA

Avi Fischer, MD, FACC, FHRS
Vice President, Global Education and Medical Director
St. Jude Medical
Austin, Texas, USA

Peter S. Fischbach, M.D., M. A.
Pediatric Electrophsysiologist
Emory University, Children's Healthcare of Atlanta
Associate Professor of Pediatrics
Emory University School of Medicine
Atlanta, Georgia, USA

Steven Fishberger, M.D.
Pediatric Electrophysiologist
Nicklaus Children's Hospital
Miami , Florida, USA

Jonathan Kaltman, M.D.
Chief, Heart Development and Structural Disease Branch
National Heart, Lung, and Blood Institute
Bethesda, Maryland, USA

Ronald J. Kanter, M.D.
Director, Pediatric Electrophysiology
Nicklaus Children's Hospital
Miami, Florida, USA

Ian Law M.D.
Director, Division of Pediatric Cardiology
University of Iowa Children's Hospital
Clinical Professor of Pediatrics
University of Iowa College of Medicine
Iowa City, USA

Barry Love, M.D.
Assistant Professor of Pediatrics
Assistant Professor of Medicine
Icahn School of Medicine
Director of Pediatric Electrophysiology
Director of Adult Congenital Heart Disease
Mount Sinai Medical Center
New York, USA

Jeffrey Moak, M.D.
Director, Electrophysiology and Pacing
Children's National Health System
Professor, Pediatrics
George Washington University
Washington, DC, USA

Kara S. Motonaga, M.D.
Pediatric Electrophysiologist
Lucile Packard Children's Hospital
Clinical Assistant Professor
Stanford University
Palo Alto, CA, USA

Akash R Patel, M.D.
Electrophysiologist, Pediatric and Congenital
Arrhythmia Center
University of California - San Francisco Benioff
Children's Hospital
Assistant Professor of Pediatrics
University of California - San Francisco
San Francisco, CA, USA

John R. Phillips, M.D.
Chief, Division of Pediatric Cardiology
Robert C. Byrd Health Sciences Center
Professor of Pediatrics
West Virginia University
Morgantown, WV

Larry Rhodes, M.D.
Chair, Department of Pediatrics
Robert C. Byrd Health Sciences Center
Professor of Pediatrics
West Virginia University
Morgantown, WV

Pamela S. Ro, M.D.
Pediatric Electrophysiologist
North Carolina Children's Heart Center
North Carolina Children's Hospital
Associate Professor of Pediatrics
The University of North Carolina at Chapel Hill
Chapel Hill, North Carolina, USA

Elizabeth Vickers Saarel, M.D.
Ronald and Helen Ross Distinguished Chair
Pediatric Cardiology
Cleveland Clinic
Professor of Pediatrics
Cleveland Clinic Lerner College of Medicine of Case
Western Reserve University
Cleveland, Ohio, USA

Maully Shah, M.B.B.S, F.A.C.C., F.H.R.S.

Medical Director, Cardiac Electrophysiology
The Children's Hospital of Philadelphia
Professor of Pediatrics
Perelman School of Medicine, University of Pennsylvania
Philadelphia, Pennsylvania, USA

Anoop Singh, M.B.B.Ch.

Director, Cardiac Electrophysiology
Children's Hospital of Wisconsin
Assistant Professor
Medical College of Wisconsin
Milwaukee, Wisconsin, USA

Karen Smoots BA, BSN, RN, CCDS

Electrophysiology Device Nurse
The Cardiac center
The Children's Hospital of Philadelphia
Philadelphia, Pennsylvania, USA

Elizabeth A. Stephenson, M.D., MSc.

Staff Cardiologist
The Hospital for Sick Children
Associate Professor of Pediatrics
The University of Toronto
Toronto, ON

Ronn E. Tanel, M.D.

Director, Pediatric and Congenital Arrhythmia Service
University of California-San Francisco Benioff
Children's Hospital
Professor of Clinical Pediatrics
University of California-San F School of Medicine
San Francisco, CA

R. Lee Vogel, M.D.

Staff Cardiologist
The Children's Hospital of Philadelphia
Professor of Clinical Pediatrics
Perelman School of Medicine, University of Pennsylvania
Philadelphia, PA

Ilana Zeltser, M.D.

Pediatric Electrophysiologist
Children's Medical Center of Dallas
Associate Professor of Pediatrics
University of Texas Southwestern School of Medicine
Dallas, Texas, USA

Frank Zimmerman, M.D.

Co-Director, Pediatric Electrophysiology Service
Advocate Children's Hospital
Clinical Associate Professor
University of Chicago
Oak Lawn, Illinois, USA

Preface

This book is written to address the unique issues of pacemaker, resynchronization and defibrillation therapy in children and young adults with special emphasis on patient size, growth, development, lifestyle, and co-existent congenital heart disease (CHD). The first functional external battery operated pacemaker was implanted in a child with post-operative heart block following repair of a ventricular septal defect in 1957. During the ensuing six decades, the field of cardiac pacing has seen ground-breaking innovations that have served as a foundation for other advanced life saving device therapies such as implantable cardioverter defibrillator (ICD) and cardiac resynchronization therapy (CRT). Although current devices and leads are designed and marketed predominantly for an adult patient population, the myriad applications in pediatric patients are well accepted. As pediatric cardiologists, we recognize that a child is not a miniature adult and we must therefore continue to pioneer, modify, and adapt techniques in accordance with the specific characteristics of our patients. Clearly, there is still significant opportunity for the scientific, engineering and regulatory organizations to manufacture cardiac rhythm devices and leads that are more suitable and efficacious for the pediatric patient.

This book addresses the need for articulation of current concepts, principles and clinical practices that underlie device management in children and patients with CHD. It is our hope that this book will serve as a comprehensive and informative resource to trainees as wells as practicing cardiologists and electrophysiologists, especially those involved in the care of CHD patients with rhythm disorders. We also hope that this book will serve as a guide to physicians who are faced with the challenges of pediatric device implantation and management in parts of the world where pediatric electrophysiologists are scarce.

The content of the book follows a logical progression starting with a brief history describing the brilliant innovations of several inventors to create the first implantable pacemaker. From there we proceed to the fundamental principles of pacing and defibrillation, a description of clinical concepts and indications, device implantation techniques, and subsequent management with detailed sections on troubleshooting, complications and follow-up. We have briefly included new technologies such as the totally sub-cutaneous ICD and the leadless pacemakers. Instructive device electrograms recordings and x-ray images are presented throughout the book. Finally, the website version has select videos and chapters 2–18 have interactive multiple choice questions.

This book could not have been completed without the encouragement and enthusiastic support of its contributors and several others. Contributors have been eager and motivated from the start and we thank them for their time, patience, and expertise. The staff at Wiley-Blackwell Publishing Company, especially Thomas V. Hartman who initiated the project and Claire Bonnett who facilitated its completion, deserve our thanks for the efficiency and meticulous care they have brought to the book's preparation. Carrie Stackhouse has been an intellectual and technical resource whom we cannot thank enough for her constant readiness to tackle difficult device programming and troubleshooting questions. Our trainees continue to inspire us with their thirst for knowledge. In many ways this book is a testament to our passion for teaching and learning with them. Most important, we thank the countless patients and families who have entrusted us with their care. It has been our privilege to learn something from each and every one of them.

Maully Shah
Larry Rhodes
Jonathan Kaltman

About the Companion Website

This book is accompanied by a companion website:

www.wiley.com/go/shah/cardiac_pacing

The website includes:

- Interactive multiple choice questions (MCQs)
- Videos

PART 1
Introduction

CHAPTER 1

History of cardiac pacing and defibrillation in the young

Larry Rhodes[1] and Robert Campbell[2]

[1]Chair, Department of Pediatrics, Robert C. Byrd Health Sciences Center, Professor of Pediatrics, WVU School of Medicine, Morgantown, WV, USA

[2]Pediatric Cardiologist, Children's Healthcare of Atlanta, Sibley Heart Center Cardiology, Professor of Pediatrics, Emory University School of Medicine, Atlanta, GA, USA

The earliest years of cardiac pacing predate the birth of many current pediatric cardiac electrophysiologists. An old saying states that "failure to understand history dooms one to repeat it." In contrast, understanding this history of successful collaboration between pioneering physicians and engineering partners allows us to marvel at the developments that were to follow rapidly over the next 50 years, and potentially repeat this formula in years to come.

Benjamin Franklin harnessed electricity from lightning using a kite in 1752. An early "medical" use of electricity was not to augment life but to document the end of it with patients receiving an electrical shock to prove they were dead. In 1774, electrical energy was applied to resuscitate a child using a transthoracic approach.[1] As early as 1899, the *British Medical Journal* published a report of experiments demonstrating that application of electrical impulses to the human heart would lead to ventricular contractions.[2] In 1926, Dr. Mark C. Lidwell and physicist Edgar H. Booth of Sydney developed a device with pacing rates of 80–120 bpm and outputs varying from 1.5 to 120 V.[3] This "pacer" was described as being a portable device

"plugged into a lighting point." One pole was connected to a pad soaked in strong salt solution and applied to the skin and the other, "a needle insulated except at its point, was plunged into the appropriate cardiac chamber." In 1928, this apparatus was used to revive a stillborn infant whose heart continued to beat after 10 minutes of stimulation.[4]

During the 1930s, Dr. Albert Hyman noted that the success of intracardiac delivery of medications for cardiac arrest was likely independent of the medication but was instead related to the needle stick leading to alteration in electrical potentials and myocardial contraction. Knowing that multiple needle sticks would be impractical and dangerous, he developed a generator to deliver electrical impulses via needle electrodes.[5]

Following World War II there was a significant interest in pacemakers generated by investigations in the use of general hypothermia for cardiac surgery. Cardiac arrest was noted during hypothermia and adequate heart rate was required to maintain adequate hemodynamics during rewarming. John A. Hopps, an engineer at the National Research Council of Canada developed a pacemaker that produced impulses at a desired rate

Cardiac Pacing and Defibrillation in Pediatric and Congenital Heart Disease, First Edition.
Edited by Maully Shah, Larry Rhodes and Jonathan Kaltman.
© 2017 John Wiley & Sons Ltd. Published 2017 by John Wiley & Sons Ltd.
Companion Website: www.wiley.com/go/shah/cardiac_pacing

through an electrode placed in the area of the sinus node.[6]

In 1952 Dr. Paul M. Zoll used an external pacemaker coupled with transcutaneous needle electrodes to rescue a patient suffering from Stokes-Adams attacks following a myocardial infarction.[7,8] The patient continued to experience ventricular asystole despite being administered 34 intracardiac injections of adrenaline over a 4-hour period. Dr. Zoll applied "external electrical stimulation" and successfully paced this patient's heart over the next 25 minutes.[8] The patient developed cardiac tamponade secondary to perforation of a cardiac vein during the intracardiac injections. Dr. Zoll then successfully paced a 65-year-old man with episodes of ventricular standstill for 5 days by external electrical stimulation at which time he developed an idioventricular rhythm at 44 bpm and was discharged.[9]

In the mid-1950s, open heart surgery was becoming a reality. Although for the first time in history, intracardiac palliation of structural heart disease was possible, the complication of surgical heart block was a significant morbidity. Dr. W. Lillehei, Dr. W. Weirich, and others at the University of Minnesota demonstrated that pacing could be performed by connecting a pulse generator to a wire electrode attached directly to the heart of a dog.[10,11] In January 1957, Lillehei used this pacing system in the first human patient, a child with post-operative heart block following repair of a ventricular septal defect. The pacer was programmed to a pulse width of 2 ms and a voltage ranging from 1.5 to 4.5 V (Figure 1.1).[12]

The generators used by both Zoll and Lillehei were devices which transformed alternating current into direct current to pace the heart. In 1957, following a power failure in Minneapolis in which patients could not be paced, Dr. Lillehei enlisted the help of Earl Bakken and Medtronic for battery backup for AC pacemakers. Silicon transistors had become commercially available in 1956 leading to the potential for development of smaller and more practical pacemakers. The original transistorized, zinc oxide battery-powered external pacemaker was developed by Mr. Bakken in 1957; the device was smaller and thus applicable for pediatric patients.[13,14] This, the first wearable external pacemaker, was housed in a small plastic

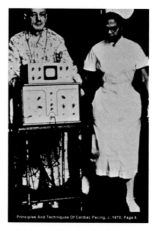

Figure 1.1 *Patient pushing pacemaker cart (1958). (Source: Reproduced with permission of Medtronic, Inc.)*

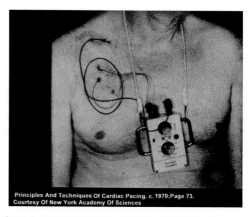

Figure 1.2 *Wearable pulse generator (1958). (Source: Reproduced with permission of Medtronic, Inc.)*

box, with controls to allow adjustment of pacing rate and voltage (Figure 1.2).

Although novel and potentially lifesaving, the advances described here were not a long term solution in that there was a significant risk of infection and external pacing was uncomfortable and impractical. There was a definite need for implantable pacing systems. Ake Senning, a Swedish surgeon, in collaboration with engineer Rune Elmqvist, developed a permanent implantable pulse generator with the first clinical implantation in 1958.[15] This device failed after three hours. A second device was implanted and lasted 2 days. The patient, Arne Larsson, went on to receive 26 different pacemakers until his death in 2001 at the age of 86 (Figure 1.3).[16]

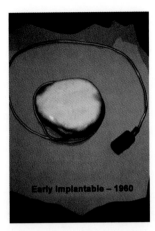

Figure 1.3 *History – First "permanent" implantable pacemaker and bipolar Hunter–Roth lead (1958). (Source: Reproduced with permission of Medtronic, Inc.)*

During that same year, Seymour Furman introduced temporary transvenous pacing using the recently described Seldinger technique.[17] In 1962 Ekestrom, Johannson, and Lagergren reported the first non-thoracotomy pacemaker implantation by introducing the electrode transvenously into the right ventricle.[18]

By the end of 1960 virtually all pacemakers used mercury-zinc cells as the power supply, but battery life expectancy was generally less than 2 years on average. A greater problem was that because the batteries emitted hydrogen gas, the pulse generator could not be sealed to protect from contamination with body fluids.[19] Dissatisfaction with this power source generated interest in alternatives that included, but were not limited to, bioenergy sources (using piezoelectric transducers that generated electricity based on the expansion and contraction of the abdominal aorta, or motion of the diaphragm), nuclear generators, and, by the mid-1970s, lithium batteries.[20] There was significant interest in the use of nuclear powered pacers because they offered a remarkable lifespan (10–20 years) and reliability. A number of drawbacks related to radiation exposure in case of a capsule leak and disposal hindered their acceptance.

Lithium-iodide power sources persist as the battery of choice today. Voltage output of the lithium-iodine cell showed gradual decline rather than the abrupt drop associated with the mercury zinc during battery depletion. This new battery

generated no gas byproduct allowing the entire pulse generator to be hermetically sealed in a titanium case, which was initially accomplished in 1969 by Telectronics and then by Cardiac Pacemakers, Inc., (Minneapolis, MN), in 1972. Battery life was significantly increased to greater than 5 years on average.

Leads

In the early 1960s it became routine practice to manage patients with temporary transvenous leads and an external pulse generator to relieve congestive heart failure. These served as a bridge to a thoracotomy for placement of a permanent pacemaker and lead system. Permanent transvenous pacing, which first appeared in the early 1960s, gained widespread acceptance by the end of the decade.[21,22] Initial leads were unipolar in design, but gradually gave way to a bipolar preference. Coaxial leads allowed for smaller lead diameter and greater durability. Smaller surface electrodes were designed to reduce energy consumption. Greater surface areas were achieved allowing improved lead function. Steroid-eluting leads were designed as a mechanism to reduce fibrosis at the epicardium-electrode interface, thus avoiding chronic rise in stimulation thresholds. Lead fixation, using passive or active mechanisms, were designed to prevent the previously high incidence of lead dislodgement. Silicone insulation gradually gave way to a preference for polyurethane. These newer leads had a generally smaller diameter than previous silicone leads, which facilitated the introduction of the implantation of two leads through a single vein, associated with the implementation of dual chamber pacing.

Pacing modes

The first implanted pacemakers were fixed rate ventricular systems, which competed with intrinsic ventricular activation. Unfortunately, the theoretical risk of inadvertent induction of ventricular fibrillation was in fact documented electrocardiographically.[23] Additionally, studies determined that fixed rate asynchronous pacing at times had an adverse hemodynamic impact on patients with myocardial dysfunction. Thus, the impetus for development of a demand pacemaker which could sense intrinsic ventricular activity was heralded. Virtually simultaneously, two companies debuted demand ventricular pacemakers. In 1966 the Medtronic system functioned in a true demand mode, with inhibition of ventricular pacing during sensed intrinsic ventricular activity.[24] The Cordis "standby" pacemaker functioned in the ventricular triggered mode, such that a sensed R-wave triggered the pacer stimulus with no AV delay so that it fell within the refractory period of the intrinsic QRS complex.[25] These modes were, respectively, termed VVI and VVT, both non-competitive modes.

The first pacemakers to permit atrial synchronization with the ventricle depended upon new sensing technology to detect intrinsic atrial activity,[26] and the triggering of a paced ventricular response after a programmed AV interval. These devices were bulky because of the complexity of the circuitry, and also demonstrated a significant reduction in battery life. Problems with erratic sensing of the intrinsic atrial activity and abrupt drops in pacing rates that occurred when upper rate limits were reached also limited the acceptance of these early dual chamber systems.

In the early 1980s a third generation of dual chamber pacemakers was introduced. These generators had long-lived lithium batteries and generally incorporated new dual endocardial leads. Pacemaker systems were able to both sense and pace in both the atrium and ventricle allowing physiologic rates and AV synchrony. The development of leads which could be used for atrial stimulation, as well as atrial sensing, enhanced the functionality of these early dual chamber systems.

Rate adaptive pacing, for patients with chronotropic incompetence, permitted rate responsive pacing that augmented heart rate response when intrinsic sinus node function was inadequate.[27] A more recent breakthrough mode was anti-tachycardia pacing, applicable especially for postoperative congenital heart disease patients with recurrent medically-refractory intraatrial reentry tachycardias.[28]

Non-invasive programmability

Seymour Furman and associates reported in 1969 the first techniques for routine transtelephonic monitoring of pacemaker function.[29,30] Subsequent advances included the ability of the system to estimate battery longevity. Continuous advancement in these non-invasive technologies has finally led to the ability to provide non-invasive electrogram analysis for tachycardia detection, tachycardia termination, and antitachycardia defibrillation systems.

Multiprogrammability

By the mid-1960s, the early non-invasively programmable pacemakers had advanced to multi-programmable units dependent upon bidirectional telemetry. In 1978, Intermedics introduced a pacemaker for whom pacing rates, pulse width, and sensitivity could be programmed; this system was a result of collaboration between engineer Robert Brownlee and physician G. Frank Tyers.[31] Dual chamber pacemakers also permitted programmability of pacing mode, in the event of recovery of intrinsic AV nodal function (allowing atrial pacing alone) or ventricular pacing only in the event of failure of the atrial lead (pacing and/or sensing capabilities).

Miniaturization

Initial external pacemaker systems required portable carts (Figure 1.1). By the early 1960s when permanent implantable systems were in place, the pulse generators were still bulky. Advanced pacemaker and software technologies allowed further miniaturization, but often at the expense of battery life. Smaller generators had a unique implant role for the smallest of neonates and pediatric patients, but required frequent generator changes due to battery depletion. Further decrease in lead size allowed implantation of multiple leads within a single vein, even in the smallest patients, but electrodes were still relatively large. Even these small lead systems were associated with a high incidence of venous obstruction/occlusion.

Pacemaker codes

The Inter-Society Commission for Heart Disease Resources (ICHD)[32] proposed a three-position "conversational" pacemaker code in 1974 to distinguish pacemakers according to three fundamental attributes:

Position 1. Chamber or chambers paced:
  V – ventricle paced
  A – atrium paced
  D (dual) – both atrium and ventricle paced
  O – neither atrium or ventricle paced

Position 2. Chamber or chambers in which native cardiac events were sensed:
  V – ventricle sensed
  A – atrium sensed
  D (dual) – both atrium and ventricle sensed
  O – neither atrium or ventricle sensed

Position 3. Pacemaker response to sensing a spontaneous chamber depolarization:
  T – triggered
  I – inhibited
  D (dual) – both triggered and inhibited
  O – none

Subsequent revisions paralleled development of pacemaker capabilities. The most recent revision of this original three-position code was published in 2000 incorporating a five-position code.[33] Position 4 is used only to indicate the presence (R) or absence (O) of a rate adaptive mechanism, used to compensate for patients with chronotropic incompetence. Position 5 indicates whether multi-site pacing is present in none of the cardiac chambers (O); in one or both of the atria (A) with stimulation sites in each atrium or more than one stimulation site in either atrium; in one or both of the ventricles (V), the stimulation sites in both ventricles or more than one stimulation in either ventricle; or in dual chambers (D), in one or both of the atria and in one or both of the ventricles. This most recent coding was endorsed by both the North American Society for Pacing and Electrophysiology (NASPE), (now known as the Heart Rhythm Society: HRS), and the British Pacing and Electrophysiology Group (BPEG).

Guidelines for implantation of cardiac pacemakers and antiarrhythmia devices

The first guidelines were introduced in 1984 through a joint subcommittee of the American College of Cardiology and the American Heart Association.[34] Pediatric cardiac pacing was represented by Dr. Paul Gillette. Guidelines were grouped according to the following classifications – class 1: conditions for which there is general agreement that permanent pacemakers and antitachycardia devices should be implanted; class 2: conditions for which permanent pacemakers and antitachycardia devices are frequently used but there is a divergence of opinion with respect to the necessity of their insertion; class 3: conditions for which there is general agreement that permanent pacemakers and antitachycardia devices are unnecessary. Multiple revisions have occurred, coincident with advances in technologies of these devices. The most recent guidelines were issued in 2008 through the American College of Cardiology, American Heart Association, and Heart Rhythm Society, and were developed in collaboration with the American Association for Thoracic Surgery and the Society of Thoracic Surgeons.[35] Guidelines for pediatric pacing were generated with the input of Dr. Mike Silka. In addition to the class 1, 2, and 3 indications for pacemaker implantation, guidelines were also rated according to evidence to support the guidelines. Levels of evidence A: data derived from multiple randomized clinical trials or meta-analysis; B: data derived from a single randomized trial or nonrandomized studies; and C: only consensus opinion of experts, case studies, or standard of care. These guidelines continue to dynamically evolve, but are widely regarded by consensus as detailing the appropriate use of devices in both adult and pediatric patients.

North American Society of Pacing and Electropysiology (NASPE)

Senior pacing physicians during the 1970s founded the *Journal of Pacing and Clinical Electrophysiology* (*PACE*) and organized a supporting professional society, NASPE.[36,37] NASPE arose out of a concern for the growing complexity of pacemaker systems and implantation techniques, the maintenance of quality control and good manufacturing practices by companies, and the proper post-implantation care of an ever expanding patient population. As lead technology advanced, the non-invasive transmission of intracardiac electrograms allowed increased patient diagnostic surveillance and treatment, and paralleled the explosive development of intracardiac electrophysiologic testing in advance of cardiac ablative therapies. NASPE (HRS since 2004) currently has over 5400 cardiac pacing and electrophysiology professionals worldwide and is the international leader in science, education and advocacy for cardiac arrhythmia professionals and patients, and the primary information resource on heart rhythm disorders. Its mission is to improve the care of patients by promoting research, education, and optimal health care policies and standards.

The implantable cardioverter defibrillator (ICD)

Prior to discussing the history of implantable cardioverter defibrillators, a brief review of defibrillation is in order. At the turn of the twentieth century, Prevost and Batelli researched ventricular fibrillation in dogs describing methods to fibrillate the heart using alternating (AC) and direct (DC) electrical currents. They noted it took stronger currents to defibrillate than to fibrillate the heart.[38] In 1947, Dr. Claude Beck performed the first successful human defibrillation using internal cardiac paddles on a 14-year-old boy who developed VF during elective chest surgery.[39] The device used on this patient, made by James Rand, had silver paddles the size of large tablespoons that could be directly applied to the heart. In 1956, Paul Zoll used a more powerful unit to perform the first closed-chest defibrillation of a human.[40]

The remarkable technical advances that occurred in clinical electrophysiology and pacemaker technologies through the 1960s and 1970s established the groundwork for the development of the implantable cardioverter defibrillator (ICD). External cardiac defibrillation was proven to be an effective method for terminating potentially life-threatening cardiac rhythm disturbances, including unstable ventricular tachycardia and ventricular fibrillation. In contrast to the pioneering collaborative efforts of multiple teams of physicians and engineers responsible for pacemaker development through the 1960s and 1970s, the development of the ICD is attributed almost single-handedly to the unwavering determination of Dr. Michael Mirowski in Baltimore, and his

engineering collaborator, Dr. Morton Mower. In a 1970 publication, Mirowski and Morton described the elements of an early ICD device, which would be required to quickly diagnose and treat ventricular fibrillation using a unit small enough for subcutaneous implantation.[41] Extended battery life would be a key component given the high output demands anticipated. Ventricular fibrillation detection techniques were initially dependent upon right ventricular pressure transducers, with a drop in blood pressure in post myocardial infarction patients triggering the device.[42] This unreliable sensing method was upgraded to the use of an intracardiac electrogram feature and a complex probability density algorithm distinguishing ventricular fibrillation from sinus rhythm. Initial device design used a hybrid endocardial and epicardial lead system with a single right ventricular transvenous lead and a subcutaneous defibrillation patch in the anterior chest wall. Subsequent iterations included a shock vector from a superior vena cava coil to apical patch. A completely transvenous system ultimately consisted of a right ventricular apical coil electrode with a second electrode in the superior vena cava or right atrium.

Initial animal studies demonstrated the efficacy of the device to terminate electrophysiologic induced ventricular fibrillation. Despite initial encouraging published results, there were vigorous dissenters who disqualified the device and the concept of the approach. The first human implantation occurred in 1980 at Johns Hopkins Hospital.[43] The device was non-programmable, committed, and had no telemetry capabilities. There was also no antitachycardia pacing option for patients with unstable ventricular tachycardia. Second generation defibrillators incorporated an epicardial right ventricular electrode for ventricular tachycardia detection.

Generator device and battery advancements have continuously developed. A significant design modification resulted in a new lead design in 1988, allowing for the first complete transvenous implantation[44] consisting of proximal and distal shocking coils.

The concept of tiered therapy was introduced in the early 1990s. A progressive therapy for ventricular tachycardia allowed for initial programmed bursts of antitachycardia pacing, followed by a low

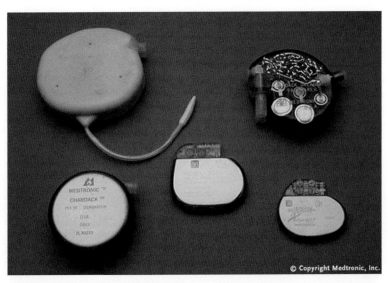

Figure 1.4 *Early implantable single chamber device to current dual chamber Kappa. (Source: Reproduced with permission of Medtronic, Inc.)*

energy shock for unstable VT, culminating in a high energy shock for unstable VT not terminated using step 2 or for tachycardia that had degenerated to ventricular fibrillation.

Advancement in devices and patches has allowed the successful implantation of ICD therapy in even young patients, and those with complex congenital heart disease anatomy limiting ICD lead placement (endocardial and/or epicardial) and generator positioning (thoracic or abdominal). Current guidelines for ICD implantation are likewise detailed in the 2008 ACC/AHA/HRS Guidelines for Device Based Therapy of Cardiac Rhythm Abnormalities.[28]

Summary

It is difficult to find a better example in medicine where the development of technology was driven in large part by the needs of children than that seen in pacer therapy. This occurred secondary to the fact that symptomatic bradycardia frequently presents in childhood as congenital heart block or a consequence of congenital heart disease. The primary motivation for successful cardiac pacing paralleled the development of open heart procedures for patients with congenital heart disease. This new era of palliation of children previously doomed to a life of disability could not to be derailed by a heart rate that did not maintain an adequate cardiac output. The commitment of Dr. C. Walter Lillehei and other pioneers at the University of Minnesota in the 1950s to continue with their heroic efforts to offer these children the potential for a normal life led to Earl Balken developing what is now Medtronics in a small garage in Minnesota. Throughout the last 60 years, the needs of children relative to size and anatomy have led to the development of smaller pacers and leads that have, in turn, continued to advance the field for patients of all sizes and ages (see Figure 1.4).

References

1 Schecter DC. Early experience with resuscitation by means of electricity. *Surgery* 1971; 69: 360.

2 McWilliam JA. Electrical stimulation of the heart in man. *Br Med J.* 1889 February 16; 1(1468): 348–350.

3 Lidwell MC. Cardiac disease in relation to anaesthesia. In: *Transactions of the Third Session, Australasian Medical Congress, Sydney, Australia*, Sept. 2–7 1929; 160.

4 Mond H, Sloman J, Edwards R. The first pacemaker. Pacing and clinical electrophysiology. *PACE* 1982; 5(2): 278–282.

5 Hyman AS. Resuscitation of the stopped heart by intracardial therapy-II. Experimental use of an artificial pacemaker. *Arch Intrn Med* 1932; 50: 283–205.

6 Callaghan, JC, Bigelow WG. An electrical artificial pace-maker for standstill of the heart. *Ann Surg*. 1951; 134(1): 8–17.

7 Kirk J. The next step in cardiac pacing: The view from 1958. *PACE* 1992; 15: 961–966.

8 Zoll PM, Linenthal AJ, Norman LR, Paul MH, Gibson W. Treatment of unexpected cardiac arrest by external electric stimulation of the heart. *New Engl J Med* 1956; 254(12): 541–546.

9 Zoll PM. Resuscitation of the heart in ventricular standstill by external electric stimulation. *New Engl J Med* 1952; 247(20): 768–771.

10 Weirich W, Gott V, Lillehei C. The treatment of complete heart block by the combined use of a myocardial electrode and an artificial pacemaker. *Surg Forum* 1957; 8: 360–363.

11 Warden HE, Lillehei CW. Pioneer cardiac surgeon. *J Thorac Cardiovasc Surg* 1989; 98: 833–845.

12 Elmqvist R. Review of early pacemaker development. *Pacing Clin Electrophysiol* 1978; 1(4): 535–536.

13 Griffin JC. The implantable pulse generator-evolution, design and function. In: PC Gillette, JC Griffin, eds. *Practical Cardiac Pacing*. Baltimore, MD: Williams & Wilkins; 1986: 1–15.

14 Lillehei CW, Gott VL, Hodges PC Jr,, Long DM, Bakken EE. Transistor pacemaker for treatment of atrioventricular dissociation. *J Am Med Assoc* 1960; 172: 2006–2010.

15 Elmqvist R, Landegren J, Pettersson SO, et al. Artificial pacemaker for treatment of Adams-Stokes syndrome and slow heart rate. *Am Heart J* 1963, 65: 731–748.

16 Jeffrey K, Parsonnet V. Cardiac pacing, 1960–1885: A quarter century of medical and industrial innovation. *Circulation* 1998; 19; 97(19): 1978–1791.

17 Furman S, Robinson G. The use of an intracardiac pacemaker in the correction of total heart block, *Surg Forum*, 1958; 9: 245.

18 Luderitz B. Historical perspectives on interventional electrophysiology. *J Interv Card Electrophysiol* 2003; 9(2): 75–83.

19 Parsonnet V. Power sources for implantable cardiac pacemakers. *Chest*. 1972; 61: 165–173.

20 Schneider A, Moser J, Webb THE, et al. A new high energy density cell with a lithium anode. *Proc US Army Signal Corps Power Sources Conf*, Atlantic City, NJ, 1970.

21 Parsonnet V, Zucker IR, Asa MM. Preliminary investigation of the development of a permanent implantable pacemaker utilizing an intracardiac dipolar electrode. *Clin Res*. 1962; 10: 391.

22 Lagergren H, Johansson L. Intracardiac stimulation for complete heart block. *Acta Chir Scand*. 1963; 125: 562–566

23 Bilitch M, Cosby RS, Cafferky EA. Ventricular fibrillation and competitive pacing. *N Engl J Med* 1967; 276: 598–604.

24 Zuckerman W, Zaroff LI, Berkovits BV, Matloff JM, Harken DE. Clinical experiences with a new implantable demand pacemaker. *Am J Cardiol*. 1967; 20: 232–238.

25 Parsonnet V, Zucker IR, Gilbert L, Myers GH. Clinical use of an implantable standby pacemaker. *JAMA*. 1966; 196: 784–786.

26 Nathan DA, Center S, Wu C-Y, et al. An implantable synchronous pacemaker for the long term correction of complete heart block. *Circulation* 1963; 27: 682–685.

27 Humen DP, Kostuk WJ, Klein GJ. Activity-sensing rate-responsive pacing: Improvement in myocardial performance with exercise. *PACE* 1985; 8: 52–59.

28 Gillette PC. Antitachycardia pacing. *Pacing Clin Electrophysiol* 1997 Aug; 20(8 Pt2): 2121–2124.

29 Furman S, Parker B, Escher DJW, Schwedel JB. Instruments for evaluating function of cardiac pacemakers. *Med Res Eng*. 1967; 6: 29–32.

30 Furman S, Parker B, Escher DJW. Transtelephone pacemaker clinic. *J Thorac Cardiovasc Surg*. 1971; 61: 827–834.

31 Tyers FO, Brownlee RR. A multiparameter telemetry system for cardiac pacemakers. In: Varriale P, Naclerio EA, eds. *Cardiac Pacing: A Concise Guide to Clinical Practice*. Philadelphia, PA: Lea & Febiger; 1979: 349–368.

32 Parsonnet V, Furman S, Smyth NPD. Implantable cardiac pacemakers: Status report and resource guidelines. Pacemaker Study Group, Inter-Society Commission for Heart Disease Resources (ICHD). *Circulation* 1974; 50: A21.

33 Bernstein AD, Daubert J-C, Fletcher RD, et al. The Revised NASPE/BPEG Generic Code for antibradycardia, adaptive-rate, and multisite pacing. *PACE* 2000; 25: 260–264.

34 Frye RL, Collins JJ, DeSantic RW, et al. Guidelines for permanent cardiac pacemaker implantation, May 1984. A Report of the Joint American College of Cardiology/American Heart Association Task Force on Assessment of Cardiovascular Procedures (Subcommittee on Pacemaker Implantation). *J Am Coll Cardiol* 1984; 4: 434–442.

35 Epstein AE, DiMarco JP, Ellenbogen KA, Mark EN III,, Freedman RA, Gettes LS, et al. ACC/AHA/HRS 2008 Guidelines for Device-Based Therapy of Cardiac Rhythm Abnormalities: Executive Summary. A Report of the American College of Cardiology/American Heart Association Task Force on Practice Guidelines (Writing Committee to Revise the ACC/AHA/NASPE 2002 Guideline Update for Implantation of Cardiac

Pacemakers and Antiarrhythmia Devices) developed in collaboration with the American Association for Thoracic Surgery and Society of Thoracic Surgeons. *J Am Coll Cardiol.* 2008; 51: 2085–2105.

36 Furman S. Why a new journal? Why PACE? *PACE Pacing Clin Electrophysiol.* 1978; 1: 1. Editorial.

37 Hawthorne JW, Bilitch M, Furman S, Goldman BS, MacGregor DC, Morse DP, Parsonnet V. North American Society of Pacing and Electrophysiology [NASPE]. *PACE Pacing Clin Electrophysiol.* 1979; 2: 521–522.

38 Beck CS. Prevost and Batelli. *Ariz Med.* 1965; 22: 691–694.

39 Beck CS, Pritchard WH, Feil SA. Ventricular fibrillation of long duration abolished by electric shock. *JAMA.* 1947; 135: 985–989.

40 Zoll, PM, Linenthal AJ, Gibson W et al. Termination of ventricular fibrillation in man by externally applied electric countershock. *N Engl J Med.* Apr 19, 1956; 254(16): 727–732.

41 Mirowski M, Mower MM, Staewen WS, et al. Standby automatic defibrillator: An approach to prevention of sudden coronary death. *Arch Intern Med* 1970; 126: 158–161.

42 Mirowski M, Mower MM. Transvenous automatic defibrillator as an approach to prevention of sudden death from ventricular fibrillation. *Heart and Lung* 1973; 2: 567–569.

43 Mirowski M, Reid PR, Mower MM, et al. Termination of malignant ventricular arrhythmias with an implanted automatic defibrillator in human beings. *N Engl J Med* 1980; 303: 322–324.

44 Moser S, Troup P, Saksena S, et al. Nonthoractomy implantable defibrillator system. (abstract) *PACE* 1988; 11: 887.

CHAPTER 2

Clinically relevant basics of pacing and defibrillation

Maully Shah[1] and Erick Cuvillier[2]

[1] Medical Director, Cardiac Electrophysiology, The Children's Hospital of Philadelphia, Professor of Pediatrics, Perelman School of Medicine, University of Pennsylvania, Philadelphia, PA, USA

[2] Director, Clinical Research and Education, Medtronic, Inc., Minneapolis, MN, USA

Basic concepts in cardiac pacing

The fundamental principle of artificial cardiac pacing involves delivery of an electrical impulse of sufficient strength from an electrode to cause excitation of a critical mass of cells. Since the heart is a syncytium, once the critical volume of cells is excited, the conduction propagates to the rest of the myocardium.[1, 2] Clinically relevant pacemaker features and terminology are described next.

Stimulation threshold

The minimal energy required to produce myocardial depolarization is called *stimulation threshold*. There are two components of stimulation: *pulse amplitude* (measured in volts, V) and *pulse duration* (measured in milliseconds, ms). Current pacemaker systems are constant voltage systems and the resultant strength-duration curve is hyperbolic in shape suggesting an exponential relationship between stimulus amplitude and duration (Figure 2.1). At short pulse durations, a small change in pulse duration is associated with a significant change in pulse amplitude required to produce myocardial depolarization. At long pulse durations, a small change in the pulse duration

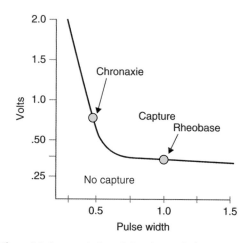

Figure 2.1 *Representation of chronic ventricular strength-duration relationships. Rheobase is the threshold at infinitely long pulse duration. Chronaxie is pulse duration at twice rheobase.*

has little effect on threshold amplitude. There are two important points on the strength-duration curve: *rheobase*, which is the smallest amplitude that stimulates the myocardium at infinitely long pulse duration and *chronaxie*, which is the threshold pulse duration at twice the stimulation amplitude. The latter approximates the point of

Cardiac Pacing and Defibrillation in Pediatric and Congenital Heart Disease, First Edition.
Edited by Maully Shah, Larry Rhodes and Jonathan Kaltman.

minimum threshold energy (microjoules) required for myocardial depolarization.[1, 2]

Stimulation thresholds typically oscillate in the ensuing weeks after implantation and are highly dependent on lead design, electrode-myocardial interface and patient factors, but chronic thresholds are typically reached by 3 months. With steroid eluting pacing leads, stimulation thresholds do not rise rapidly after implantation as with earlier generation non-steroid leads, but, tend to decrease to acute threshold values following a slight initial increase.[3]

Transvenous pacing leads with acute fixation mechanisms often have relatively high immediate pacing thresholds at implantation secondary to hyperacute injury due to advancement of the screw into the myocardium and frequently decline within the first 5–30 minutes.[4] The implanter should keep this in mind and wait a few minutes and re-check thresholds before repositioning the pacing lead.

Implantation of a pacing lead results in acute injury to the myocardial cellular membrane resulting in an acute inflammatory response, and this tissue becomes fibrotic over time. As a consequence, the distance between the electrode and excitable myocardial tissue is increased and may result in increased stimulation thresholds

(typically 4–8 weeks after implantation) and a decrease in the sensed endocardial signal. This phenomenon is known as *lead maturation*. With increasing time, the size of the edematous capsule shrinks and stimulation thresholds decrease and stabilize chronically (typically by 12 weeks after implantation). Steroid eluting leads improve lead maturation by minimizing fibrous capsule formation and reducing energy consumption along with maintenance of stimulation and sensing thresholds as well as lead impedance values (Figures 2.2 and 2.3).[3, 5–9] *Exit block* is manifested by progressive rise in threshold over time due to fibrous tissue at the lead myocardial interface resulting in capture threshold that exceeds the programmed output of the pacemaker.[4]

Post implantation, stimulation thresholds may be altered by various factors. An increase in thresholds is encountered during sleep, hyperglycemia, hypoxemia, acidosis, acute illnesses, electrolyte disturbances, and certain cardiac drugs (Table 2.1).[10–17]

Pacemaker sensing

Intrinsic cardiac electrical signals are produced by electric activation in the myocardium. As the

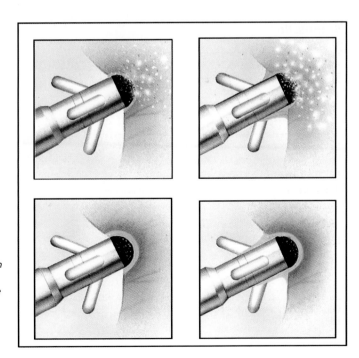

Figure 2.2 *The illustration compares a steroid eluting lead (top views) to a lead without steroid (bottom views) from the day of implant into the chronic phase. The steroid eluting from the tip of the lead suppresses each stage of the inflammatory process. The result is less inflammation, and a thinner capsule surrounding the lead tip. (Source: Reproduced with permission of Medtronic, inc.)*

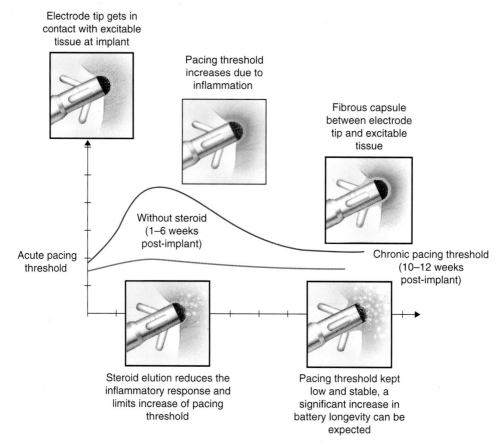

Electrode tip gets in contact with excitable tissue at implant

Pacing threshold increases due to inflammation

Fibrous capsule between electrode tip and excitable tissue

Without steroid (1–6 weeks post-implant)

Acute pacing threshold

Chronic pacing threshold (10–12 weeks post-implant)

Steroid elution reduces the inflammatory response and limits increase of pacing threshold

Pacing threshold kept low and stable, a significant increase in battery longevity can be expected

Figure 2.3 *Threshold changes are shown over a 12-week period post-implant, where a comparison is made between non-steroid and steroid-eluting electrode. Traditionally, implant stimulation thresholds are relatively low. Non-steroid-eluting electrodes exhibit a peaking phase (red curve); steroid-eluting electrodes exhibit virtually no peaking (blue curve). The pacing threshold increase is due to inflammation caused by the activity of phagocytes at the electrode-tissue interface that release many different inflammatory mediators. (Source: Reproduced with permission of Medtronic, Inc.)*

Table 2.1 *Effect of anti arrhythmic drugs on pacemaker stimulation thresholds*

Increase stimulation threshold	Decrease stimulation threshold
• Class IA: e.g., Quinidine, Procainamide	• Corticosteroids
• Class IC: e.g., Flecainide, Proprafenone	• Sympathomimetics: e.g., Epinephrine, Ephedrine, Isoproterenol

wavefront of activation approaches the electrode, it becomes positively charged and the signal is recorded as a positive deflection in the intracardiac electrogram. When the activating wavefront passes directly underneath the electrode, a negative deflections is recorded which is referred to as the *intrinsic deflection*. The analog signal of intrinsic electrical activity is amplified and filtered and then converted to a digital signal and processed by the pacemaker. Atrial electrogram frequency densities are generally in the range of 10–30 Hz and ventricular electrogram are in the range of 80–100 Hz. Based on these frequencies, filtering systems of pulse generators are designed to attenuate signals outside these ranges such as myopotentials, EMI and non-cardiac signals, although, overlap may still exist.[2, 18, 19] The minimum atrial or ventricular intracardiac signal amplitude required to inhibit a demand pacemaker is known as the *sensing threshold* and is expressed in millivolts (mV).

The maximal rate of change of the electrical potential between the sensing electrodes is known as the *slew rate*.[2, 10] The slew rate is the first derivative of the electrogram (dV/dt). An acceptable slew rate in the atrium or ventricle should be at least 0.5 V/s. Higher the slew rate, the more likely the signal will be sensed. T waves typically generate slow broad signals and a low slew rate and are therefore less likely to be sensed.

Impedance

Impedance describes the impediment to current flow of electrons within the entire pacing system. In pacemaker technology, Ohm's law (V = I × R, V = voltage, I = current, and R = resistance) is used for determining impedance but it should be noted that technically, impedance and resistance are separate entities. Factors that contribute to impedance include lead conductor resistance, electrode resistance, electrode-tissue interface and polarization. All current pacemakers are constant voltage systems, and according to Ohm's law, the higher the pacing impedance the lower the current flow. Reduced current flow can reduce pacemaker battery drainage.

Engineering aspects of transvenous pacemaker leads and generators

The following section will discuss key features of pacemaker lead and generators including designs and components.

Pacemaker lead construction and components

The main components of a pacing lead include the electrodes, fixation mechanism, conductor, insulation, and connector. Figure 2.4 shows the components of an atrial passive fixation lead.

Cardiac pacing requires a tip electrode and an indifferent electrode to complete the electrical circuit. When one of the electrodes is in contact with the heart and the other is away from the heart, the configuration is described as *unipolar*. When both electrodes are in the same chamber of the heart and contained on the pacing lead, the configuration is *bipolar*. The electrode in contact with the heart is the *stimulating* electrode and the

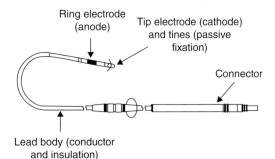

Figure 2.4 *Representation of the main components of a pacing lead which include the electrodes, fixation mechanism (passive fixation in this example) lead body and connector. (Source: Reproduced with permission of Medtronic, Inc.)*

one away from the heart is the *indifferent* electrode. The indifferent electrode is usually larger compared to the stimulating electrode to lower the resistance of the stimulation configuration. When the stimulating electrode is negative with respect to the indifferent electrode, stimulation is called *cathodal* and when the stimulating electrode is positive, it is called *anodal* stimulation.[1] In a unipolar pacing system, the tip electrode of the lead functions as the cathode and the pulse generator as the anode. The pacing pulse travels from the generator to the tip electrode to stimulate the myocardium and returns to the pulse generator through the chest tissues to complete the circuit (Figure 2.5).

In a bipolar pacing system, the tip electrode functions as the cathode and the lead ring electrode functions as the anode. The pacing pulse travels from the generator to the tip electrode and then to the ring electrode (anode) and returns

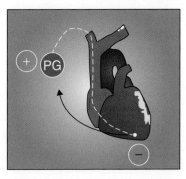

Figure 2.5 *In a unipolar pacing system the cathode (–) is on the lead and the anode (+) is the pacemaker.*

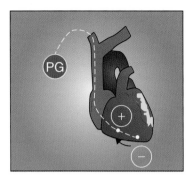

Figure 2.6 *In a bipolar pacing system both the anode (+) and the cathode (−) are contained on the pacing lead. The move away from unipolar offers better detection of spontaneous cardiac signals.*

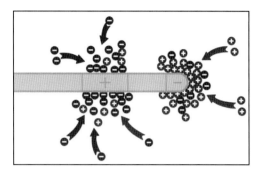

Figure 2.7 *Illustration of the polarization concept: the cathode is negatively charged when the current is flowing; as a result, positive ions are attracted at the tip electrode (the amount of positive charge is directly proportional to the pulse duration and inversely proportional to the functional electrode size).*

to the generator via the second conductor wire (Figure 2.6).

Bipolar leads have a greater external diameter and are stiffer than the unipolar leads because each coil must be electrically separated by insulating material. In general, bipolar pacing and sensing is preferred due to a lower probability of extra-cardiac stimulation and sensing of myopotential and far field signals. Unipolar leads have a lower likelihood of short circuiting in case of an insulation breach when compared to bipolar leads.

The primary purpose of the tip electrode (cathode) is to act as a long-term interface between the lead and the myocardium. Electrode materials currently in use are platinum-iridium, platinized titanium coated platinum, iridium oxide and platinum. Current cathode sizes range from 1.2–8.5 mm^2. In pacing systems, current is carried by electrons in the electronic device and leads and by ions inside the patient's body. When electrical current flows, the tip electrode attracts positively charged ions and a charged layer surrounds the electrode. This build-up of charge on the electrode is called *polarization* (Figure 2.7). When polarization is excessive, less current is available for myocardial stimulation and capture threshold increases. By altering the electrode surface to be more porous and irregular in texture, the surface area is increased and the polarization voltage is decreased (Figure 2.8). Ideally, an electrode should have high resistance to minimize current drain, large surface area to minimize polarization and small radius to increase current density and reduce

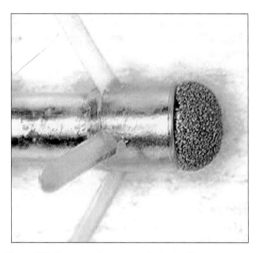

Figure 2.8 *Close-up of a porous electrode. (Source: Reproduced with permission of Medtronic, Inc.)*

voltage threshold. This has been accomplished in the manufacturing process by using either microscopic pores, wire filament mesh, microsphere, and fractal coatings.[20]

Passive fixation (Figure 2.9) lead tips are held in position by the lead tip being "trapped" in myocardial trabeculae and no part of the lead tip is embedded in the endocardium. *Active fixation* (Figure 2.10) leads have a fixed or extendable-retractable helix that is extended into the endocardial tissue resulting in a current of injury. An adequate current of injury at the time of an active fixation lead placement correlates with adequate lead fixation.[9] In the pediatric and

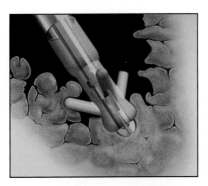

Figure 2.9 *Illustration of a passive fixation endocardial lead with times at the tip entrapped in the myocardial trabeculae. (Source: Reproduced with permission of Medtronic, Inc.)*

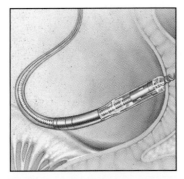

Figure 2.10 *Illustration of an active fixation endocardial lead screwed into the heart wall. (Source: Reproduced with permission of Medtronic, Inc.)*

congenital heart disease population, active fixation leads are preferred due to variable anatomy, presence of myocardial scar, need for alternative pacing sites and long-term stability.

Lead *conductors* are wires that carry electrical pulses from the device to the heart via the distal tip electrode and transmit intrinsic signals from the heart to the device (Figure 2.4, Figure 2.5). Currently, the most commonly used alloy in conductors is MP35N® (a nickel-cobalt alloy with the following nominal composition: 35% nickel, 35% cobalt, 20% chromium, and 10% molybdenum). Advantages of this alloy are tensile strength, ductility, and corrosion resistance. Other alloys with superior qualities include MP35N® silver cored conductor and 35N LT®.[20]

Conductors can be unifilar or multifilar. A unifilar conductor is a single wire coil that is

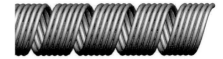

Figure 2.11 *Hexafilar conductor coil. (Source: Reproduced with permission of Medtronic, Inc.)*

wound around a central axis in a spiral manner. A multifilar conductor consists of two or more wire coils wound in parallel together around a central axis (Figure 2.11). Coiling the wire facilitates flexibility and fatigue resistance and allows a stylet to be placed through the central lumen of the coil. A disadvantage is that they are susceptible to crush fractures. In current pacing leads, a multifilar coil is surrounded by insulation in unipolar leads and bipolar leads are constructed in a coaxial or co-radial fashion where an insulated layer separates the multifilar conductor coils.

Another type of lead construction involves a cable conductor which consists of two or more filaments that are twisted together and then bundled with other strands around each other. Cable conductors do not have a lumen but allow for a smaller sized lead body and are less prone to crush fractures. An example of this type of lead is the Medtronic SelectSecure™ (model 3830, Medtronic Inc., Minneapolis MN), frequently used in the pediatric population that has a cable type inner conductor[21] (Figure 2.12).

Lead *insulation* is non conducting material that prevents electrical current from escaping into surrounding tissue. The predominant materials in lead insulation are silicone and polyurethane and emerging materials such as fluoropolymers and

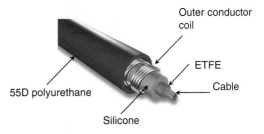

Figure 2.12 *Cross-section showing a SelectSecure™ lead body construction. This pacing lead bears no lumen and thus no guiding stylet. Its insertion and endocardial positioning is facilitated by a steerable guiding catheter. (Source: Reproduced with permission of Medtronic, Inc.)*

Table 2.2 *Advantages and disadvantages of lead insulation materials*

Type of Insulation	Silicone	Polyurethane	Fluoropolymers
Advantages	• Biostable	• High tear strength	• Inert
	• Flexible	• Low friction coefficient in blood	• High tensile strength
	• Inert	• Less thrombogenic	
	• Long standing performance	• High cut resistance	
		• Superior compressive properties	
		• Allows thinner lead diameter	
Disadvantages	High friction coefficient in blood	Susceptible to environmental stress cracking (P80A)	Relatively stiff
	• Low cut resistance	• Susceptible to metal ion oxidation (P80A)	• Susceptible to "pinholes" and subsequently metal ion oxidation
	• More thrombogenic	• Relatively stiff (55D)	• Susceptible to creep
	• Abrades and tears easily	• Susceptible to cautery heat damage	
	• Cold flow failure	• Manufacturing process sensitive	

copolymers, all of which are biocompatible. Some of the advantages and disadvantages are presented in Table 2.2.

Ideally, insulation material should be flexible, durable and have low friction. However, transvenous leads are subjected to a variety of loading forces leading to insulation damage. *Environmental stress cracking* is an oxidative condition that manifests as cracking of polyurethane insulation resulting in a frosty white surface appearance. In *metal ion oxidation,* peroxides produced by macrophage cells degrade polyurethane insulation and oxygen molecules mix with the metal ions from the conductor. *Compression set* is the permanent deformation of insulation material from compressive forces over time (Figure 2.13). This can be seen where the lead is wrapped under the pulse generator in the pocket, underneath the pectoralis muscle in sub-muscular pockets or between the rib and the clavicle. Leads rubbing against each other or against the generator or ligaments can

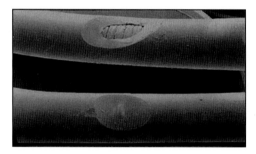

Figure 2.13 *Deformation of insulation from compressive force.*

cause *abrasions.* A *crush* injury from compression between the first rib and clavicle may result in disruption of the insulation. *Cold flow* is a time dependent dimensional change usually resulting in thinning due to movement of a polymer under load.[20] Copolymers have been developed to combine the biostability and flexibiity of silicone and durability and abrasion resistance of polyurethane.

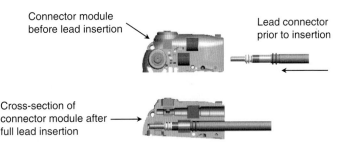

Connector module
before lead insertion

Lead connector
prior to insertion

Figure 2.14 *Illustration of an IS-1 connector assembly. (Pacemaker connector module and lead connector.)*

Cross-section of
connector module after
full lead insertion

One such proprietary product is Optim™ used on several models of St. Jude medical cardiac leads (St. Jude Medical, St. Paul, MN).

The lead body includes one or more electrodes at the distal end and a *connector* having a similar number of electrical elements for connection to the pulse generator at the distal end (Figure 2.14). Current low profile IS-1 in line lead connectors are 3.2 mm in diameter, have sealing rings, and a short connector pin.[22]

Some patients with older functioning 5–6 mm unipolar leads require *adaptors* when connected to current generators. In 2010, the International Organization for Standardization (ISO) approved a four-pole connector system (ISO 27186) (Figure 2.15). Its specifications apply to both low-energy (IS-4) and high-energy (DF-4) leads. The connector port cavity design of the IS-4/DF-4 connector consists of an epoxy header with a cylindrical bore opening.

Pacemaker generator construction and components

The key components of all generators include a battery, circuitry for sensing and pacing, telemetry, microprocessor, memory, and sensors, which are

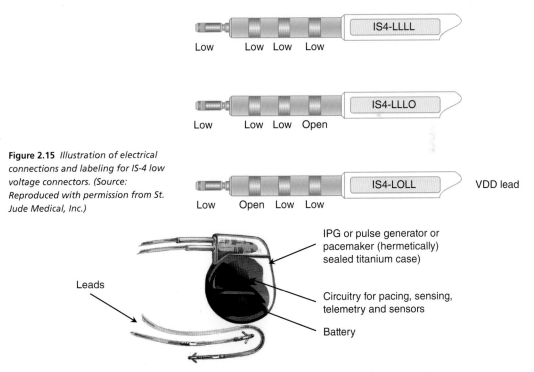

IS4-LLLL

Low   Low Low   Low

IS4-LLLO

Low   Low Low   Open

Figure 2.15 *Illustration of electrical connections and labeling for IS-4 low voltage connectors. (Source: Reproduced with permission from St. Jude Medical, Inc.)*

IS4-LOLL   VDD lead

Low   Open Low   Low

IPG or pulse generator or pacemaker (hermetically) sealed titanium case)

Leads

Circuitry for pacing, sensing, telemetry and sensors

Battery

Figure 2.16 *Illustration of a pacing system. (Source: Reproduced with permission of Medtronic, Inc.)*

encased in a titanium can with a header having standardized connectors for lead attachment (Figure 2.16).

Contemporary pulse generators utilize lithium iodine cells for the energy source where Lithium is the anodal element that supplies the electrons and iodine is the cathodal element that accepts the electrons. Pacemakers with antitachycardia pacing and implantable defibrillators that support high current drain utilize lithium-silver-oxide-vanadium compositions. For lithium iodine batteries, cell voltage is 2.8 V at beginning of life and decreases to 2.4 V when approximately 90% usable battery life has been reached and internal cell impedance increases. The voltage exponentially declines to 1.8 V at end of life. When the elective replacement indicator (ERI) or recommended replacement time (RRT) has been has been reached, approximately 180 days remain before end of service (EOS) or end of life (EOL). At end of life, for safety reasons, the pulse generator reverts to a fixed high output mode and loses telemetry and programmability. Magnet rates characteristic of battery status vary with manufacturer. Battery longevity is determined by size, composition, stimulation frequency, stimulation amplitude, pulse duration, stored diagnostic information, current required for circuitry, amount of internal discharge, and voltage decay. Longevity of battery can be determined by the formula: $114 \times$ (battery capacity (A-HR)/current drain (µA). Ampere Hours (A-HR) is specified by the manufacturer.[2]

In addition to the battery, other components of the pulse generator include internal circuits, and discrete components such as capacitors, diodes, inductors, and transmission coils (Figure 2.17). The internal circuits and discrete components are mounted on a sheet of polymer and along with the battery occupy 80–90% of the pacemaker space.

There is an output circuit for delivery of pacing pulses that involves charging and discharging of the output capacitor to the pacing electrodes. Contemporary generators deliver a constant voltage pulse throughout the pulse duration with some voltage drop occurring at the leading and trailing edges of the impulse. The output wave front is followed by the afterpotential, which is determined by the polarization of the electrode at its tissue interface (Figure 2.7). Newer pacemakers use the output

circuit to discharge the afterpotential quickly to lower afterpolarization sensing and eliminate inappropriate pacemaker inhibition.[1, 2]

The intracardiac electrogram signal is conducted from the myocardium to the sensing circuit via the pacing leads and subsequently amplified and filtered. The sensing circuit uses bandpass filtering, time domain sampling, and amplitude threshold comparison in order to distinguish the P- and R-waves of the signal from other noise. After filtering, the electrogram signal is compared to the programmed sensitivity setting. Signals with an amplitude within or higher than this reference voltage are sensed as true intracardiac signals and are forwarded to the timing circuit whereas signals below the reference voltage are regarded as extracardiac signals.

The timing circuit is the control center of the pacing circuit. It regulates the pacing cycle length, thresholds, AV delays, blanking and refractory periods. A crystal oscillator circuit, which serves as a basic timing clock for the entire pacing circuit, is connected to the digital controller/timer circuit. This circuit produces a voltage of a very stable frequency by utilizing a crystal of a tightly-controlled size and thickness between two electrodes. When a voltage source is applied to the crystal, it resonates at a stable characteristic frequency due to the piezoelectric effect. This stable frequency can be used for timing events carried out by the digital controller/timer circuit.

The pacemaker also includes a rate-responsive circuit that detects increased bodily movement and adjusts the pacing of the heart appropriately in order to increase the heart rate during exercise. This is accomplished using a piezoelectric force sensor attached to the housing unit encasing the device

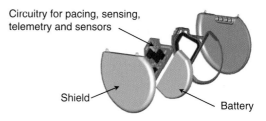

Figure 2.17 *Illustration of components inside a pacemaker (connector module not shown). (Source: Reproduced with permission of Medtronic, Inc.)*

and an activity circuit for processing the sensor signals.[23] Other types of sensors are discussed in Chapter 6.

The microcomputer circuit includes a micro-processor, a system clock, and Random-access memory (RAM)/Read only memory (ROM) chips. ROM is used to operate sensing and output functions and RAM is used in diagnostic operations. Parameter values and execution instructions are stored in the microcomputer and sent as commands to the digital controller/timer circuit in the pacing circuit. The microcomputer also stores recorded data to relay back when the device is interrogated.[1, 2]

External telemetry is included in all implantable devices and information between the programmer and pulse generator is transmitted via radiofrequency, which is exclusive to the manufacturer. The most recent advance in telemetry is that of remote or "wireless" capability that allow for bidirectional exchange of information without the programming "wand" continuously positioned over the pulse generator.

MRI conditional pacemakers

Recent advances in pacemaker technology include the introduction of Magnetic Resonance Imaging (MRI) conditional pacemakers as well as leadless pacemakers. MRI has been a long standing contraindication for patients with pacemakers. The increasing importance of MRI as a diagnostic tool and the limitations imposed by conventional pacemakers has prompted a large amount of research and efforts to develop devices suitable for use in this environment. Gathering the knowledge collected in *in vitro*, animal, and human studies, pacemaker manufacturers introduced a significant number of modifications to their devices to make them MRI "conditional." These include reduction in ferromagnetic components, replacement of the reed switch by a Hall sensor, changing the winding pattern of the filaments of the inner lead coil to limit conducted radiofrequencies, lead tip coating and generator shielding to minimize electromagnetic interference and injury, special filters to reducing risk of damage to the internal power supply and circuitry and programmable "MRI mode."[24, 25] Specific pacing leads (e.g., CapSureFix Novus 5076 Lead, Medtronic Inc., Minneapolis,

MN) that have not been specifically been modified for MRI compatibility are also considered MRI conditional (Chapter 3).

Leadless pacemakers

Recently, a leadless endocardial pacemaker has been introduced to potentially overcome some of the short- and long-term complications associated with pacing leads. The pulse generator and sensing/pacing electrodes are fully contained within a single unit which is delivered transvenously (Figure 2.18). Short term safety, feasibility of implantation, and pacing performance data are encouraging. However, further follow-up is required to assess the intermediate- and long-term safety (e.g., risk of embolization, proarrhythmia, and other unanticipated adverse events) and performance (e.g., battery longevity, pacing thresholds over time, and rate response function) of this device.[26, 27]

Basic concepts in ICDs

Ventricular fibrillation (VF) is the most common cause of sudden death. VF ensues when there is an increased amount of inhomogeneity of the electrophysiology properties between adjacent myocardial cells together with local reentry resulting in characteristic, random, uncoordinated excitation wavefronts. For a defibrillation shock to succeed, it must extinguish existing VF activations throughout the myocardium or in a critical mass, as well as not initiate new fibrillatory wavefronts. Conceptually, defibrillation can be considered to be a two-step process. Firstly, the applied shock drives currents that traverse the myocardium and cause complex polarization changes in transmembrane potential distribution.[28] Secondly, post-shock active membrane reactions are invoked that eventually result either in termination of VF in the case of shock success, or in re-initiation of fibrillatory activity in the case of shock failure. Furthermore, shocks that result in induction of arrhythmia are bound by a minimum and a maximum strength, termed the lower and upper limits of vulnerability (Chapter 7), suggesting that the mechanisms of induction and termination of VF may be similar.[29, 30] Despite the impressive clinical success and efficacy of current ICD

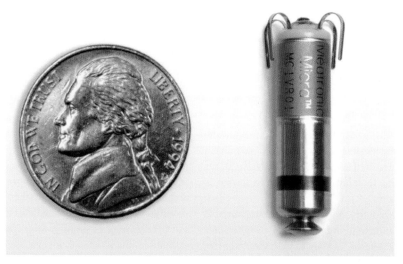

Figure 2.18 *Leadless Pacemaker: Micra transcatheter pacing system from Medtronic., Inc. (Source: Reproduced with permission of Medtronic, Inc.)*

devices, the biophysical underpinnings of defibrillation mechanisms have not been definitively elucidated.[31–35]

Excessively high energy shocks can theoretically lead to myocardial damage.[36] Conventional ICDs are designed for adult cohorts for whom ICD therapy is indicated. There are limited data regarding efficacious defibrillation doses in pediatric patients using conventional ICDs but low defibrillation thresholds (DFT) have been reported in a series of patients <60 kg.[37] Antiarrhythmic and other cardiovascular drugs can affect DFTs and examples of anti-arrhythmic drugs are shown in Table 2.3.[2]

Engineering aspects of transvenous ICD leads and generators

The ICD has evolved to a multi-functional therapeutic and monitoring device that can incorporate atrial and ventricular pacing and sensing, atrial and ventricular defibrillation, arrhythmia monitoring and thoracic impedance measurements for fluid status estimations. In addition to bradycardia pacing the ICD can also provide anti-tachycardia pacing.

ICD lead construction and components

ICD leads, similar to pacing leads can be categorized by their fixation methods: active fixation,

Table 2.3 *Effect of anti-arrhythmic agents on DFTs*

Increase in DFT	No change in DFT	Decrease in DFT
• Class I B,C: Lidocaine, Flecainide, Mexilitene	• Class IA: Procainamide, Disopyramide	• Class III: Sotalol (mixed effect) Ibutilide, Dofetilide
• Class II (minimal ↑): Atenolol Metoprolol, Carvedilol	• Class IC: Propafenone	
• Class III : Amiodarone (mixed effect)		
• Class IV: Diltiazem, Verapamil		

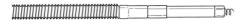

Figure 2.19 *Active fixation design. (helix electrode extended.)*

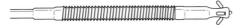

Figure 2.20 *Passive fixation design.*

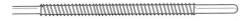

Figure 2.21 *No fixation mechanism.*

passive fixation and no fixation (Figures 2.19–2.21). The latter is usually added as a high voltage electrode that "floats" in the SVC or in the coronary sinus in patients with high DFTs (Figure 2.22).

Except for the standardized connector, the lead bodies, conductors and electrodes vary among manufacturers. The international Organization for Standardization (ISO) approved an "in-line" four pole connector system (ISO 27186) with pacing, electrogram sensing, and defibrillation functions for ICDs in 2010 (Figure 2.23A and B). This is referred to as the DF-4 high voltage connector.

The DF-4 connector is a relatively novel industry standard for the connection of a defibrillator lead to the generator. It aims at reducing the bulk created

by two or three pins at the proximal end of the defibrillator lead and its corresponding ports at the header of the device. Having only one connection port between the lead and the device reduces the material in the pocket, eliminates the risk of lead-to-port mismatch and makes the implantation procedure a little easier since only one set screw is required. The idea was also to design a connector system that has the sealing rings placed inside a connector module and not on the lead connector anymore.

Its predecessor, the DF-1 connector is bifurcated for single coil ICD leads to accommodate the IS-1 pace/sense connector and the DF-1 high voltage connector (Figure 2.24) or trifurcated for dual coil ICD leads to accommodate the IS-1 pace/sense connector and two DF-1 high voltage connectors (Figure 2.25).

The electrodes on the lead are the helix, ring, RV coil, and, if present, SVC coil electrodes. In *true bipolar pace/sense configuration*, there is a separate tip and ring electrode designed for sensing and pacing, similar to pacing leads. The impulse flows from the lead tip electrode (cathode) to the myocardium and returns to the ring electrode. In an *integrated pace/sense bipolar configuration*, there is a single tip electrode and the anode is integrated into the RV coil electrode. The electrograms

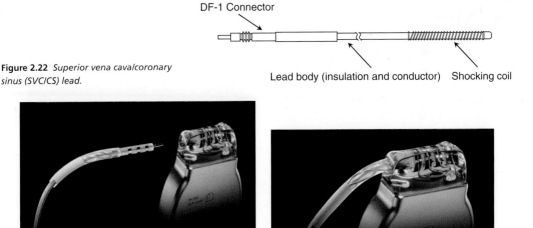

Figure 2.22 *Superior vena cava/coronary sinus (SVC/CS) lead.*

Figure 2.23 *(A) and (B) The DF-4 connector system offers physicians simplicity and speed of implant by reducing defibrillation connections from three to one and by minimizing the number of set screws. (Source: Reproduced with permission of St. Jude Medical, Inc.)*

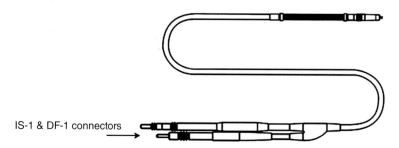

IS-1 & DF-1 connectors

Figure 2.24 *Single coil active fixation lead (tripolar). (Source: Reproduced with permission of Medtronic, Inc.)*

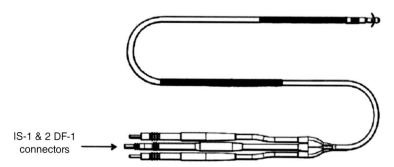

IS-1 & 2 DF-1 connectors

Figure 2.25 *Dual coil passive fixation lead (tripolar). (Source: Reproduced with permission of Medtronic, Inc.)*

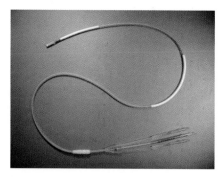

Figure 2.26 *Coil electrodes covered with GORE-TEX® (ePTFE) sleeve. (Source: courtesy of Boston Scientific.)*

obtained from the integrated bipolar lead may have a more "unipolar" appearance due to the larger surface for sensing. Coil electrodes are made of platinum/iridium or platinum-clad tantalum and offer a large surface area creating a large electric field. Some lead designs incorporate sleeves of polytetrafluoroethylene (ePTFE) GORE-TEX® with the goal of preventing tissue ingrowth and facilitating lead extraction (Figure 2.26). Another design utilized for preventing tissue ingrowth between and around coil wires is to backfill the

coil with silicone rubber and/or to utilize a flat shocking coil construction (Figures 2.27 and 2.28).

High voltage transvenous leads can be built on a single lumen, coaxial or multi-lumen platform. A single lumen design has a central conductor surrounded by insulation. Coaxial construction has conductors embedded within concentric layers of insulation and a multi-lumen design allows. Multi-lumen designs have multiple isolated compression lumens that insulate the conductors from each other.[38–40] The coaxial construction results in a greater lead body diameter and stiffness. Multi lumen designs allow for smaller lead diameters and have been implemented recently (Figures 2.29–2.32).[21, 41]

However, current lead designs for downsizing leads have led to premature lead fractures in adults and children and have resulted in recall of the Sprint Fidelis (Medtronic, Inc., Minneapolis, MN) and the St. Jude Riata and Riata ST leads (St. Jude Medical, Sylmar, CA).[42, 43]

In designing the Sprint Fidelis (SF) lead (Medtronic Inc., Minneapolis, MN) engineers achieved a 23% reduction in diameter by replacing the multiple isolated compression lumens used in

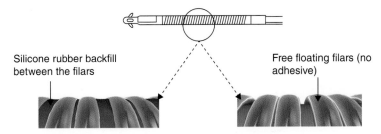

Figure 2.27 *Coil electrode construction. (Source: Reproduced with permission of Medtronic, Inc.)*

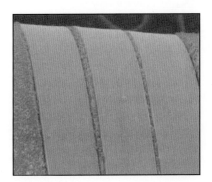

Figure 2.28 *Flat shocking electrode construction. (Source: Reproduced with permission of St. Jude Medical, Inc.)*

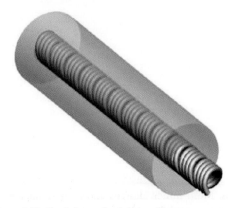

Figure 2.29 *Single lumen lead design. (Source: Reproduced with permission of Medtronic, Inc.)*

their standard ICD leads with an integrated compression lumen around conductor wires.[44] Riata leads (SJM Inc., St. Paul, MN) were designed to be true bipolar leads, with downsized components and a silicone core structure with 3 or 4 lumens. With body diameters of 6.7–7.6 Fr., these were the first ICD models capable of introduction through an 8-F sheath. The Riata ST lead represented further downsizing to a 6.3-F body, by reducing the central lumen and moving the conductor cables closer to the lead central axis, without changing the diameter of the outer silicone insulation. In addition, Riata ST models incorporated flat wire shocking electrodes, backfilled with silicone.[45] After reports of premature lead failures in the Riata and Riata ST leads secondary to inside-out abrasion of the silicone inner core of the lead, the Riata ST Optim™ lead was created. Similar in design to its predecessor, the most notable difference was the addition of an outer coating made of a silicone and polyurethane co polymer (Optim™, St. Jude medical Inc., St. Paul, MN), designed to improve abrasion resistance. The Durata lead builds further on the Riata ST Optim™ design, with the addition of a soft silicone tip and a slightly curved RV coil, both efforts to improve lead tip-endocardium interface and prevent myocardial perforations. Since recognition of premature failure of Riata and Riata ST leads, these models have been recalled, and the only remaining small-diameter defibrillation lead on the market is the St. Jude Durata.[44–48]

Use of dual-coil ICD leads are frequently selected, possibly due to the lower energy requirement during DFT testing, but no significant difference in ICD treatment efficacy has been shown between single and dual coil ICDs in the clinical setting.[49–52] In a small cohort of pediatric patients, we found no significant difference in the defibrillation energy requirement or clinical efficacy in dual coil versus single coil leads.[51] Dual-coil ICD leads have a more complicated lead structure and add hardware burden to patients. The presence of a proximal SVC defibrillation coil may in fact add an additional risk in transvenous lead extraction.[52] This factor should be considered particularly in children with transvenous ICDs implanted at a young age who have the potential to

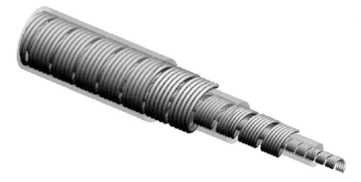

Figure 2.30 *Coaxial construction (lead body diameter tends to be high for the multiple layers of insulation, body stiffness is also substantial). (Source: Reproduced with permission of Medtronic, Inc.)*

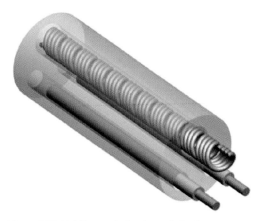

Figure 2.31 *Multilumen design (extruded polymer insulates the conductors from one another). (Source: Reproduced with permission of Medtronic, Inc.)*

develop significant scar tissue and fibrous binding due to tissue ingrowth in coils. When possible, a simpler single-coil ICD lead system should be considered for improvement in the long-term survival of lead systems and relative ease of lead extraction, especially in patients with long life expectancy.

ICD generator construction and components

The energy that an ICD must deliver is significantly higher than a pacemaker (an average of 30 J over a few milliseconds versus 1–10 microjoules with a pacemaker). Therefore, ICD battery size and material differs from that of a pacemaker in that low resistance battery compounds such as lithium-vanadium oxide or lithium-silver-vanadium oxide are used in ICDs. The key components of an ICD generator are shown in Table 2.4 and Figure 2.33.

ICD therapies

Antitachycardia pacing

Antitachycardia pacing (ATP) refers to the use of pacing stimulation techniques for termination of tachyarrhythmias. Such techniques can be automatically applied using ICDs and offer the potential for painless termination of ventricular tachycardia (VT). VT with a reentrant mechanism is often susceptible to termination with ATP. The anatomic substrate for reentry is the interweaving of viable myocardium and scar. The reentry wavefront circulates around areas of functional or anatomically fixed conduction block. Areas of fixed conduction block are most often due to inexcitable scar tissue due to prior myocardial infarction, surgical incisions, prosthetic material, or anatomic barriers. In a reentrant circuit, the tissue in front of the leading edge of the wavefront must have recovered to create an excitable gap so that it the tachycardia can perpetuate itself. ATP delivered as a series of pacing impulses at rates faster than the tachycardia rate can terminate tachycardia by depolarizing tissue in the excitable gap so that the tissue in front of the advancing tachycardia wavefront becomes refractory preventing arrhythmia perpetuation, (Figure 3.34).[53] ICD ATP algorithms include burst pacing, which may be rate adaptive or fixed rate. In rate adaptive algorithms, the pacing rate is determined by the tachycardia rate and generally a percentage of that rate (usually 95–70% of tachycardia rate). The following terminology is often used for programming ATP therapies for atrial and ventricular tachycardia.

- *Burst* – train of pulses delivered at a fixed cycle length that is a percentage of the tachycardia rate

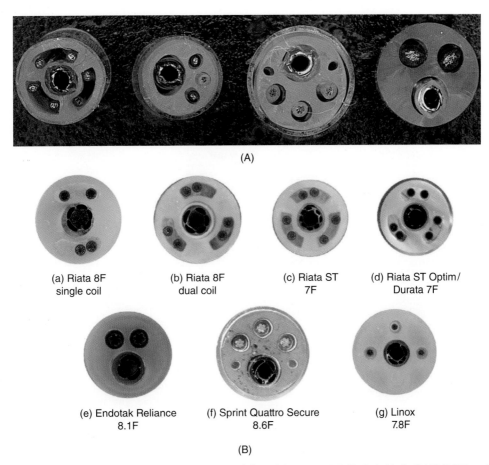

(A)

(a) Riata 8F
single coil

(b) Riata 8F
dual coil

(c) Riata ST
7F

(d) Riata ST Optim/
Durata 7F

(e) Endotak Reliance
8.1F

(f) Sprint Quattro Secure
8.6F

(g) Linox
7.8F

(B)

Figure 2.32 *(A) Cross sections of multilumen designs. From left to right: Durata 7 Fr (St. Jude Medical), Fidelis 7 Fr and Sprint Quattro 9 Fr (Medtronic) and Reliance 9 Fr (Boston Scientific). (Source: Reproduced with permission of St. Jude Medical, Inc. (B) Cross sections of multilumen designs (to scale).)*

Table 2.4 *ICD generator components and functions*

ICD Component	Function
Battery	Powers generator
Capacitor	Energy storage
Transformer	Generates high voltage
Microprocessor based circuitry	Diagnostic data storage, software for ICD algorithms implementation
Sensing circuits and amplifiers	Sensing of input signals, automatic sensing threshold, and amplitude gain adjustment
Generator header block	Connection of sealed internal circuitry to lead system

- *Burst+* – burst followed by two extrastimulus at the end of the train
- *Ramp* – begins with coupling interval that is a percentage of the tachycardia rate and is followed by decremental coupling intervals throughout the train
- *Scan* – series of ramps that decrement in starting coupling interval between each train.

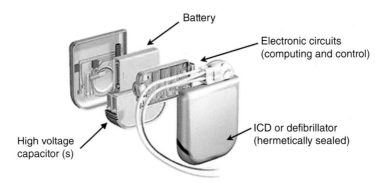

Battery

Electronic circuits
(computing and control)

High voltage
capacitor (s)

ICD or defibrillator
(hermetically sealed)

Figure 2.33 *Illustration of an ICD generator.*

ATP can be programmed in the VF zone in many current ICDs to deliver therapy before capacitor charging or during capacitor charging. Numerous studies in adult cohorts and a smaller pediatric case series have demonstrated that ATP terminates 78–94% of ventricular tachycardias (VTs) < 200 bpm with a 2–4% risk of acceleration.[54] If ATP fails, the device can be programmed to deliver a cardioversion or defibrillation shock. Of note, the PainFREE Rx III prospective randomized trial demonstrated that empirical ATP is safe and effective compared with shocks for fast VT (FVT) and that ATP terminated 73% of FVT episodes (cycle length (CL) < 320 ms) with a low risk of VT acceleration and syncope and there was no difference in mortality. These observations, combined with the established efficacy of ATP for slower VT, reposition the ICD as primarily an ATP device with only occasional backup defibrillation.[54, 55] The role of ATP for termination of VT in children with ICDs also seems to be promising.[55]

Cardioversion

Monomorphic ventricular tachycardia can be terminated by synchronized cardioversion shocks. Sometimes, even low energy (≤5 J) are effective in terminating VT. However, weak shocks that are unsuccessful in VT termination could risk degeneration of VT into VF and programming of higher energy cardioversion shocks may be preferred. It should be noted that shock pain in not dependent on shock strength and ICD charge time to deliver a higher energy shock may not be clinically relevant.

Defibrillation

The classic waveform used for defibrillation is truncated and characterized by the initial voltage (Vi), the final voltage (Vf) and the pulse width or tilt. In a monophasic shock, the shock is given in only one direction from one electrode to the other. In a biphasic shock, initial direction of shock is reversed by changing the polarity of the electrodes in the latter part of the shock being delivered. Biphasic shocks are more effective than monophasic shocks and need lesser energy.[38–40] All currently available ICDs utilize biphasic waveforms. The "dose" of defibrillation is usually given in units of energy (joules) and can be described as stored or delivered energy. Since the waveforms are truncated approximately 10% of stored energy is not delivered. In most ICDs, pulse widths and waveform tilt (defined as percentage of initial voltage drawn from a capacitor) for defibrillation are pre-set values with tilts ranging from 50–65% for phase 1 and phase 2. Some devices also permit individualization of pulse widths which can be optimized for patients with high defibrillation thresholds.[56, 57] Alteration in polarity configuration can also affect defibrillation thresholds. In transvenous lead systems, the distal (RV) electrode can be used as the anode or the cathode. Defibrillation thresholds with monophasic shocks have been shown to be ~30% lower with the distal electrode as the anode but the results with biphasic shocks are mixed.[58–60] However, when polarity effect has been demonstrated, waveforms with a first phase in which the RV coil electrode is the anode seem to be more effective. Due to individual variations, it makes sense to test the opposite polarity during

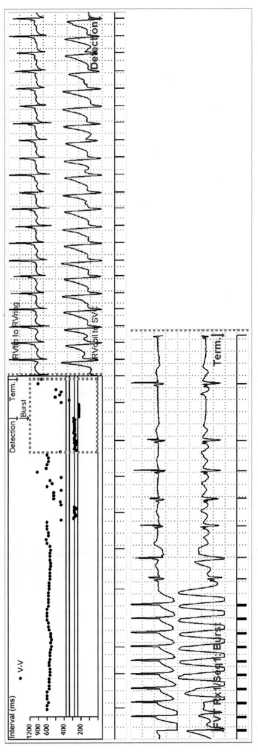

Figure 2.34 A remote monitoring transmission from a 13-year-old patient with Arrhythmogenic Right Ventricular Cardiomyopathy shows appropriate detection of monomorhic ventricular tachycardia (CL 240 ms). Programmed ATP is delivered using a burst pacing protocol at a CL of 200 ms which terminates VT. Top channel shows near near field EGMs, middle channel shows far field EGMs and the marker channel is shown at the bottom.

defibrillation threshold testing (DFT) when an adequate safety margin is not obtained. Due to the large surface area of the ICD generator shell, it can be used as an active electrode and reduces the biphasic DFT by 30% compared with that of a dual coil defibrillation lead.[61] Finally, defibrillation energy programming is usually based on an objective determination of defibrillation efficacy during testing in an individual patient (Chapter 7).

ICD monitoring, algorithms, and alerts

ICDs and pacemakers share many monitoring features such as battery status, lead impedance measurements, pacing thresholds, sensed signal amplitudes, rate histograms, percentage of pacing, arrhythmia detection with recorded electrograms, and noninvasive EPS capability. Some other features specific to ICDs include, capacitor charge time, defibrillation impedance measurements, arrhythmia detection in rate defined zones, and arrhythmia discrimination (SVT vs VT).

Some ICDs have additional manufacturer specific algorithms. Both single and dual chamber ICDs have algorithms to discriminate between SVT and VT. The right ventricular (RV) Lead Noise Discrimination algorithm differentiates RV lead noise from VT/VF by comparing a far field EGM signal to near field sensing. If lead noise is identified, VT/VF detection is withheld, shock therapy is not delivered and an RV Lead Noise alert is triggered by the device (Figure 3.35).[62] In order to prevent inappropriate ICD shocks due to oversensing of T waves, discrimination features are designed to withhold therapy if there is evidence that a "fast" ventricular rate is due to T wave oversensing.[63] The algorithm operates on the assumption that R waves and T waves have different waveform characteristics. R waves are generally higher frequency waveforms than T waves. The algorithm utilizes a differential frequency filter that enables R-T pattern recognition and withholds detection and averts an inappropriate shock if a consistent pattern of T wave oversensing is detected. The LIA™ (Lead Integrity Alert) is a manufacture specific audible alert designed to detect early lead failure, ideally, prior to an adverse clinical event

such as multiple inappropriate shocks. It is triggered if at least two of the following three criteria are met within the past 60 days of each other:[64]

- Abnormal RV lead impedance (defined as impedance that is significantly higher or lower than a calculated baseline impedance level).
- Two or more high-rate-nonsustained VTs with intervals that are shorter than 220 ms.
- At least 30 short V-V interval counts within 3 consecutive days.

ICD technology has expanded to incorporate intrathoracic impedance measurements to detect fluid status changes in heart failure patients. Using the RV Coil to ICD Can pathway, which passes through the tissue within the thoracic cavity, daily average impedances are recorded. If the daily impedance falls below the reference impedance, it may indicate fluid accumulation in the patient's thoracic cavity and this data may be useful in patient management.[65]

Currently, available ICD alert features also warn the patient (via an audible or vibratory alert) in case of low battery voltage, excessive capacitor charge time, and out of range lead impedances. An alert may be triggered if VF detection and/or three or more VF therapies are programmed off inadvertently. An alert may also be triggered if anywhere from one to six high voltage shocks occur during one single episode or if all device therapies within one tachycardia detection zone are delivered.

Remote monitoring

Transtelephonic monitoring for pacemakers has been available for many years, but provided only basic information on battery status, sensing, and lead capture. More recently, home transmitters are available from most major device companies that are able to interrogate the pacemakers and ICDs, automatically using wireless technology.[66] The data downloaded from the device by the transmitter is then sent to the physician, using either the landline phone or the GSM network. Many current pacemakers and ICDs are able to automatically execute an entire device interrogation and a large portion of the testing that is otherwise performed manually at a clinic visit. Data acquired automatically on a pre-defined periodic basis by the device can then be sent from the patient's home to the physician

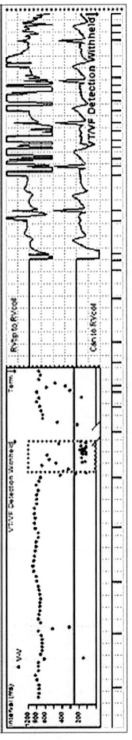

Figure 2.35 *A 15-year-old patient with an ICD lead failure. The top channel shows electrograms obtained from an integrated bipolar lead recorded between the RV tip and RV coil. The middle channel shows far field electrograms recorded between the Can and RV coil. The marker channel shows that there are more markers than the far field ventricular electrograms. However, VT/VF detection was withheld and no shock therapy was delivered due to appropriate recognition of lead noise by the RV Lead Noise Discrimination algorithm in the ICD.*

using the transmitter. Patients and physicians are notified if any device alerts are triggered.

References

1 Mehra R, Belk P. Fundamental of cardiac stimulation. In: Saksena S, Camm AJ, eds. *Electrophysiology Disorders of the Heart*, 2nd Edn. Philadelphia, PA: Elsevier Saunders, 2005: 173–185.

2 Bunch TJ, Hayes DL, Friedman PA. Clinically relevant basics of pacing and defibrillation. In: Hayes, DL, Friedman PA, eds. *Cardiac Pacing, Defibrillation and Resynchronization*, 2nd Edn. Oxford, UK: Wiley-Blackwell, 2008: 1–42.

3 Mond H, Stokes K, Helland J, et al. The porous titanium steroid eluting electrode: a double blind stud assessing the stimulation threshold effects of steroid. *Pacing Clin Electrophysiol* 1988; 11: 214–219.

4 Kay GN, Anderson K, Epstein AE, Plumb VJ. Active fixation atrial leads: randomized comparison of two lead designs. *Pacing Clin Electrophysiol* 1989; 12: 1355–1361.

5 Schwabb B, Frohlig G, Berg M, Schwerdt H, Schieffer H. Five year follow up of a bipolar steroid eluting ventricular pacing lead. *Pacing Clin Electrophysiol* 1999; 22: 1226–1228.

6 Wiegand UK, Portratz J, Bonnemeier H, et al. Long term superiority of steroid elution in atrial active fixation platinum leads. *Pacing Clin Electrophysiol* 2000; 23: 1003–1009.

7 King DH, Gillette PC, Shannon C, Cuddy TE. Steroid eluting endocardial pacing lead for treatment of exit block. *Am Heart J* 1983; 106: 1438–1440.

8 Timmins G, Helland J, Westveer D. The evolution of low threshold leads. *Clin Prog Pacing Electrophysiol* 1983; 1: 313–314.

9 Saxonhouse SJ, Conti JB, Curtis AB. Current of injury predicts adequate active lead fixation in permanent pacemaker/defibrillation leads. *J Am Coll Caridiol* 2005;45: 412–417.

10 Hayes DL. Electromagnetic interference, drug-device interactions, and other practical considerations. In: Furman S, Hayes DL, Holmes DR, eds. *A Practice of Cardiac Pacing*. 3rd Edn. New York: Futura, 1993; 665–684.

11 Reiffel JA, Coromolas J, Zimmerman JM, et al. Drug-device interactions: clinical considerations. *PACE* 1985; 8: 369–373.

12 Hayes DL. Effects of drugs and devices on permanent pacemakers. *Cardiology* 1991; 1: 70–75.

13 Gay RJ, Brown DF. Pacemaker failure due to procainamide toxicity. *Am J Cardiol* 1974; 34: 728–732.

14 Hellestrand KJ, Burnett PJ, Milne JR. Effect of the antiarrhythmic agent flecainide acetate on acute and chronic pacing thresholds. *PACE* 1983; 6: 892–899.

15 Bianconi L, Boccadamo R, Toscano S, et al. Effects of oral propafenone therapy on chronic myocardial pacing threshold. *PACE* 1992; 15: 148–154.

16 Kruse IM. Long-term performance of endocardial leads with steroid-eluting electrodes. *PACE* 1986; 9: 1217–1219.

17 LeVick CE, Mizgala HF, Kerr CR. Failure to pace following high dose antiarrhythmic therapy-reversal with isoproterenol. *PACE* 1984; 7: 252–256.

18 Furman S, Hurzeler P, DeCaprio V. The ventricular endocardial electrogram and pacemaker sensing. *J Thorac Cardiovasc Surg* 1977; 73: 258–266.

19 Kleinert M, Elmquvist H, Strandberg H. Spectral properties of atrial and ventricular endocardial signals. *Pacing Clin Electrophysiol* 1979; 2: 11–19.

20 Cuvillier E. Pacing lead terminology and technology. In: *Handbook of Leads for Pacing, Defibrillation and Cardiac Resynchronization*, 2nd Edn, 2011; 39–49.

21 Cantù F, Filippo P, Gabbarini F, Borghi A, Brambilla R, Ferrero P, et al. Selective-site pacing in paediatric patients: a new application of the Select Secure system. *Europace* 2009; 11(5): 601–606.

22 Calfee RV, Saulson Sh. A voluntary standard for 3.2 mm unipolar and bipolar pacemaker leads and connectors. *Pacing Clin Electrophysiol* 1986; 9: 1181–1185.

23 Anderson, Kenneth M., et al. Rate adaptive pacer. Medtronic, Inc., assignee. Patent 4,428,378. 31 Jan. 1984. Web. 15 Dec. 2010.

24 Ferreira AM, Costa F, Tralhão A, Marques H, Cardim N, Adragão P. MRI-conditional pacemakers: current perspectives. *Med Devices (Auckl)* 2014; 7: 115–124.

25 Shinbane JS, Colletti PM, Shellock FG. MR imaging in patients with pacemakers and other devices: engineering the future. *JACC Cardiovasc Imaging* 2012; 5: 332–333.

26 Knops RE, Tjong FV, Neuzil P, Sperzel J, Miller MA, Petru J, et al. Chronic performance of a leadless cardiac pacemaker: 1-year follow-up of the LEADLESS trial. *J Am Coll Cardiol*. 2015 Apr 21; 65(15): 1497–1504.

27 Ritter P, Duray GZ, Steinwender C, Soejima K, Omar R, Mont L, et al. and the Micra Transcatheter Pacing Study Group. Early performance of a miniaturized leadless cardiac pacemaker: the Micra Transcatheter Pacing Study. *Eur Heart J*. 2015 June 4; 36(37): 2510–2519.

28 Zipes DP, Fischer J, King RM, Nicoll AD, Jolly WW. Termination of ventricular fibrillation in dogs by depolarizing a critical amount of myocardium. *Am J Cardiol* 1975; 36: 37–44.

29 Mazeh N, Roth BJ. A mechanism of the upper limit of vulnerability. *Heart Rhythm*. 2009; 6(3): 361–367.

30 Chen PS and Lin SF. Upper limit of vulnerability and heterogeneity. *Heart Rhythm*. 2009 March; 6(3): 368–369.

31 Moore EN, Spear JF. Ventricular fibrillation thresholds physiological and pharmacological importance. *Arch Intern Med.* 1975; 135(3): 446–453.

32 Trayanova N. Defibrillation of the heart. Insights into mechanisms from modeling studies. *Exp Physiol.* 2006 Mar; 91(2): 323–337.

33 Dosdall D, Fast V, Ideker R. Mechanisms of defibrillation. *Annu. Rev. Biomed. Eng.* 2010; 12: 233–258.

34 Ideker RE, Chattipakorn TN, Gray RA. Defibrillation mechanisms: the parable of the blind men and the elephant. *J Cardiovasc Electrophysiol.* 2000 Sep; 11(9): 1008–1013.

35 Dillon SM, Kwaku KF. Progresive depolarization: a unified hypothesis for defibrillation and fibrillation induction by shocks. *J Cardiovasc Electrophysiol* 1998; 9: 529–552.

36 Yee R, Klein GJ, Guiraudon GM, et al. Initial clinical experience with the pacemaker-cardioverter-defibrillator. *Can J Cardiol.* 1990; 6: 147–156.

37 Radbill AE, Triedman JK, Berul CI, Walsh EP, Alexander ME, Webster G, Cecchin F. Prospective evaluation of defibrillation threshold and postshock rhythm in young ICD recipients. *Pacing Clin Electrophysiol* 2012; 35: 1487–1493.

38 Swerdlow CD. ICD waveforms: what really matters? *Heart Rhythm.* 2006 Sep ;3(9): 1060–1062.

39 Hwang GS, Tang L, Joung B, Morita N, Hayashi H, Karagueuzian HS, et al. Superiority of biphasic over monophasic defibrillation shocks is attributable to less intracellular calcium transient heterogeneity. *J Am Coll Cardiol.* 2008 Sep 2; 52(10): 828–835.

40 Shepard RK, DeGroot PJ, Pacifico A, Wood MA, Ellenbogen KA. Prospective randomized comparison of 65%/65% versus 42%/42% tilt biphasic waveform on defibrillation thresholds in humans. *J Interv Card Electrophysiol.* 2003 Jun; 8(3): 221–225.

41 Medtronic, Inc. *Medtronic Technical Concept Paper: Insights on Sprint Design Enhancements.* June 2004.

42 St. Jude Medical, Inc. St. Jude Medical ICD Lead Design and Long-Term Performance. May 2013.

43 Rordorf R, Poggio L, Savastano S, et al. Failure of implantable cardioverter-defibrillator leads: a matter of lead size? *Heart Rhythm* 2013; 10: 184–190.

44 Janson CM, Patel AR, Bonney WJ, Smoots K, Shah MJ. Implantable cardioverter-defibrillator lead failure in children and young adults: a matter of lead diameter or lead design? *J Am Coll Cardiol.* 2014 Jan 21; 63(2): 133–140.

45 Atallah J, Erickson CC, Cecchin F, Dubin AM, Law IH, Cohen MI, et al. and the Pediatric and Congenital Electrophysiology Society (PACES). Multi-institutional study of implantable defibrillator lead performance in children and young adults: results of the Pediatric Lead Extractability and Survival Evaluation (PLEASE) study. *Circulation.* 2013 Jun 18; 127(24): 2393–2402.

46 Rordorf R, Canevese F, Vicentini A, et al. Delayed ICD lead cardiac perforation: comparison of small versus standard-diameter leads implanted in a single center. *Pacing Clin Electrophysiol* 2011; 34: 475–483.

47 Ellis CR, Rottman JN. Increased rate of subacute lead complications with small-caliber implantable cardioverter-defibrillator leads. *Heart Rhythm* 2009; 6: 619–624.

48 Cairns JA, Epstein AE, Rickard J, Connolly SJ, Buller C, Wilkoff BL, et al. Prospective long-term evaluation of Optim-insulated (Riata ST Optim and Durata) implantable cardioverter-defibrillator leads. *Heart Rhythm.* 2014 Dec; 11(12): 2156–2162.

49 Kutyifa V, Huth Ruwald AC, Aktas MK, Jons C, McNitt S, Polonsky B, et al. Clinical impact, safety, and efficacy of single- versus dual-coil ICD leads in MADIT-CRT. *J Cardiovasc Electrophysiol.* 2013 Nov; 24(11): 1246–1252.

50 Neuzner J, Carlsson J. Dual- versus single-coil implantable defibrillator leads: review of the literature. *Clin Res Cardiol.* 2012 Apr; 101(4): 239–245.

51 Patel A, Chang PM, Smoots K, Shah MJ. Clinical defibrillation efficacy of single coil transvenous ICD leads in children and young patients with congenital heart disease. *Heart Rhythm* 8(5): S98.

52 Cooper JM, Stephenson EA, Berul CI, Walsh EP, Epstein LM. Implantable cardioverter defibrillator lead complications and laser extraction in children and young adults with congenital heart disease: implications for implantation and management. *J Cardiovasc Electrophysiol.* 2003 Apr; 14(4): 344–349.

53 Peinado R, Almendral JM, Rius T, et al. Randomized, prospective comparison of four burst pacing algorithms for spontaneous ventricular tachycardia. *Am J Cardiol.* 1998; 82: 1422–1425.

54 Wathen MS, DeGroot PJ, Sweeney MO, Stark AJ, Otterness MF, Adkisson WO, et al. Prospective randomized multicenter trial of empirical antitachycardia pacing versus shocks for spontaneous rapid ventricular tachycardia in patients with implantable cardioverter-defibrillators. pacing fast ventricular tachycardia reduces shock therapies (PainFREE Rx II) *Trial Results. Circulation.* 2004 Oct 26; 110(17): 2591–2596.

55 Kalra Y, Radbill AE, Johns JA, Fish FA, Kannankeril PJ. Antitachycardia pacing reduces appropriate and inappropriate shocks in children and congenital heart disease patients. *Heart Rhythm.* 2012 Nov; 9(11): 1829–1834.

56 Irnich W. How to program pulse duration or tilt in implantable cardioverter defibrillators. *Pacing Clin Electrophysiol.* 2003 Jan; 26(1 Pt 2): 453–456.

57 Natarajan S, Henthorn R, Burroughs J, Esberg D, Zweibel S, Ross T, et al. "Tuned" defibrillation waveforms outperform 50/50% tilt defibrillation waveforms: a randomized multi-center study. *Pacing Clin Electrophysiol.* 2007 Jan; 30 Suppl 1: S139–142.

58 Strickberger SA, Hummel JD, Horwood LE, Jentzer J, Daoud E, Niebauer M, et al. Effect of shock polarity on ventricular defibrillation threshold using a transvenous lead system. *J Am Coll Cardiol.* 1994 Oct; 24(4): 1069–1072.

59 Strickberger SA, Man KC, Daoud E, Neary MP, Horwood LE, Niebauer M, et al. Effect of first-phase polarity of biphasic shocks on defibrillation threshold with a single transvenous lead system. *Am Coll Cardiol.* 1995 Jun; 25(7): 1605–1608.

60 Olsovsky MR, Shorofsky SR, Gold MR. Effect of shock polarity on biphasic defibrillation thresholds using an active pectoral lead system. *J Cardiovasc Electrophysiol.* 1998 Apr; (4): 350–354.

61 Gold MR, Foster AH, Shorofsky SR. Lead system optimization for transvenous defibrillation. *Am J Cardiol* 1997; 80: 1163–1167.

62 Koneru JN, Kaszala K, Bordachar P, Shehata M, Swerdlow C, Ellenbogen KA. Spectrum of issues detected by an ICD diagnostic alert that utilizes far-field electrograms: Clinical implications. *Heart Rhythm.* 2015 May; 12(5): 957–967.

63 Almehairi M, Somani R, Ellenbogen K, Baranchuk A. Inappropriate detection of ventricular fibrillation in the presence of T-wave oversensing algorithm. *Pacing Clin Electrophysiol.* 2015 Mar; 38(3): 407.

64 Swerdlow CD, Gunderson BD, Ousdigian KT, Abeyratne A, Sachanandani H, Ellenbogen KA. Downloadable software algorithm reduces inappropriate shocks caused by implantable cardioverter-defibrillator lead fractures: a prospective study. *Circulation.* 2010 Oct 12; 122(15): 1449–1455.

65 Gula LJ, Wells GA, Yee R, Koehler J, Sarkar S, Sharma V, et al. A novel algorithm to assess risk of heart failure exacerbation using ICD diagnostics: validation from RAFT. *Heart Rhythm.* 2014 Sep; 11(9): 1626–1631.

66 Reynolds DW, Jayaprasad N, Francis J, et al. Remote monitoring of implantable cardioverter defibrillator. *Indian Pacing Electrophysiol J.* 2006; 6: 186–188.

PART 2
Clinical Concepts

CHAPTER 3

Indications for permanent pacing, device, and lead selection

Philip M. Chang[1], Christopher Carter[2], and Yaniv Bar-Cohen[3]

[1] Pediatric Electrophysiologist, Medical Director, Adult Congenital Heart Disease Care Program, Keck Medical Center of University of Southern California, Assistant Professor of Clinical Medicine, Keck School of Medicine of University of Southern California, Los Angeles, CA, USA

[2] The Children's Heart Clinic of Minnesota and North Dakota, Pediatric Electrophysiologist, Minneapolis, MN, USA

[3] Director, Cardiac Rhythm Devices, Children's Hospital Los Angeles, Associate Professor of Clinical Pediatrics and Medicine, University of Southern California, Los Angeles, CA, USA

Introduction

Permanent pacing has become a standard part of the therapeutic armamentarium in the care of rhythm disturbances in pediatric and congenital heart disease (CHD) patients. Structural abnormalities, acquired disease, and functional disturbances can involve any part of the conduction system, making permanent pacing necessary in a variety of circumstances. Great care must be taken to evaluate the specific need for and expected benefit from pacemaker implantation. This requires an awareness of the potential short- and long-term complications of pacing as well an understanding of the available pacing hardware and features.

The following chapter is divided into three primary sections: implantation guidelines, lead decisions, and generator selection. In the first section, a comprehensive discussion of the accepted and expanding indications for permanent pacing in pediatric and CHD patients will be presented. Subsequently, specific considerations involving the selection of leads and pulse generators will be discussed. The aim of the chapter is to provide the implanting physician with a practical framework to properly approach patients who may require and benefit from pacemaker implantation.

Section 1: indications for permanent pacemaker implantation

Indications for permanent pacemaker implantation in the pediatric and CHD population are in many ways similar to those in adults. However, special consideration needs to be given to several unique attributes of this group that affect these indications. Unlike adults, the majority of pacing indications in children and individuals with CHD arise in the setting of congenital rhythm abnormalities or intrinsic or acquired rhythm disturbances related to CHD and its associated interventions. Furthermore, criteria that rely on absolute values of heart rate or pause duration need to be considered cautiously when extrapolated to children.

Cardiac Pacing and Defibrillation in Pediatric and Congenital Heart Disease, First Edition.
Edited by Maully Shah, Larry Rhodes and Jonathan Kaltman.
© 2017 John Wiley & Sons Ltd. Published 2017 by John Wiley & Sons Ltd.
Companion Website: www.wiley.com/go/shah/cardiac_pacing

The indications for permanent pacing in the pediatric population have continued to expand as evidenced by the most recent updated ACC/AHA/HRS recommendations published in 2012 (see Table 3.1).[1] These recommendations are classified based on the presumed benefit versus risk of each indication. Class I indications have a benefit that is clearly demonstrated in the literature. Class IIa indications are felt to be beneficial but further research is still needed for absolute clarification. Class IIb recommendations may be beneficial but more information is needed. In general, class IIb recommendations can be considered but are generally not indicated. Class III indications are

Table 3.1 *Recommendations for permanent pacing in children, adolescents, and patients with congenital heart disease. Class I – indicated, Class IIa – probably indicated, Class IIb – may be considered. Level of evidence in parentheses: A – multiple populations evaluated, B – limited populations evaluated, C – very limited populations evaluated. AV – atriventricular, CHD – congenital heart disease, SND – sinus node dysfunction, IART- intraatrial reentrant tachycardia. Source: Epstein 2013. Reproduced with permission of Wolters Kluwer[1]*

Class I	
1	Symptomatic *SND* during age inappropriate bradycardia
2	Symptomatic bradycardia in conjunction with any degree of *AV block* or with ventricular arrhythmias presumed to be due to AV block
3	Advanced second or third degree AV block with symptomatic bradycardia, ventricular dysfunction or low cardiac output
4	Congenital third degree AV block with wide QRS escape rhythm, complex ventricular ectopy or ventricular dysfunction
	Postoperative high-grade second- or third-degree AV block that is not expected to resolve or persists ≥ 7 days after cardiac surgery
	Congenital third degree AV block in an infant with ventricular rate < 55 bpm or with CHD and ventricular rate < 70 bpm.
Class IIA	
1	Sinus or junctional bradycardia for the prevention of recurrent IART in CHD
2	Congenital third degree AV block beyond the first year of life with an average heart rate <50 bpm, abrupt pauses in ventricular rate that are 2 or 3 times the basic cycle length, or associated with symptoms due to chronotropic incompetence
3	Sinus bradycardia with complex congenital heart disease with a resting heart rate less than 40 bpm or pauses in ventricular rate longer than 3 s
4	CHD and impaired hemodynamics due to sinus bradycardia or loss of AV synchrony
5	Unexplained syncope in the patient with prior congenital heart surgery complicated by transient complete heart block with residual fascicular block after a careful evaluation to exclude other causes of syncope
Class IIB	
1	Transient postoperative third-degree AV block that reverts to sinus rhythm with residual bifascicular block.
2	Congenital third-degree AV block in asymptomatic children or adolescents with an acceptable rate, a narrow QRS complex and normal ventricular function
Class III	
1	Pacing is not indicated for transient postoperative AV block with return of normal AV conduction in the otherwise asymptomatic patient
2	Pacing is not indicated for asymptomatic bifascicular block with or without first-degree AV block after surgery for CHD in the absence of prior transient complete AV block
3	Pacing is not indicated for asymptomatic type I second-degree AV block
4	Pacing is not indicated for asymptomatic sinus bradycardia with the longest relative risk interval less than 3 s and a minimum heart rate more than 40 bpm

those where risk is felt to outweigh benefit and are therefore not recommended.

Acquired heart block

There are a number of reasons for acquired heart block in the pediatric population. The most common etiology is as a complication of procedures to correct CHD. This accounts for about 55% of all pediatric patients receiving pacemakers in one series.[2] Heart block complications are usually encountered following CHD surgery, but catheter-based procedures, such as device closure of lesions, can also result in AV block. Catheter ablation procedures for the treatment of arrhythmias can also contribute, but these complications are less common since the widespread use of cryoablation.

Surgical corrections involving ventricular septal defect (VSD) repair have a higher incidence of post-operative AV block, as do surgeries that can impact the left ventricular outflow such as the Ross-Konno procedure, subaortic membrane resection, or mitral valve replacement. While the incidence has decreased over the years with improved surgical technique, permanent AV block still occurs in up to 3% of pediatric cardiac surgeries.[3,4] The long-term prognosis of untreated permanent post-operative heart block is very poor. Prior to the advent of permanent pacing, mortality associated with post-operative heart block was estimated to be between 28–100%.[5–8]

While loss of conduction can be due to permanent injury to the conduction system, it can also be transient. Postoperative heart block resolves with conservative management and observation in 43–92% of cases.[5–10] Temporary pacing is usually required in the interim as the slower rates and the loss of atrioventricular synchrony can lead to hemodynamic instability. Based on the poor outcomes of untreated postoperative heart block, high grade second degree or third degree AV block that persists for longer than 7 days is a class I indication for pacemaker implantation.[1] This 1-week waiting period is based on the natural history of post-operative complete heart block, where the majority of those that resolve do so within that time.[4,7–9]

While patients who recover AV conduction after an initial period of post-operative AV block have traditionally been considered low risk and have not undergone pacemaker implantation, more recent data suggests a need for some caution with this group of patients.[4,10,11] In one study monitoring the long-term follow-up of patients with repaired tetralogy of Fallot (TOF), 40% of patients with transient post-operative complete heart block that persisted past the third post-operative day experienced late sudden death during follow-up thought to possibly be due to heart block.[12] Other studies have attempted to identify features that may predispose patients to late heart block. Those with initial complete heart block who recover conduction but have persistent bifascicular block appear to have a higher risk of recurrence of late heart block when compared to patients with bifascicular block without initial complete heart block.[11] Due to the possible risk of late heart block, pacemaker implantation can be considered, but is not necessarily indicated, in patients with bifascicular block after recovery of conduction (class IIb indication). In patients with residual fascicular block and unexplained syncope, the risk may be higher and a class IIa indication has been advised. While syncope in this setting with no other etiology is felt to be an indicator of late onset heart block,[13,14] a thorough workup should be performed to rule out other potential etiologies before device implantation.

Other rare etiologies of acquired heart block also need to be considered and include medication toxicities, infection, and complications of systemic disease. Common medications causing heart block include cardiac glycosides, beta blockers, and calcium channel blockers. Classic infections causing heart block include Lyme disease, Rocky Mountain spotted fever, Chagas disease, rheumatic fever, and viral myocarditis. Systemic diseases such as Kawasaki disease, sarcoidosis, and amyloidosis may also result in heart block.[15] Many of these may be transient depending on response to medical therapy or removal of the offending agent. Any persistent complete heart block with symptomatic bradycardia, decreased ventricular function or low cardiac output meets a class I indication for pacemaker placement.[1]

Patients with progressive neuromuscular disorders are approached more conservatively when permanent pacing is considered. These disorders include myotonic muscular dystrophy, Becker muscular dystrophy, Kearns–Sayre syndrome, and peroneal muscular atrophy. Patients with these conditions can acquire progressive conduction system disease that progresses in a rapid fashion.[16–19] Any degree of AV block associated with these disorders, including first degree, is considered a class IIb indication for consideration of pacemaker placement, while complete or advanced second degree AV block in this population is a class I indication.[1]

Congenital heart block

Congenital complete heart block is seen in infants with or without associated CHD. In infants with structurally normal hearts, congenital heart block is primarily due to maternal connective tissue disease. Specifically, infants of mothers with anti-SSA/Ro antibodies are at particular risk. The maternal autoantibodies cross the placenta and attack the conduction system of the fetus resulting in inflammation and fibrosis and subsequent heart block. It is estimated that in seropositive mothers, the incidence of complete heart block is 1–2% of live births.[20,21] In infants born to mothers with a previous child with congenital heart block the chance of heart block is increased from 10 to 16%.[22–24] When these infants are born with first or second degree AV block, progression to complete heart block can still occur and should be followed very closely.[24]

The association of certain congenital defects with complete heart block is also well established.[25,26] In up to 53% of fetuses found to have complete heart block prenatally, associated CHD can be demonstrated.[27] The most common defect in this group is left atrial isomerism, often with an associated AV septal defect.[28,29] Prior to the widespread use of prenatal echocardiographic screening, however, the most common lesion associated with AV block was congenitally corrected transposition of the great arteries (CCTGA).[30,31] In patients with CCTGA who have intact atrioventricular conduction at birth, there is a 2% per year lifetime risk of acquiring heart block. These patients require lifelong observation.[32]

Symptomatic bradycardia or symptoms due to AV dissociation are a class I indication for pacing in any patient with congenital heart block.[1] However, many patients with congenital heart block remain asymptomatic due to physiologic adaptation to AV dissociation and slower escape rates. Regardless,

the large majority will meet criteria for pacing at some point during childhood or adolescence and undergo pacemaker placement.[33] In children less than a year of age, studies have demonstrated that symptoms and mortality are greater with lower resting heart rates.[30,31,33] Based upon this data, the current class I recommendation is for any infant in the first year of life with a resting heart rate of less than 55 bpm to have a permanent pacemaker placed.[1] It is important to note that these studies considered mean resting heart rate, not minimum heart rate, which can be lower in these patients. In the setting of CHD with congenital AV block mortality is higher due to the additional hemodynamic consequences of their disease.[27–29] Consequently the mean resting rate below which a pacemaker is recommended is 70 bpm in this subgroup of patients.[1]

The escape rate in patients with congenital heart block slows with increasing age, and the recommendations for pacemaker placement adjust accordingly.[31,34–36] In children older than 1 year with average heart rates below 50 bpm or with pauses in the ventricular rate that are greater than two to three times the basic cycle length, pacemaker implantation has been given a class IIa recommendation. Symptoms due to chronotropic incompetence are also a IIa indication for permanent pacing in children older than 1 year of age.[1,34,37]

Escape rhythms in congenital heart block patients often arise high in the conduction system and result in a narrow QRS complex. These are felt to be somewhat reliable escape rhythms and often provide sufficient chronotropic competence. However, wide QRS escape rhythms are felt to be less predictable and often have slower rates with chronotropic incompetence. Prognosis based upon the duration of the QRS complex remains unclear.[34–36] In addition, the presence of complex ventricular ectopy, such as polymorphic premature ventricular contractions, or ventricular tachycardia is also an indication for pacemaker placement.[36,38] Lastly, any decrease in ventricular function in these patients is an indication for pacemaker implantation.[39] All of these findings have received a class I indication for pacemaker placement.[1]

Despite the absence of any of the findings described here, it may still be reasonable to implant a permanent pacemaker in congenital heart block patients with acceptable rates, normal ventricular function and a narrow QRS escape rhythm as a class IIb recommendation.[1] However, many practitioners attempt to delay implantation if possible in the very young. If pacing can be delayed to allow for patient growth, epicardial systems can often be avoided and a transvenous system can instead be placed. Some patients can make it well into adolescence or even adulthood before pacing becomes necessary.

Sinus node dysfunction

Sinus node dysfunction (SND) accounts for 7–18% of the pediatric indications for pacemaker insertion.[40–42] Kardelen et al. noted that among 26 patients with SND treated with pacemaker implantation, nearly 70% had associated cardiovascular disease including CHD, myocarditis, and dilated cardiomyopathy. Additionally, 11 of the 26 patients (35%) developed SND following cardiac surgery.[41] SND is particularly common in procedures with extensive atrial dissection and suturing such as the Mustard, Senning, and Fontan operations. Certain intrinsic anatomic abnormalities can also predispose patients to sinus node dysfunction, such as left atrial isomerism.[43] With increasing understanding of the genetic basis of disease, there is greater recognition that certain channelopathies can also cause SND, such as congenital long QT syndrome and other sodium channel defects.[44–46]

Patients can develop symptoms with SND due to low heart rates, extended pauses, chronotropic incompetence, or lack of atrio-ventricular coordination during junctional escape rhythms. While many patients remain asymptomatic, the only class I indication for pacemaker placement in SND is symptoms documented during an age-inappropriate bradycardia.[1] The difficulty in these cases is that symptoms such as fatigue, presyncope, and exercise intolerance are subjective and can be difficult to quantify. Furthermore, other potentially reversible systemic diseases, such as anemia or hypothyroidism, can cause similar symptoms and should be excluded. It can be helpful to perform exercise testing with or without metabolic measurements to help make this distinction, especially in the CHD population.

In patients with CHD, altered hemodynamics can be seen in the baseline state, but when impaired hemodynamics are believed to be directly due to bradycardia or loss of AV synchrony, pacemaker implantation is given a class IIa recommendation.[1] One particularly important subset of patients in this group are those with protein losing enteropathy (PLE), seen predominantly in single ventricle patients after a Fontan operation. These patients may have junctional rhythms at acceptable rates but the loss of AV synchrony results in increased right sided pressures which are thought to contribute to the development of PLE. Restoration of AV synchrony through pacing has been shown to be of some benefit in selected patients.[7] In the patient with SND without obvious symptoms, there are additional indications for pacemaker placement. Those with complex CHD and a resting heart rate below 40 bpm or pauses in the ventricular rate greater than 3 seconds have a class IIa indication for pacemaker placement.[1] Complex CHD includes single ventricle lesions, transposition of the great vessels, truncus arteriosus, TOF and other abnormalities of atrioventricular or ventriculoarterial connections. Asymptomatic patients after biventricular or corrective repair with the same rhythm criteria carry a class IIb indication for pacemaker implantation, related to more favorable hemodynamics and ability to tolerate slower sinus rates or chronotropic incompetence. Recent recommendations for permanent pacing in adults with congenital heart disease are shown in Table 3.2.[48]

Intraatrial Reentrant Tachycardia (IART)

Late onset intraatrial reentrant tachycardia (IART) is not uncommon in patients who have complex CHD.[49–51] It can occur following any surgical procedure incorporating atriotomies and complex atrial dissections due to the eventual development of scars and fibrosis of the atrial tissue. Increased ventricular filling pressures with subsequent atrial stretch and atrial remodeling may also contribute to the arrhythmia burden in these patients.[52,53]

Rapid ventricular response rates and loss of consistent AV synchrony with IART can result in significant morbidity and mortality. Treatment options include antiarrhythmic medications, anticoagulation, close monitoring, cardioversion,

Table 3.2 *Recommendations for permanent pacing in adults with congenital heart disease. Class I – indicated, Class IIa – probably indicated, Class IIb – may be considered. Level of evidence in parentheses: A – multiple populations evaluated, B – limited populations evaluated, C – very limited populations evaluated. AV – atriventricular, CHD – congenital heart disease, SND – sinus node dysfunction, IART – intraatrial reentrant tachycardia*

Class I	
1	Symptomatic *SND*, including documented sinus bradycardia or chronotropic incompetence that is intrinsic or secondary to required drug therapy
2	Symptomatic bradycardia in conjunction with any degree of *AV block* or with ventricular arrhythmias presumed to be due to AV block
3	Complete AV block and a wide QRS escape rhythm, complex ventricular ectopy, or ventricular dysfunction
4	Postoperative high-grade second- or third-degree AV block that is not expected to resolve
Class IIA	
1	Sinus bradycardia/loss of AV synchrony causing impaired hemodynamics,
2	Sinus or junctional bradycardia for the prevention of recurrent IART
3	Complete AV block and an average daytime resting heart rate <50 bpm
4	Awake resting heart rate <40 bpm or ventricular pauses >3 s in complex CHD
Class IIB	
1	Awake resting heart rate <40 bpm or ventricular pauses >3 s in moderate CHD
2	History of transient postoperative complete AV block, and residual bifascicular block
Class III	
1	Pacing is not indicated in asymptomatic patients bifascicular block with or without first-degree AV block in the absence of a history of transient complete AV block
2	Endocardial leads are generally avoided in presence of intracardiac shunts

repeat surgical procedures and ablation.[51,52] Despite these modalities, IART remains particularly challenging in the setting of complex CHD. One review demonstrated IART treatment success in only 50–70% of Fontan cases.[54]

First line therapy for IART is often the use of medications to gain rhythm control, such as amiodarone and sotalol. Some patients can develop significant sinus bradycardia or an exacerbation of underlying SND due to these antiarrhythmic medications. As a result, pacemaker implantation to treat bradycardia caused by these medications allows for more appropriate management of their IART and has been given a class IIa recommendation. At the same time, native SND frequently coexists in what may be described as "tachycardia-bradycardia syndrome" and the bradycardia itself may be a stimulus for the initiation of IART. For these patients, atrial pacing can potentially prevent episodes of IART. Furthermore, the rate adaptive abilities of pacemakers may play an important role in preventing

IART since chronotropic incompetence in addition to the bradycardia seems to predispose patients to IART.[55,56]

In addition to bradycardia pacing, automatic and manual antitachycardia pacing (ATP) can be delivered through devices as therapy for breakthrough episodes of IART. Results have shown some promise but vary widely in range of success with reported conversion rates between 53–96% of detected episodes meeting criteria for therapy.[57,58] Rhodes et al. noted a high rate of successful ATP conversion (96%) among implanted patients, likely related to the fact that all patients received an individually tailored ATP program through repeated induction and termination testing following device implantation, highlighting the importance of proper device programming if this treatment option is going to be offered.[58] In patients with pacemakers without ATP capabilities, rhythm converting interventions cannot be automatically programmed, but the device can still be used to overdrive pace a patient out of IART once medical attention is sought, rather than proceeding to DC-cardioversion.[59]

Long QT syndrome

Permanent pacing in conjunction with standard medical therapy may be indicated in individuals with significant QT prolongation related to congenital or acquired etiologies. Pacing provides consistent heart rates, thereby potentially minimizing the risk of pause-dependent ventricular arrhythmias. Pacing may also help decrease QT dispersion and could potentially shorten QT intervals as well.[60,61] For these reasons, patients with long QT syndrome and pause-dependent ventricular tachycardia have an indication for pacemaker implantation. Select patients with inherent bradycardia and slow heart rates on beta blockers may benefit from long-term pacing.[1]

Vasovagal syncope

Vasovagal syncope is a common cause of syncope in the pediatric population. These syncopal episodes can be due to a vasodepressor response with hypotension; a cardioinhibitory response with sinus pauses or AV block; or a combination of the two. In patients with a predominant vasodepressor response without significant bradycardia or pause, a pacemaker is not indicated, although differentiating the exact cause of symptoms can be difficult. Likewise, patients with syncope that can be managed medically or by situational avoidance should not receive a pacemaker.

Several studies in the adult population have contributed to the current indications for pacemaker placement.[62–64] These studies suggest a class I indication for recurrent syncope in patients with pauses longer than 3 s with carotid sinus pressure, a class IIa indication for patients with syncope without provocative events who have pauses longer than 3 s and a class IIb indication for patients with significantly symptomatic vasovagal syncope and bradycardia at the time of tilt table testing.

The difficulty with these studies is that they were retrospective, observational or unblinded. Conflicting data has arisen out of double-blinded studies that did not demonstrate a significant effect in similar patient populations.[65,66] In these double-blinded studies, all patients underwent permanent pacemaker implantation but both patients and physicians were blinded to whether the devices were programmed to active or inactive pacing. No significant benefit was seen in either study and patients who simply knew that a pacemaker was implanted appeared to experience improvements, suggesting what has been labeled as an "expectation" effect. This also raises the question of whether this effect was present in other studies that supported permanent pacemaker placement for vasovagal syncope.[67]

The vast majority of pediatric patients can be medically managed and few at baseline have debilitating recurrent syncope. In addition, vasovagal syncope seems to cluster during adolescence with significant improvement in symptoms by adulthood making permanent pacing and its attendant risks potentially unnecessary.[68] Furthermore, it should be noted that there are no studies in the pediatric population that have been performed indicating pacemaker placement is beneficial. In our experience, the need for pacing in patients with vasovagal syncope is extremely rare.

Section 2: lead selection

In order to optimize pacemaker implantation, careful assessments and consideration of the various lead options is imperative. These assessments pertain to lead diameter and length, steroid versus non-steroid electrodes, active versus passive fixation mechanisms, as well as other factors influencing lead placement. When pacemaker implantation is contemplated, however, perhaps the most important decision regarding lead selection is whether epicardial or transvenous leads will be implanted. This decision often relates to the indication for pacing in the first place since the feasibility of transvenous implantation may influence the decision for pacemaker placement. Specifically, when the absolute need for pacing is less certain, the ability to implant a transvenous system may sway the decision towards permanent pacing, while the necessity of an epicardial approach may result in a decision to delay pacing therapy.

Epicardial versus transvenous pacing

Epicardial lead placement is considered more invasive than the transvenous (or endocardial)

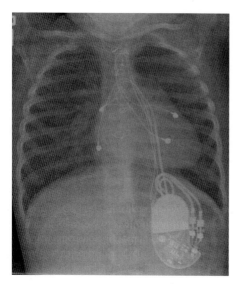

Figure 3.1 *Chest X-ray of a child with an epicardial lead system. Bipolar leads have been sewed to the epicardial surface of the atrium (A) and ventricle (V), and the pacemaker device was placed in the abdomen.*

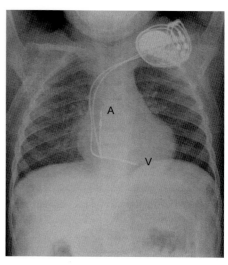

Figure 3.2 *Chest X-ray of a child with a transvenous pacing system. Active-fixation, bipolar transvenous leads have been implanted into the atrium (A) and ventricle (V) with the pacemaker device in the left pectoral region.*

technique since it requires surgical access to the epicardial surface of the heart, and hence a sternotomy, thoracotomy or subxiphoid approach (Figure 3.1). These surgical procedures mandate an inpatient stay and recovery times are generally longer. In addition, the longer surgical scars from epicardial pacemaker placement can have important psychological ramifications, depending on the individual. Lastly, epicardial leads are generally considered less effective than transvenous leads as described next, but advances in lead technology have minimized these differences. Most agree that transvenous pacemaker implantation is preferable (Figure 3.2), with the epicardial approach reserved for patients in whom transvenous lead placement is not considered advisable.

Small patient size accounts for a large majority of patients undergoing epicardial lead systems. Although implantation of a transvenous system is generally technically possible at any age,[69] most prefer to avoid transvenous leads until the child is "large enough." Defining that threshold, however, remains somewhat controversial and is generally institution-specific. In general, there is a desire to avoid transvenous lead placement in younger children in order to preserve the veins for future use. Furthermore, transvenous leads generally require

device placement in the pectoral region where inadequate subcutaneous tissue could result in complications such as skin erosion and infection.[70] Finally, the tremendous amount of future growth expected in very young children likely has negative consequences for lead longevity. We generally use 10–15 kg as the lower limit for transvenous lead placement, although others have implanted transvenous systems in far smaller children. In a study by Kammeraad et al. describing the outcome of 39 infants ≤10 kg with transvenous pacing systems, complications were somewhat frequent, including 3 (8%) with initial wound closure problems, 2 (5%) with wound or lead related infection, and 4 (11%) with asymptomatic venous occlusion found during lead extraction.[71] While such studies suggest that transvenous lead placement may be an option for those under 10 kg, we would advise caution in placement of transvenous lead systems in those under 10–15 kg.

Another common reason for epicardial lead placement is the presence of an intracardiac shunt. The potential for paradoxical systemic thromboemboli arising from transvenous leads has generally made placement of a transvenous pacing system in those with intracardiac shunts inadvisable. More recently, Khairy et al. sought to better define this risk in a study of 202 patients with intracardiac shunts (excluding a patent foramen ovale), 64 of which had transvenous leads. The presence of an intracardiac shunt was an independent predictor for systemic thromboembolism with a hazard ratio of 2.6 (p = 0.03).[72] Interestingly, the presence of a confirmed right-to-left shunt did not modulate the thromboembolic risk, and anticoagulation with neither aspirin nor warfarin could be proven to be protective. The results of this study showing a greater than twofold systemic thromboembolic risk is consistent with previous concerns, and the authors advocated efforts to eliminate shunting prior to transvenous lead implantation, with epicardial leads recommended if that is not feasible. We agree with this premise and avoid transvenous lead placement in patients with intracardiac shunts whenever possible.

The last common indication to avoid transvenous lead placement relates to restricted superior vena caval access to the heart. While such restricted access could result from unusual anatomic variants or occur due to previous lead or line placement in the systemic veins, this issue is most commonly encountered in those who have undergone the Fontan procedure. With the classic Fontan procedure as well as the lateral tunnel variant, transvenous access to the atrium can still be achieved for adequate atrial pacing.[73,74] This is rarely possible, however, with the extracardiac Fontan approach. Furthermore, while atrial pacing (AAI or AAIR) may be adequate for many Fontan patients with SND, a transvenous approach is not advisable in Fontan patients requiring ventricular pacing since this necessitates a lead in the systemic circulation (although placement of a ventricular lead through the coronary sinus is theoretically possible). Before placement of a transvenous atrial lead, the presence of shunting should be closely investigated, especially since these shunts are obligatorily right to left in the Fontan circulation.

Rarely, the presence of tricuspid valve pathology needs to be factored into transvenous ventricular lead placement and may necessitate an epicardial system. While case reports have suggested feasibility of placing a transvenous lead through a bioprosthetic tricuspid valve or tricuspid annuloplasty ring,[75–77] placement of a transvenous lead through a mechanical tricuspid valve is not advised due to the risk of dangerous valve dysfunction. In general, transvenous lead placement in a patient with significant tricuspid valve pathology should be approached with extreme caution, but placement of a left ventricular lead through the coronary sinus may be considered.[78–80]

Epicardial leads have generally been considered to be less effective than transvenous leads. The change to steroid-eluting leads has minimized this difference (see next), but studies continue to show lower myocardial capture thresholds with transvenous leads over epicardial leads. Fortesque et al. compared 521 leads (265 epicardial versus 265 transvenous) and found pacing thresholds to be higher at implant and during follow-up for both epicardial atrial and ventricular leads.[81] In order to standardize measurements across different pulse widths and impedances, "threshold energy" (TE) was calculated using the voltage threshold, the pulse width and the resistance. When combining all time points, transvenous leads had lower TEs than epicardial leads for both atrial leads (0.6 vs 1.0 µJ, p < 0.001) and ventricular leads (0.8 vs 1.6 µJ, p = < 0.001). Bipolar epicardial leads had lower TEs than unipolar epicardial leads, but comparing only bipolar epicardial and transvenous leads continued to show statistically significantly higher TEs for epicardial leads at implant, but not at late follow-up. Both sensing thresholds and lead failures, on the other hand, were found to be equivalent across lead types.

Odim et al. studied steroid eluting epicardial and transvenous leads and also demonstrated higher capture thresholds for epicardial leads.[82] Transvenous leads had lower mean stimulation thresholds than epicardial leads for both atrial leads (0.74 vs 1.61 µJ, p = 0.0005) and ventricular leads (0.49 vs 1.83 µJ, p = 0.0001). Lead impedance was significantly lower for epicardial leads, but sensing thresholds were similar between the two groups. The relative hazard of endocardial versus epicardial site for lead failure was 0.408 (p = 0.038), but when adjusting for other factors (including CHD, single ventricle physiology, and age), the relative hazard was no longer statistically significant. Our own experiences as well as others[83] are also consistent with the observation that epicardial leads have higher thresholds than transvenous leads. Unfortunately, this difference in thresholds ultimately leads to higher pacing outputs, a shorter battery life and a need for more frequent pacemaker replacements in epicardial systems (Chapter 10).

Steroid eluting leads

The advent of steroid-eluting epicardial leads has greatly improved epicardial lead longevity (and pacing thresholds). Steroid elusion has been incorporated into a variety of lead types, including both epicardial and transvenous, and studies have shown that the post-implant increase in stimulation thresholds is attenuated with these steroid-eluting leads. For example, at a 10 years' follow-up, the mean energy requirement for steroid-eluting leads was 1.2 µJ compared to 4.4 µJ for non-steroid eluting leads (P < 0.05).[85] In fact, chronic thresholds for steroid-eluting leads did not differ significantly from the values at time of lead implantation. Today, nearly all leads implanted incorporate a steroid-eluting component. For active fixation transvenous leads, a steroid-eluting collar surrounds the screw; for tined leads and sew-on epicardial leads, a silicone rubber plug is impregnated with glucocorticoids and sits within the electrode. The steroid releases very slowly, and residual local steroid has been proven to be present at 10 years' follow-up (and presumed to be present as late as 20 years).[86]

Active versus passive fixation

Studies comparing passive to active fixation leads in children are rare. Ceviz et al. compared 20 children with active fixation ventricular leads to 21 children with passive fixation ventricular leads.[87]

While mean pacing thresholds were similar for the two lead types at implant, after one week of pacing, mean thresholds were lower for the active fixation leads (P < 0.05) (Figure 3.3). Sensing amplitudes were similar between the groups, but impedance was lower for the active fixation leads (557 ± 92 Ω) compared to passive fixation (664 ± 160 Ω, P < 0.05). Although this study and others have not shown differences in dislodgement rates,[88] we generally advocate for active fixation given the ease of lead implantation at a variety of sites and the theoretical ability to unscrew the lead if extraction becomes necessary.

Unipolar versus bipolar configurations

All pacing is by definition "bipolar" (from cathode pole to anode pole), but for the purposes of cardiac pacing, a distinction is made between unipolar and bipolar pacing. Due to the need for two separate electrodes and wires in the bipolar configuration, bipolar transvenous pacing leads were thicker than unipolar leads when originally developed. As a result of the larger French size, higher fracture rates due to lead complexity and more technical difficulty with implantation,[88] unipolar leads were initially more popular. As advances in lead technology have allowed reliable bipolar leads in a thinner profile, bipolar leads have gradually become more popular and are now standard for transvenous systems. In epicardial pacing systems, bipolar leads require a second implantation site on the epicardium, so placement of a bipolar epicardial lead requires more time and effort for implantation.

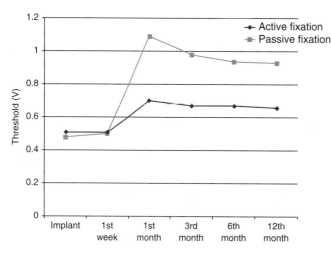

Figure 3.3 *Comparison of ventricular capture thresholds over time for passive and active fixation transvenous leads in children (adapted from Ceviz et al.).[85] (Source: Mond (1996). Reproduced with permission of John Wiley & Sons, Ltd.)*

Table 3.3 *Summary of differences between unipolar and bipolar leads. Source: Cate 2002. Reproduced with permissions of BMJ[83]*

	Bipolar	Unipolar
Lead size		+
Lead repair		++
Stimulation threshold	0	
Cardiac myopotential sensing	+	
Far-field sensing	++	
Cross-talk	+++	
Skeletal myopotential oversensing	+++	
Extracorporeal oversensing	++	
Local skeletal muscle stimulation	+++	
Stimulus artifact size		+++
Programming flexibility	+++	

0 = no significant difference,
+ not significant but preferable,
++ significant but not an important preference,
+++ significant and important preference

As a result, the decision to implant unipolar versus bipolar epicardial leads remains at the discretion of the surgeon.

Table 3.3 summarizes features of bipolar and unipolar configurations, but in our experiences these differences are not of significant importance in current pacemaker lead decisions. Since transvenous leads are nearly always bipolar, understanding these differences is mostly relevant for epicardial systems. Probably most importantly, it is not clear that significant clinical differences exist for stimulation and sensing thresholds between unipolar and bipolar leads.[81,89] Unfortunately, such comparisons between unipolar and bipolar leads in the literature are nearly exclusive to transvenous systems since modern epicardial systems are rarely implanted in adults. A direct comparison of modern bipolar and unipolar epicardial leads in children is therefore less clear. Bipolar leads are thought to minimize extracardiac stimulation, myopotential oversensing, far-field signals and electromagnetic interference.[88] In our experience, however, we have seen several instances of bipolar epicardial systems manifesting oversensing of a ventricular electrogram immediately after ventricular pacing. While this is rarely clinically important, the over-sensed

R-wave can restart the timing before the next P-wave can be sensed (due to the programmed PVARP) and limit the upper rates in DDD pacing. While this has been difficult to correct by increasing the ventricular sensing value during bipolar sensing, this problem has been easily eliminated by programming to ventricular unipolar sensing. In general, we do not have a strong opinion regarding bipolar versus unipolar epicardial pacing leads. While placement of a bipolar lead allows for the flexibility of reprogramming to unipolar later, the extra time and effort involved in placing a second electrode can be more than trivial.

Lead size

Lead size relates to both length and thickness and is most important in transvenous systems where the caliber of the accessed vein as well the size of the pacemaker pocket can be very important. Most leads are available in a variety of lengths, and lead pacing and sensing properties are not greatly affected by the relatively small changes in wire length. In general, determining the most appropriate lead length relates to placing the right amount of slack in the system without an abundance of "extra lead" to remain in the pacemaker pocket. In larger children with ample subcutaneous tissue, placing a lead that is too long is of minimal consequence since an extra loop of lead can be accommodated by the pacemaker pocket. In small children, however, choosing the "right" lead length is more important since fitting an extra loop of lead in the pacemaker pocket can impact the cosmetic appearance of the pocket and result in more dermal tension. In general, we strive to choose individual atrial and ventricular lead lengths that result in both leads having similar loops of excess leads. This selection results in easier device placement and less acute bends on the leads when placed into the pacemaker pocket.

In our experience, the appropriate lead length is easiest to calculate at the time of sheath placement, when the introducer wire is in the heart. The length of this wire is clearly labeled on the sheath packaging (usually ~45 cm), and by inferring how far into the body the wire needs to be to reach the expected implantation site, one can estimate how much wire would be left over in the pocket. Once a first lead is implanted, estimations of lead lengths for further leads are more obvious. In general, the younger the child and the more expected future growth, the more extra slack should be placed. While this slack can be expected to decrease over time as the child grows, fibrosis and adherence of the lead to the vascular tissue is not uncommon, so that even significant slack will be irrelevant if it is proximal to any future adhesion. As a result, care should be taken to avoid leaving too much slack, especially since looping of the lead in the heart may result in tricuspid valve distortion and possible later difficulty with lead extraction.

Thinner leads are usually preferred due to a general desire to minimize the amount of vascular space that is taken up by the leads. Furthermore, thinner leads require thinner sheaths, which are usually easier to place. Earlier studies had suggested that larger and multiple leads were associated with a higher chance for future venous stenosis. Figa et al. defined a lead INDEX (total cross sectional area of leads indexed to body surface area at implantation) and found a higher mean INDEX in patient with venous obstruction (assessed by clinical findings or echocardiography) compared to those without obstruction.[90] Furthermore, an INDEX of > 6.6 predicted future obstruction with a sensitivity of 90% and specificity of 84%. While the argument that more and thicker leads are associated with a higher risk for future venous stenosis appears intuitive, a later study by Bar-Cohen et al. did not find this association.[91] In fact, patient age, body size, lead size, number of leads, and lead INDEX were not predictive of venous stenosis in this population more vigorously screened for obstruction with angiography. While the exact role of lead size in the risk for future venous obstruction may not be completely clear, we nonetheless aim to implant the thinnest leads possible, as long as reliability and the technical ease of implantation are not sacrificed.

The majority of lead manufacturers supply leads that can be introduced into 6 French (Fr) or 7 Fr sheaths, and we generally use the smallest sheaths possible for our pediatric implants (6 Fr sheaths for the large majority). The advent of the lumenless transvenous lead (SelectSecure, Medtronic, Inc., Minneapolis, MN) has allowed for implantation of an even thinner 4.1 Fr lead. Since a lumen is not present in these leads, lead positioning is generally performed using a larger (8.4 Fr) steerable sheath.

Several reports, however, have demonstrated the feasibility of implanting these leads through a 5 Fr peel-away sheath, although this is not advocated for the majority of cases.[92,93]

Lumenless leads

The SelectSecure lead allows for controlled placement of a thin (4.1 Fr) lead, usually through a larger deflectable sheath. The lead construction consists of a lumenless lead with a non-retractable helix electrode that has a surface area of 3.6 mm^2, a tip to ring spacing of 9 mm, and a ring electrode surface area of 16.9 mm^2. While placement of a lead at the right ventricular apex can be performed via standard stylets, a large amount of data suggests that apical pacing may lead to impaired cardiac function and arrhythmias in a subset of patients.[94] Similarly, while standard J-type stylets can guide an atrial lead to the right atrial appendage, pacing from the appendage can result in intra-atrial dyssynchrony, possibly resulting in atrial arrhythmias or atrial hemodynamic dysfunction.[95] The preformed and steerable sheaths in the SelectSecure pacing system allow reliable implantation at sites outside of the right ventricular apex and right atrial appendage.[96] The small lead size, however, as well as the ability to navigate through the more complex anatomies of many patients with CHD makes this lead possibly appealing to pediatric and other CHD indications.

Several studies have demonstrated the safety and effectiveness of the SelectSecure system in pediatric and CHD patients.[97–99] Khan compared the Select-Secure lead (n = 91) to traditional stylet-driven transvenous leads (n = 80) over a 5-year period. The lumenless leads had lower thresholds and impedances with similar sensed electrograms at implantation, although there were no significant differences in any of these parameters at 4–5-year follow-up.[99] Lead dislodgement, however, occurred in five patients (6%) with traditional stylet-driven leads versus only one patient (1%) with the lumenless lead. The authors concluded that the lumenless lead offers an improved design option for cardiac pacing in pediatrics and CHD.

A smaller lead size is preferable in very young children, as is a smaller implanting sheath diameter. While the 8.4 Fr sheath is generally advocated for placement of the SelectSecure lead, several investigators have described placement of the lumenless lead through a 5 Fr delivery system. Kenny described placement of the lumenless lead through a standard 5 Fr tearaway sheath (13 cm in length).[92] After advancing the lead to the IVC, it was deflected off the wall of the IVC to create a loop allowing access to the right atrial appendage or right ventricle. LaPage et al. used a long sheath to reach the site of desired implantation.[93] The valved end of the sheath was then cut off, and the SelectSecure lead delivered through a modified long sheath. Successful implantation was achieved with both techniques. While long term data on these leads is not yet available, the availability of this thin and reliable lead appears quite promising for pediatric and CHD applications.

The VDD lead

VDD lead (also known as a single-pass lead) allows for atrial sensing and ventricular sensing and pacing through a single transvenous lead, thereby allowing adequate AV synchrony in patients with heart block but without SND. The lead is constructed such that when the lead tip is fixed in the right ventricular myocardium, a set of proximal electrodes are positioned inside the right atrial chamber without being directly implanted into the atrial myocardium. While theoretically useful, in reality there are few indications for this approach in children. Currently, only a small number of VDD leads are commercially available, and these leads need to be implanted through a relatively large sheath (at least 9 Fr). A VDD lead may be considered in a relatively small patient, where there is a preference to avoid placing multiple leads through the innominate vein, but in whom AV synchrony is desired to augment cardiac output.[100] In these same small patients, however, placement of a relatively large implanting sheath (9 Fr) is generally not desirable either. As a result, in smaller children a decision is often made to implant a single ventricular lead (for VVI or VVIR pacing) and delay AV synchrony until a future system upgrade at an older age. Since it is not clear that AV synchrony provides a clear clinical benefit in many patients,[101] placing a single ventricular lead is reasonable for a large majority of these smaller children. In the rare patient with a clear need for AV synchronous pacing, but with a desire for a single transvenous lead (either due to small size or stenosed/limited venous access), a VDD lead may be indicated.

While VDD systems in children may be useful, some data suggests that the VDD leads should generally be avoided in pediatrics. Five of twelve children (41.7%) studied by Sudkamp et al. (21 months to 14.5 years at implant), required reoperation due to severe traction on the leads.[102] This was felt to be mostly related to the sensing ring being in contact with endocardial tissue and inducing endocardial fixation of the lead at the atrium or SVC. With natural growth of the patient, this caused a pull on the ventricular aspect of the lead, leading to the need for reoperation. Others have shown somewhat more encouraging data. Seiden demonstrated a diminution in both P-wave and R-wave amplitude during follow-up of these leads while two leads required repositioning or replacement due to inadequate ventricular capture.[103] Atrial sensing, however, remained adequate at last follow-up (mean of 16 months after implant) in all seven patients with Holter monitoring.

Section 3: device selection

Similar to the array of currently available pacemaker leads, a wide variety of pacemaker pulse generators exists. In deciding which pacing device to implant in pediatric and CHD patients, several factors need to be considered. The basic functions of current pacemakers across all manufacturers are fairly similar and any of the available models can be implanted in patients to address the majority of pacing needs. However, certain conditions may favor implantation of one device model over another based on more specialized and specific pacemaker features.

General device considerations

When choosing a pulse generator, the implanting physician must consider the site for implantation, the need for single or dual chamber pacing, and the size of the pulse generator itself. In addition, consideration of specific functions and features of the various available devices should be made when selecting devices for patients with certain conditions.[104] Table 3.4 summarizes the dimensions, basic features, and some advanced features

Table 3.4 *Currently available pacemaker pulse generators from three major manufacturers: St. Jude Medical, Medtronic, and Boston Scientific. "Both" refers to single- and dual-chamber models available*

Manufacturer	St. Jude Medical				Boston Scientific	Medtronic		
Model	Accent	Identity	Zephyr	Microny	Altrua	Adapta	EnRhythm	Revo
Dimensions (mm)	52×52×6*	44×52×6**	44×52×6**	33×33×6	49×43×8$^\alpha$	50×48×7.5$^\beta$	45×51×8	45×51×8
Mass (gm)	23	23.5	23.5	12.8	29.6	28.5	21	21.5
Weight (cc)	12.8	11	11	5.9	12.1	14.2	13	12.7
Single, dual, or both	Both	Both	Both	Single	Both	Both	Dual	Dual
Maximum upper track rate (bpm)	170	170	170	160	185	210	150	150
Rate response	Yes	Yes	Yes	Yes	Yes	Yes	Yes	Yes
Automatic capture adjustment	Yes	Yes	Yes	Yes	Yes	Yes	No	No
Preferential intrinsic conduction	Yes	No	Yes	No	No	Yes	Yes	Yes
Additional features	RF capable			Smallest available device			ATP capable	MRI compatible

* Dual chamber model
** XL model
α Extended battery model
β ADDR06 model
RF radiofrequency wireless communication

of the available pacemaker pulse generators from three major device manufacturers.

Size considerations

In infants and small children, the generator size may be critical given the proportionately larger footprint that the same generators will have in this patient group compared to older and larger patients. Additionally, the thinner skin, fat, and muscle layers in smaller patients make generators more prone to erosion and migration.[104] Sites in the subcutaneous and submuscular layers of the chest and abdomen have been used for generator placement. An axillary approach has been applied to permit alternate access to the subpectoral space while offering a cosmetic advantage by hiding the incision scar under the axilla. However, placement in the axilla may be less comfortable for patients and could increase risk of device migration. Less conventional sites for implantation have included the extrapleural intrathoracic space and the left renal fossa superior to the peritoneum.[105,106] The ideal site should provide stable generator position, maximum patient comfort, and low risk for infection, pocket erosion, and device impingement on other organs. Presently, the most common location for generator placement in small patients is either the pectoral region (either between the pectoral fascia and muscle or submuscular) or abdominal wall (generally sub-rectus). Careful pocket creation is important to avoid migration, possible impingement, and obstruction of bowel and to minimize superficial tension which could lead to wound dehiscence, poor healing, and pocket erosion. The reported incidence of sterile pocket erosion is approximately 5% with an additional 2–4% of patients with erosion of the skin and soft tissues overlying the proximal leads. Pocket infection rates have been reported to be as high as 12%, but are less frequent today due to improved implant techniques and meticulous wound care.[107] A more recent review of endocardial systems in children showed pocket erosion or infection as the cause for system failure in only 2 out of 117 patients.[108]

Foregoing dual chamber pacing may be necessary in order to minimize generator size in the smallest patients. In this context, single-chamber pacing may be viewed as a bridge to permit patient growth, with the expectation of adding a second lead for dual-chamber pacing at the time of a future generator change. The St. Jude Medical Microny generator is the smallest available pacemaker generator on the market today. At just under 6 cc of weight and 13 g of mass, it only allows single chamber pacing, but still affords rate responsive pacing as well as automatic pacing capture adjustment. Battery longevity is very reasonable (often greater than 5 years) and is usually long enough to allow sufficient patient growth for future upgrade to a dual chamber system.

Single versus dual chamber pacing

Generator choice is significantly influenced by the dominant pacing needs in any given patient. For some patients, single chamber pacing is sufficient. These include patients with exclusive SND without evidence of current or anticipated AV nodal or His–Purkinje disease and those with only the rare need for pacing to prevent ventricular pauses. In patients with heart block, the decision of single-chamber (ventricular) or dual-chamber pacing can be more challenging. While single-chamber pacing introduces less overall hardware, dual-chamber pacing affords the ability to maintain AV synchrony and allows for ventricular pacing at an individual's intrinsically desired rate provided sinus node function is preserved.

A meta-analysis of adult trials comparing single-chamber (ventricular) and dual-chamber pacing for heart block and SND demonstrated a trend toward reducing stroke, heart failure, and mortality and statistically significant prevention of atrial fibrillation with dual chamber pacing.[109] In pediatric and CHD patients, however, the data is conflicting. Horenstein et al. evaluated the impact of single- and dual-chamber pacing on left ventricular function by echocardiographic assessment.[110] Patients with congenital or acquired heart block (all with corrected biventricular physiology) were initially VVIR paced for a mean duration of 10.2 years prior to being upgraded to dual-chamber devices and paced in DDDR or VDD modes for a mean duration of 0.7 years of follow-up. No significant changes were seen in the short term following conversion to dual-chamber pacing; however, all patients had preserved LV functional parameters prior to device upgrade. Among Fontan patients, Fishberger et al. noted a trend toward improved survival among patients who received dual-chamber devices (15 of 19 patients) compared to VVI pacemakers (4 of 9 patients).[111]

Placement of a second pacing lead for dual-chamber pacing, either through the transvenous or open surgical route, does introduce a higher potential for complications, particularly in very small and young patients and in those who have previously undergone extensive cardiac surgery. The ultimate decision for the type of pacing system that will be implanted in a patient with heart block, however, depends on a variety of specific patient factors including underlying anatomy and hemodynamics, potential for SND and patient size. In general, we advocate for placement of a dual-chamber system in our heart block patients, except in very small children with transvenous implants or those with restricted venous access.

MRI compatibility

The growing application of magnetic resonance imaging (MRI) in the diagnosis and management of cardiac and non-cardiac conditions must be considered when pacemaker decisions are made. A 2005 study estimated a 50–75% probability of a patient with an implanted cardiac device being recommended for an MRI over the device lifetime.[112] Given the rising application of MRI for multiple disorders and in multiple organ systems, and particularly the rising importance of cardiac MRI in the management of CHD patients, the probability in pediatric and CHD patients may be even higher than this estimate. In 2004, the American College of Radiology published an update to their MR Safe Practice Guidelines recommending that the presence of implanted cardiac devices be made a contraindication to routine MR imaging.[113] Magnetic fields can result in a variety of pacemaker issues: inadvertent changes to asynchronous pacing modes, alterations in pacing thresholds and lead impedances, inappropriate over- or under-sensing, and device resetting.[112] The magnetic field within the MR scanner may physically result in movement of components of the implanted device system, resulting in patient discomfort and possibly lead dislodgement. Additionally, the electromagnetic interference from the pulsed RF field in the MRI environment could result in sufficient current in the lead system to cause thermal injury at the tissue/myocardial interface. The controversy over the safety of implanted cardiac devices during MR imaging has resulted in efforts to alter the MR imaging environment in order to diminish its effect on implanted cardiac devices. This has included changing the MRI bore location relative to the pacemaker, imaging in lower magnetic fields (1.5 Tesla), and altering image acquisition protocols that yield less interference with pacemakers. Additionally, pacemakers are often re-programmed prior to the MR study to minimize the potential for undesired functionality changes.

The AHA Scientific Statement on safety of MRI in patients with cardiovascular devices published in 2007 recommended that MR imaging be discouraged in non-pacemaker dependent patients and only considered if there is strong clinical indication and when the benefit clearly outweighs risks. The statement goes on to recommend against MRI studies in pacemaker-dependent patients unless there are "highly compelling circumstances" along with a favorable risk:benefit ratio.[114] While several investigators have demonstrated the possible safe use of MRI in adults with pacemakers,[115,116] far less data is available in children. Pulver et al. published a small prospective study evaluating the safety of MRI studies in pediatric and CHD patients with pacemakers and the quality of the acquired MRI images.[117] They evaluated patient and device safety and MRI quality in eight non-pacemaker-dependent CHD patients. A total of 11 MRI studies were performed, four of which were cardiac-specific. Devices were programmed to asynchronous sensing modes (OAO, OVO, ODO) during the MRI study. Devices were assessed prior to and after the MR studies, and patients were monitored closely during scans. The results showed that diagnostic quality MRI studies could be safely performed in this small cohort of patients.

The MRI conditional pacing system includes a generator and leads specifically designed to minimize problems of pacing within MRI environments. The hardware components were designed to resist heating, vibration, and movement that can be associated with MRI-device interactions. The system is marketed for MRI studies above the C1 level or below the T12 level of the spine; that is, the system is not approved for chest and cardiac MR studies, where there remains a continued risk of significant lead heating. Only scanners with a static 1.5 Tesla magnetic field can be used with the Revo SureScan system. In addition, the SureScan programming must be activated prior to the MR scan and results in asynchronous pacing that is expected to resist changes within the MR imaging environment.

Basic device features

Most pacemaker pulse generators across the majority of manufacturers incorporate similar basic functions for antibradycardia pacing. Generators are programmable for all variations of single or dual chamber pacing and sensing. Rate responsive pacing, high rate event recording, and pacing mode switch function are all part of a standard function set for most pulse generators.

Rate responsive pacing

Rate responsive pacing is available as a standard feature on most pulse generators and can be very useful in patients with chronotropic incompetence. Cabrera et al. described results demonstrating safe application and benefit of VVIR over standard VVI pacing in 14 patients who underwent cardiopulmonary exercise testing.[118] Patients programmed with VVIR pacing exhibited a 51% increase in peak heart rate and 16% increase in exercise duration and maximum oxygen uptake along with a 27% decrease in peak oxygen pulse suggesting a proportionately smaller stroke volume compared to VVI paced patients. Ragonese et al. reviewed VVIR pacing in pediatric patients with complete heart block.[119] Ten patients were selected to undergo treadmill exercise testing in both the VVI and VVIR modes. While exercise tolerance was normal in these patients in either pacing mode, maximum achieved heart rates and systolic blood pressures were significantly higher when paced VVIR (p < 0.0013) corresponding to a more appropriate response to exercise. These results suggested that rate-responsive pacing yielded better physiologic responses to exercise than standard VVI pacing and that careful programming of rate responsive pacing parameters could provide an alternative to dual chamber pacing in younger and smaller patients. Rate responsive pacing is most useful for patients with primary chronotropic incompetence or for heart block patients who receive single-chamber ventricular pacing devices.

Automatic pacing output adjustment

Automatic pacing output adjustment is a valuable tool that may aid in the conservation of device battery longevity. The feature goes by various names depending on manufacturer: Capture Management (Medtronic), Autocapture (St. Jude Medical), and Automatic Capture (Boston Scientific). With this feature, the device determines the underlying pacing capture threshold and automatically adjusts its pacing output to be slightly higher. In the St. Jude Medical and Boston Scientific features, adequate capture is confirmed on a beat-by-beat basis while Medtronic's Capture Management system measures a threshold several times per day and automatically sets its output at a certain multiple above this threshold (usually 1.5–times). With any of these features, much lower pacing outputs are theoretically possible, thereby extending battery longevity and decreasing the frequency of generator changes. However, capture may not be adequately confirmed in some patients, which makes this feature unusable. Studies have demonstrated the safety and battery-prolonging benefit of automatic pacing output adjustment in pediatric patients. Bauersfeld et al. showed early stability of this feature in 12 pediatric patients who were implanted with AutoCapture-capable Pacesetter Microny and Regency devices.[120] Pacing thresholds remained low at 18 months of follow-up without adverse events. Calculated service life was substantially longer in the devices with AutoCapture programmed on compared to the same generators programmed in conventional settings (21 years versus 7.2 years for Regency generators, 7.8 years

vs 4.8 years for Microny generators). Tomaske et al. reviewed an additional 56 pediatric patients with AutoCapture-capable devices.[121] Fifty-three of 56 patients maintained this feature over a median follow-up time of 3 years. Calculated battery life was increased up to 15% over conventional settings (p = 0.008) and up to 30% in a subgroup of patients with ventricular pacing thresholds greater than 1.5 V at 0.5 ms pulse duration (p < 0.001).

Mode switching

In dual chamber devices, most generators have the ability to automatically change pacing modes if certain arrhythmia detection criteria are reached. For heart block patients with dual chamber pacemakers, this typically occurs when an atrial tachyarrhythmia is detected. The automatic switching of the pacing mode (also known as "mode switching") permits continued ventricular pacing at a desired rate (often in a VVI or DDI mode) instead of rapidly tracking the atrial rate. After the arrhythmia subsides, the pacing mode resumes its previous baseline setting. The mode switching feature is frequently used in adults with paroxysmal forms of atrial arrhythmias and atrial fibrillation and can be a valuable tool for CHD patients with intra-atrial reentrant tachycardia.

Advanced device features

While there is generally little difference in the basic features across the majority of available pacemaker pulse generators, advanced features of certain pulse generators may need to be considered when selecting a device for certain subsets of patients. Several of these features may also aid in battery conservation.

Rate-adaptive AV delay adjustment

Automatic adjustment of the AV delay is a useful feature incorporated into most current dual chamber pacemaker generators and may provide more physiological AV coordination during activity. The goal of this feature is to mimic the intrinsic acceleration in AV nodal conduction in response to increased catecholaminergic tone. Rate adaptive AV delay adjustment functions by shortening the AV delay during periods of faster intrinsic or paced atrial rates, which presumably correspond to higher levels of circulating catecholamines.

Re-programming of the AV delay and automatic AV delay adjustment has been studied more within the context of AV optimization and cardiac resynchronization therapy and its overall benefit in that context remains debatable.[122] There are currently no published studies on the impact of rate-adaptive AV delay adjustments in permanent pacing for pediatric and CHD patients.

Sleep mode and hysteresis rates

The ability to selectively pace at lower heart rates can both conserve battery voltage and provide for more physiologic pacing. With sleep modes, the device is programmed with a lower basal rate during presumed hours of sleep, thereby following the usual diurnal heart rate variation more closely. Additionally, this may conserve battery life by providing periods of relatively lower pacing (and energy) requirement. The feature theoretically would work best in individuals with a consistent daily sleep pattern.

A hysteresis rate is a rate below the lower rate of the device that must be reached before pacing at the lower rate initiates. For example, if a lower pacing rate of 60 bpm were programmed, but with a hysteresis rate of 50 bpm, intrinsic heart rates could drift below the 60 bpm limit. If the intrinsic rate falls below 50 bpm, however, pacing commences at the programmed basal rate of 60 bpm. Hysteresis provides longer potential periods of intrinsic and physiologic rates. At the same time, it may conserve battery life since the overall pacing burden would theoretically be less.

Preferential intrinsic ventricular conduction

Preferential intrinsic ventricular conduction is a feature that can be incorporated in patients with primary SND or in patients with intermittent heart block. With this feature, the pacemaker will preferentially withhold ventricular pacing and permit intrinsic AV node conduction. The feature allows a longer AV interval before ventricular pacing, but once ventricular pacing becomes necessary, a shorter AV interval is actually used. This feature is available as Managed Ventricular Pacing (MVP) or Search AV+ (SAV+) in Medtronic devices, Ventricular Intrinsic Preference (VIP) in St. Jude Medical devices, and AV Search Hysteresis in Boston Scientific models.

While these manufacturer-specific features differ algorithmically, the overall intent is the same and the benefit of this function is twofold. First, preferential intrinsic conduction allows for the normal depolarization of the ventricles through the His–Purkinje system, which may result in a more synchronized depolarization and contractile pattern. Second, preferential intrinsic conduction conserves battery life as less energy is consumed when ventricular pacing is avoided. Kaltman et al. reported a multicenter retrospective review in pediatric and CHD patients comparing standard DDD rate responsive pacing with DDD pacing incorporating Medtronic's MVP feature.[123] A total of 62 patients (64% with CHD) had MVP devices with an observed cumulative percentage of ventricular pacing of only 4.3%. Subgroup analysis on patients who had previously been implanted with a DDDR device showed 67.1% ventricular pacing with DDDR pacing compared to 9.2% ventricular pacing with their MVP device (p = 0.002). Among the cohort studied, only one patient experienced symptoms due to nonconducted atrial beats during MVP programming. The study concluded that MVP could be safely applied with significant reductions in unnecessary ventricular pacing in this patient population.

Sudden bradycardia response

Permanent pacemaker implantation can be effective in minimizing symptoms and syncopal events in some patients with vasovagal syncope. Programming of hysteresis rates (as described above) has shown some benefit, but incorporation of sudden bradycardia response functions may be more effective. Sudden bradycardia response provides immediate chronotropic support in situations where intrinsic rates drop precipitously, which can occur just prior to syncope. This function is called Rate Drop Response in Medtronic devices, Advanced Hysteresis in St. Jude Devices, and Sudden Bradycardia Response in Boston Scientific devices. These algorithms sense and determine a rate drop based on counting a preselected decrease in rate within a predefined period of time. When criteria are met, pacing is initiated at a prespecified rate. Ammirati et al. compared the effectiveness of sudden bradycardia response in 20 patients with vasovagal syncope.[124] Patients were randomized to receive either DDD pacing with Medtronic's Rate Drop Response (12) or DDI pacing with rate hysteresis (8). Repeat tilt testing demonstrated a 25% incidence of syncope among those with Rate Drop Response compared to 62.5% with rate hysteresis. Additionally, over the course of study follow-up (mean duration 17.7 months), no patients with Rate Drop Response experienced clinical syncope while three of the eight patients with rate hysteresis had syncope recurrence (p < 0.05).

Atrial antitachycardia pacing

Atrial antitachycardia pacing (ATP) is available as a programmable feature in devices offered by only one manufacturer (Medtronic pacemakers such as the EnRhythm and Adapta models). This feature incorporates sensing algorithms to determine if a patient is in an atrial tachyarrhythmia and institutes rapid overdrive pacing in the atrium in a similar manner to how ATP works in terminating reentrant ventricular tachycardias (Figure 3.4). Studies have demonstrated some benefit of atrial ATP in CHD patients. The overall benefit remains debatable in general adult electrophysiology and the management of macroreentrant atrial tachyarrhythmias and atrial fibrillation in adults.[125] Kamp et al. reported that 28% of CHD patients implanted with an atrial ATP-capable device experienced successful ATP.[126] Two-ventricle physiologies, atrial switch surgery, and documented atrial tachyarrhythmias prior to device implantation were associated with a higher rate of successful ATP therapy. Stephenson et al. reported a 54% success rate with atrial ATP in 167 tachycardia events among 28 CHD patients implanted with the Medtronic AT500 pacemaker.[57] The incorporation of a patient-activated ATP

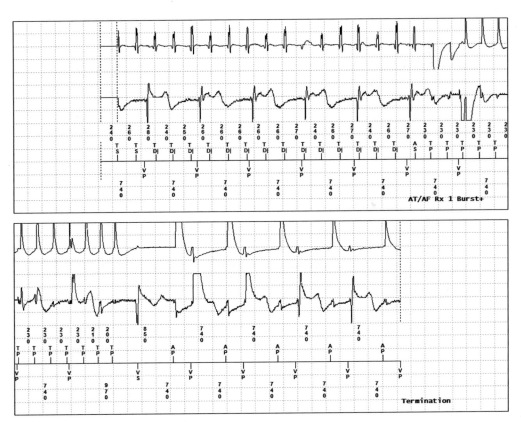

Figure 3.4 *Intra-atrial reentrant tachycardia (IART) at an average cycle length of 260 ms was detected in a patient with repaired tetralogy of Fallot and a dual chamber pacemaker with automatic atrial ATP therapy capability originally implanted for sinus and AV node dysfunction. In this example, ATP with a Burst + protocol is effective in terminating IART. (Source: Dr. Maully Shah, Division of Cardiology, The Children's Hospital of Philadelphia, U.S.A. Reproduced with permission of Dr. Maully Shah.)*

system has also been described and allows activation of ATP therapy via an external device when the patient experiences symptomatic tachycardia.[127] Based on the authors' experience, implantation of atrial ATP devices has the highest likelihood of success when the atrial lead is positioned close to the reentrant circuit itself and when atrial overdrive pacing by other means has previously been successful. For example, in some atrial switch patients, reentrant circuits often involve the cavotricuspid isthmus. Since transvenous atrial leads are frequently implanted in the leftward aspect of the systemic atrial baffle or the remnant left atrial appendage, failure to terminate atrial tachycardia in these patients may be due to overdrive pacing from an area too distant from the reentrant circuit, thereby limiting the ability to interrupt the circuit. Additionally, patients who have received successful ATP through transesophageal, temporary transvenous, or previously placed permanent transvenous leads during noninvasive programmed stimulation (NIPS) would likely be better candidates for implantation of an ATP-capable device than those who have failed with these modalities.

Conclusions

Standard and well accepted indications guide the implanting physician in selecting pediatric and CHD patients who are most likely to benefit from permanent pacemaker implantation. While recommendations have been extensively discussed, the decision for implantation must still be approached on a case-by-case basis due to the extreme heterogeneity of functional and anatomical abnormalities in these patients. The implanting physician must pay close attention to the unique patient characteristics as well as the presently available pacemaker hardware in order to appropriately select the right leads and generators. Ultimately, pacemaker implantation should be performed in a manner that minimizes the risk of short- and long-term complications while maximizing quality of life and functional status.

References

1 Epstein AE, DiMarco JP, Ellenbogen KA, Estes NA 3rd, Freedman RA, Gettes LS, et al. and American College of Cardiology Foundation; American Heart Association Task Force on Practice Guidelines; Heart Rhythm Society. 2012 ACCF/AHA/HRS focused update incorporated into the ACCF/AHA/HRS 2008 guidelines for device-based therapy of cardiac rhythm abnormalities: a report of the American College of Cardiology Foundation/American Heart Association Task Force on Practice Guidelines and the Heart Rhythm Society. J Am Coll Cardiol. 2013 Jan 22; 61(3): e6–75.

2 Welisch E, Cherlet E, Crespo-Martinez E, Hansky B. A single institution experience with pacemaker implantation in a pediatric population over 25 years. *Pacing Clin Electrophysiol.* 2010; 33: 1112–1118.

3 Bonatti V, Agnetti A, Squarcia U. Early and late postoperative complete heart block in pediatric patients submitted to open-heart surgery for congenital heart disease. *Pediatr Med Chir.* 1998; 20: 181–186.

4 Weindling SN, Saul JP, Gamble WJ, Mayer JE, Wessel D, Walsh EP. Duration of complete atrioventricular block after congenital heart disease surgery. *Am J Cardiol.* 1998; 82: 525–527.

5 Lillehei CW, Sellers RD, Bonnabeau RC, Eliot RS. Chronic postsurgical complete heart block. With particular reference to prognosis, management, and a new P-wave pacemaker. *J Thorac Cardiovasc Surg.* 1963; 46: 436–456.

6 Hofschire PJ, Nicoloff DM, Moller JH. Postoperative complete heart block in 64 children treated with and without cardiac pacing. *Am J Cardiol.* 1977; 39: 559–562.

7 Murphy DA, Tynan M, Graham GR, Bonham-Carter RE. Prognosis of complete atrioventricular dissociation in children after open-heart surgery. *Lancet.* 1970; 1: 750–752.

8 Squarcia U, Merideth J, McGoon DC, Weidman WH. Prognosis of transient atrioventricular conduction disturbances complicating open heart surgery for congenital heart defects. *Am J Cardiol.* 1971; 28: 648–652.

9 Daicoff GR, Aslami A, Tobias JA, Miller BL. Management of postoperative complete heart block in infants and children. *Chest.* 1974; 66: 639–641.

10 Nishimura RA, Callahan MJ, Holmes DR Jr, Gersh BJ, Driscoll DJ, Trusty JM, et al. Transient atrioventricular block after open-heart surgery for congenital heart disease. *Am J Cardiol.* 1984; 53: 198–201.

11 Krongrad E. Prognosis for patients with congenital heart disease and postoperative intraventricular conduction defects. *Circulation.*1978; 57: 867–870.

12 Hokanson JS, Moller JH. Significance of early transient complete heart block as a predictor of sudden death late after operative correction of tetralogy of Fallot. *Am J Cardiol.* 2001; 87: 1271–1277.

13 Banks MA, Jenson J, Kugler JD. Late development of atrioventricular block after congenital heart surgery in Down syndrome. *Am J Cardiol.* 2001; 88: 86–89.

14 Gross GJ, Chiu CC, Hamilton RM, Kirsh JA, Stephenson EA. Natural history of postoperative heart block in congenital heart disease: implications for pacing intervention. *Heart Rhythm.* 2006; 3: 601–604.

15 Sumitomo N, Karasawa K, Taniguchi K, Ichikawa R, Fukuhara J, Abe O, et al. Association of sinus node dysfunction, atrioventricular node conduction abnormality and ventricular arrhythmia in patients with Kawasaki disease and coronary involvement. *Circ J.* 2008 Feb; 72: 274–280.

16 Petri H, Vissing J, Witting N, Bundgaard H, Køber L. Cardiac manifestations of myotonic dystrophy type 1. *Int J Cardiol.* 2012; 160(2): 82–88.

17 Akdemir R, Ozhan H, Gunduz H, Yazici M, Erbilen E, Uyan C, Imirzalioglu N. Complete atrioventricular block in Becker muscular dystrophy. *N Z Med J.* 2004; 117: U895.

18 Welzing L, von Kleist-Retzow JC, Kribs A, Eifinger F, Huenseler C, Sreeram N. Rapid development of life-threatening complete atrioventricular block in Kearns–Sayre syndrome. *Eur J Pediatr.* 2009; 168: 757–759.

19 Littler WA. Heart block and peroneal muscular atrophy. A family study. *Q J Med.* 1970; 39: 431–440.

20 Brucato A, Frassi M, Franceschini F, Cimaz R, Faden D, Pisoni MP, et al. Risk of congenital complete heart block in newborns of mothers with anti-Ro/SSA antibodies detected by counterimmunoelectrophoresis: a prospective study of 100 women. *Arthritis Rheum.* 2001; 44: 1832–1835.

21 Costedoat-Chalumeau N, Amoura Z, Lupoglazoff JM, Thi Huong du L, Denjoy I, Vauthier D, et al. Outcome of pregnancies in patients with anti-SSA/Ro antibodies: a study of 165 pregnancies, with special focus on electrocardiographic variations in the children and comparison with a control group. *Arthritis Rheum.* 2004; 50: 3187–3194.

22 Buyon JP, Hiebert R, Copel J, Craft J, Friedman D, Katholi M, et al. Autoimmune-associated congenital heart block: demographics, mortality, morbidity and recurrence rates obtained from a national neonatal lupus registry. *J Am Coll Cardiol.* 1998; 31: 1658–1666.

23 Eronen M, Siren MK, Ekblad H, Tikanoja T, Julkunen H, Paavilainen T. Short- and long-term outcome of children with congenital complete heart block diagnosed in utero or as a newborn. *Pediatrics.* 2000; 106: 86–91.

24 Brucato A, Gasparini M, Vignati G, Riccobono S, De Juli E, Quinzanini M, et al. Isolated congenital complete heart block: longterm outcome of children and immunogenetic study. *J Rheumatol.* 1995; 22: 541–543.

25 Lev M. Pathogenesis of congenital atrioventricular block. *Prog Cardiovasc Dis.* 1972; 15: 145–157.

26 Anderson RH, Wenick AC, Losekoot TG, Becker AE. Congenitally complete heart block. Developmental aspects. *Circulation.* 1977; 56: 90–101.

27 Schmidt KG, Ulmer HE, Silverman NH, Kleinman CS, Copel JA. Perinatal outcome of fetal complete atrioventricular block: a multicenter experience. *J Am Coll Cardiol.* 1991; 17: 1360–1366.

28 Machado MV, Tynan MJ, Curry PV, Allan LD. Fetal complete heart block. *Br Heart J.* 1988; 60: 512–515.

29 Crawford D, Chapman M, Allan L. The assessment of persistent bradycardia in prenatal life. *Br J Obstet Gynaecol.* 1985; 92: 941–944.

30 Pinsky WW, Gillette PC, Garson A Jr, McNamara DG. Diagnosis, management, and long-term results of patients with congenital complete atrioventricular block. *Pediatrics.* 1982; 69: 728–733.

31 Michaelsson M, Engle MA. Congenital complete heart block: an international study of the natural history. In: Brest AN, Engle MA, eds. *Cardiovascular Clinics.* Philadelphia, PA: FA Davis. 1972; 4(3): 85–101.

32 Huhta JC, Maloney JD, Ritter DG, Ilstrup DM, Feldt RH. Complete atrioventricular block in patients with atrioventricular discordance. *Circulation.* 1983; 67: 1374–1377.

33 Jaeggi ET, Hamilton RM, Silverman ED, Zamora SA, Hornberger LK. Outcome of children with fetal, neonatal or childhood diagnosis of isolated congenital atrioventricular block. A single institution's experience of 30 years. *J Am Coll Cardiol.* 2002; 39: 130–137.

34 Sholler GF, Walsh EP. Congenital complete heart block in patients without anatomic cardiac defects. *Am Heart J.* 1989; 118: 1193–1198.

35 Esscher EB. Congenital complete heart block in adolescence and adult life. A follow-up study. *Eur Heart J.* 1981; 2: 281–288.

36 Michaelsson M, Jonzon A, Riesenfeld T. Isolated congenital complete atrioventricular block in adult life. A prospective study. *Circulation.* 1995; 92: 442–449.

37 Dewey RC, Capeless MA, Levy AM. Use of ambulatory electrocardiographic monitoring to identify high-risk patients with congenital complete heart block. *N Engl J Med.* 1987; 316: 835–839.

38 Villain E, Coastedoat-Chalumeau N, Marijon E, Boudjemline Y, Piette JC, Bonnet D. Presentation and prognosis of complete atrioventricular block in childhood, according to maternal antibody status. *J Am Coll Cardiol.* 2006; 48: 1682–1687.

39 Moak JP, Barron KS, Hougen TJ, et al. Congenital heart block: development of late-onset cardiomyopathy, a previously underappreciated sequela. *J Am Coll Cardiol.* 2001; 37: 238–242.

40 Aellig NC, Balmer C, Dodge-Khatami A, Rahn M, Prêtre R, Bauersfeld U. Long-term follow-up after pacemaker implantation in neonates and infants. *Ann Thorac Surg.* 2007; 83: 1420–1423.

41 Kardelen F, Celiker A, Ozer S, Ozme S, Oto A. Sinus node dysfunction in children and adolescents: treatment by implantation of a permanent pacemaker in 26 patients. *Turk J Pediatr.* 2002; 44: 312–316.

42 Walsh CA, McAlister HF, Andrews CA, Steeg CN, Eisenberg R, Furman S. Pacemaker implantation in children: a 21-year experience. *Pacing Clin Electrophysiol.* 1988; 11: 1940–1944.

43 Ferrero P, Massa R, Amellone C, Trevi G. "Sinus node" dysfunction associated with left atrial isomerism. *J Cardiovasc Med.* 2008; 9: 953–956.

44 Kugler JD. Sinus nodal dysfunction in young patients with long QT syndrome. *Am Heart J.* 1991; 121: 1132–1136.

45 Yasuda K, Hayashi G, Horie A, Taketani T, Yamaguchi S. Clinical and electrophysiological features of Japanese pediatric long QT syndrome patients with KCNQ1 mutations. *Pediatr Int.* 2008; 50: 611–614.

46 Benson DW, Wang DW, Dyment M, et al. Congenital sick sinus syndrome caused by recessive mutations in the cardiac sodium channel gene (SCN5A). *J Clin Invest.* 2003; 112: 1019–1028.

47 Cohen MI, Rhodes LA, Wernovsky G, Gaynor JW, Spray TL, Rychik J. Atrial pacing: an alternative treatment for protein-losing enteropathy after the Fontan operation. *J Thorac Cardiovasc Surg.* 2001; 121: 582–583.

48 Khairy P, Van Hare GF, Balaji S, Berul CI, Cecchin F, Cohen MI, et al. PACES/HRS Expert Consensus Statement on the Recognition and Management of Arrhythmias in Adult Congenital Heart Disease: developed in partnership between the Pediatric and Congenital Electrophysiology Society (PACES) and the Heart Rhythm Society (HRS). Endorsed by the governing bodies of PACES, HRS, the American College of Cardiology (ACC), the American Heart Association (AHA), the European Heart Rhythm Association (EHRA), the Canadian Heart Rhythm Society (CHRS), and the International Society for Adult Congenital Heart Disease (ISACHD). *Heart Rhythm.* 2014 Oct; 11(10): e102–165.

49 Kanter RJ, Garson A Jr., Atrial arrhythmias during chronic follow-up of surgery for complex congenital heart disease. *Pacing Clin Electrophysiol.* 1997; 20: 502–511.

50 Vetter VL, Horowitz LN. Electrophysiologic residua and sequelae of surgery for congenital heart defects. *Am J Cardiol.* 1982; 50: 588–604.

51 Triedman JK. Arrhythmias in adults with congenital heart disease. *Heart.* 2002; 87: 383–389.

52 Morton JB, Sanders P, Vohra JK et al. Effect of chronic right atrial stretch on atrial electrical remodeling in patients with an atrial septal defect. *Circulation.* 2003; 107: 1775–1782.

53 Garson A Jr, Bink-Boelkens M, Hesslein PS, Hordof AJ, Keane JF, Neches WH, Porter CJ. Atrial flutter in the young: a collaborative study of 380 cases. *J Am Coll Cardiol.* 1985; 6: 871–878.

54 Cohen MI, Rhodes LA. Sinus node dysfunction and atrial tachycardia after the Fontan procedure: The scope of the problem. *Semin Thorac Cardiovasc Surg Pediatr Card Surg Annu.* 1998; 1: 41–52.

55 Drago F, Silvetti MS, Grutter G, De Santis A, Gagliardi MG, Giannico S. Use of DDDRP pacing device in prevention and treatment of tachy-brady syndrome after Mustard procedure. *Pacing Clin Electrophysiol.* 2004; 27: 530–532.

56 Silka MJ, Manwill JR, Kron J, McAnulty JH. Bradycardia-mediated tachyarrhythmias in congenital heart disease and responses to chronic pacing at physiologic rates. *Am J Cardiol.* 1990; 65: 488–493.

57 Stephenson EA, Casavant D, Tuzi J, Alexander ME, Law I, Serwer G, et al. ATTEST Investigators. Efficacy of atrial antitachycardia pacing using the Medtronic AT500 pacemaker in patients with congenital heart disease. *Am J Cardiol.* 2003; 92: 871–876.

58 Rhodes LA, Walsh EP, Gamble WJ, Triedman JK, Saul JP. Benefits and potential risks of atrial antitachycardia pacing after repair of congenital heart disease. *Pacing Clin Electrophysiol.* 1995; 18: 1005–1016.

59 Wu JM, Young ML, Wu MH, Wang JK, Lue HC. Atrial overdrive pacing for conversion of atrial flutter in children. *Zhonghua Min Guo Xiao Er Ke Yi Xue Hui Za Zhi.* 1991; 32: 1–8.

60 Eldar M, Griffin JC, Van Hare GF, Witherell C, Bhandari A, Benditt D, Scheinman MM. Combined use of beta-adrenergic blocking agents and long-term cardiac pacing for patients with the long QT syndrome. *J Am Coll Cardiol.* 1992; 20: 830–837.

61 Moss AJ, Liu JE, Gottlieb S, Locati EH, Schwartz PJ, Robinson JL. Efficacy of permanent pacing in the management of high-risk patients with long QT syndrome. *Circulation.* 1991; 84: 1524–1529.

62 Sutton R, Brignole M, Menozzi C, Raviele A, Alboni P, Giani P, Moya A. Dual-chamber pacing in the treatment of neurally mediated tilt-positive cardioinhibitory syncope: pacemaker versus no therapy: a multicenter randomized study. The Vasovagal Syncope

International Study (VASIS) Investigators. *Circulation.* 2000; 102: 294–299.

63 Ammirati F, Colivicchi F, Santini M. Syncope Diagnosis and Treatment Study Investigators. Permanent cardiac pacing versus medical treatment for the prevention of recurrent vasovagal syncope: a multicenter, randomized, controlled trial. *Circulation.* 2001; 104: 52–57.

64 Connolly SJ, Sheldon R, Roberts RS, Gent M. The North American Vasovagal Pacemaker Study (VPS). A randomized trial of permanent cardiac pacing for the prevention of vasovagal syncope. *J Am Coll Cardiol.* 1999; 33: 16–20.

65 Raviele A, Giada F, Menozzi C, Speca G, Orazi S, Gasparini G, Sutton R, Brignole M; Vasovagal Syncope and Pacing Trial Investigators. A randomized, double-blind, placebo-controlled study of permanent cardiac pacing for the treatment of recurrent tilt-induced vasovagal syncope. The vasovagal syncope and pacing trial (SYNPACE). *Eur Heart J.* 2004; 25: 1741–1748.

66 Connolly SJ, Sheldon R, Thorpe KE, Roberts RS, Ellenbogen KA, Wilkoff BL, et al. VPS II Investigators. Pacemaker therapy for prevention of syncope in patients with recurrent severe vasovagal syncope: Second Vasovagal Pacemaker Study (VPS II): a randomized trial. *JAMA.* 2003; 289: 2224–2229.

67 Sud S, Massel D, Klein GJ, Leong-Sit P, Yee R, Skanes AC, et al. The expectation effect and cardiac pacing for refractory vasovagal syncope. *Am J Med.* 2007; 120: 54–62.

68 Wagshal AB, Weinstein JM, Weinstein O, Zeldetz V, Damri E, Ilia R, Katz A. Do the recently modified pacemaker guidelines for neurocardiogenic syncope also apply to young patients? Analysis based on five-year follow-up of Israeli soldiers with syncope and a positive tilt test. *Cardiology.* 2004; 102: 200–205.

69 Stojanov PL, Savic DV, Zivkovic MB, Calovic ZR. Permanent endovenous pediatric pacing: absence of lead failure – 20 years follow-up study. *Pacing Clin Electrophysiol.* 2008 Sep; 31(9): 1100–1107.

70 Silka MJ, Bar-Cohen Y. Pacemakers and implantable cardioverter-defibrillators in pediatric patients. *Heart Rhythm.* 2006 Nov; 3(11): 1360–1366.

71 Kammeraad JA, Rosenthal E, Bostock J, Rogers J, Sreeram N. Endocardial pacemaker implantation in infants weighing < or = 10 kilograms. *Pacing Clin Electrophysiol.* 2004 Nov; 27(11): 1466–1474.

72 Khairy P, Landzberg MJ, Gatzoulis MA, Mercier LA, Fernandes SM, Côté JM, et al. Transvenous pacing leads and systemic thromboemboli in patients with intracardiac shunts: a multicenter study. *Circulation.* 2006 May 23; 113(20): 2391–2397.

73 Shah MJ, Nehgme R, Carboni M, Murphy JD. Endocardial atrial pacing lead implantation and midterm follow-up in young patients with sinus node dysfunction after the Fontan procedure. *Pacing Clin Electrophysiol.* 2004 Jul; 27(7): 949–954.

74 Takahashi K, Cecchin F, Fortescue E, Berul CI, Alexander ME, Walsh EP, et al. Permanent atrial pacing lead implant route after Fontan operation. *Pacing Clin Electrophysiol.* 2009 Jun; 32(6): 779–785.

75 Antonelli D, Freedberg NA. Endocardial ventricular pacing through a bioprosthetic tricuspid valve. *Pacing Clin Electrophysiol.* 2007 Feb; 30(2): 271–272.

76 Kistler PM, Sanders P, Davidson NC, Mond HG. The challenge of endocardial right ventricular pacing in patients with a tricuspid annuloplasty ring and severe tricuspid regurgitation. *Pacing Clin Electrophysiol.* 2002 Feb; 25(2): 201–205.

77 Pernenkil R, Wright JS. Endocardial pacing through a prosthetic tricuspid valve. *Pacing Clin Electrophysiol.* 1990 Nov; 13(11 Pt 1): 1365–1366.

78 De Kerpel F, Duytschaever M, Tavernier R. Permanent ventricular pacing via a low posterolateral cardiac vein in a patient with a mechanical tricuspid valve prosthesis and complete atrioventricular block. *Acta Cardiol.* 2004 Oct; 59(5): 565–567.

79 Demir AD, Sen N, Erbay AR, Atak R. An effective and safe alternative to epicardial pacemaker placement for permanent pacemaker implantation in a patient with mechanical tricuspid valve: stimulation of the left ventricle through the coronary sinus. *Turk Kardiyol Dern Ars.* 2011 Apr; 39(3): 244–247.

80 Lopez JA, Lufschanowski R. Transvenous bifocal left ventricular pacing after mechanical prosthetic tricuspid valve replacement with use of echocardiography to optimize pacing parameters. *J Interv Card Electrophysiol.* 2007 Apr; 18(3): 233–237.

81 Fortescue EB, Berul CI, Cecchin F, Walsh EP, Triedman JK, Alexander ME. Comparison of modern steroid-eluting epicardial and thin transvenous pacemaker leads in pediatric and congenital heart disease patients. *J Interv Card Electrophysiol.* 2005 Oct; 14(1): 27–36.

82 Odim J, Suckow B, Saedi B, Laks H, Shannon K. Equivalent performance of epicardial versus endocardial permanent pacing in children: a single institution and manufacturer experience. *Ann Thorac Surg.* 2008 Apr; 85(4): 1412–1416.

83 Udink ten Cate F, Breur J, Boramanand N, Crosson J, Friedman A, Brenner J, et al. Endocardial and epicardial steroid lead pacing in the neonatal and paediatric age group. *Heart.* 2002 Oct; 88(4): 392–36.

84 Singarayar S, Kistler PM, De Winter C, Mond H. A comparative study of the action of dexamethasone sodium phosphate and dexamethasone acetate in steroid-eluting pacemaker leads. *Pacing Clin Electrophysiol.* 2005 Apr; 28(4): 311–315.

85 Mond HG, Stokes KB. The steroid-eluting electrode: a 10-year experience. *Pacing Clin Electrophysiol.* 1996 Jul; 19(7): 1016–1020.

86 Horenstein MS, Hakimi M, Walters H 3rd, Karpawich PP. Chronic performance of steroid-eluting epicardial leads in a growing pediatric population: a 10-year comparison. *Pacing Clin Electrophysiol.* 2003 Jul; 26(7 Pt 1): 1467–1471.

87 Ceviz N, Celiker A, Küçükosmanoğlu O, Alehan D, Kiliç A, Uner A, Ozme S. Comparison of mid-term clinical experience with steroid-eluting active and passive fixation ventricular electrodes in children. *Pacing Clin Electrophysiol.* 2000 Aug; 23(8): 1245–1249.

88 Beck H, Boden WE, Patibandla S, Kireyev D, Gutpa V, Campagna F, et al. 50th Anniversary of the first successful permanent pacemaker implantation in the United States: historical review and future directions. *Am J Cardiol.* 2010 Sep 15; 106(6): 810–818.

89 Wiegand UK, Bode F, Bonnemeier H, Tölg R, Peters W, Katus HA. Incidence and predictors of pacemaker dysfunction with unipolar ventricular lead configuration. Can we identify patients who benefit from bipolar electrodes? *Pacing Clin Electrophysiol.* 2001 Sep; 24(9 Pt 1): 1383–1388.

90 Figa FH, McCrindle BW, Bigras JL, Hamilton RM, Gow RM. Risk factors for venous obstruction in children with transvenous pacing leads. *Pacing Clin Electrophysiol.* 1997 Aug; 20(8 Pt 1): 1902–1909.

91 Bar-Cohen Y, Berul CI, Alexander ME, Fortescue EB, Walsh EP, Triedman JK, Cecchin F. Age, size, and lead factors alone do not predict venous obstruction in children and young adults with transvenous lead systems. *J Cardiovasc Electrophysiol.* 2006 Jul; 17(7): 712–716.

92 Kenny D, Walsh KP. Noncatheter-based delivery of a single-chamber lumenless pacing lead in small children. *Pacing Clin Electrophysiol.* 2007 Jul; 30(7): 834–838.

93 Lapage MJ, Rhee EK. Alternative delivery of a 4Fr lumenless pacing lead in children. *Pacing Clin Electrophysiol.* 2008 May; 31(5): 543–547.

94 Tops LF, Schalij MJ, Bax JJ. The effects of right ventricular apical pacing on ventricular function and dyssynchrony implications for therapy. *J Am Coll Cardiol.* 2009 Aug 25; 54(9): 764–776.

95 Zanon F, Svetlich C, Occhetta E, Catanzariti D, Cantù F, Padeletti L, et al. Safety and performance of a system specifically designed for selective site pacing. *Pacing Clin Electrophysiol.* 2011 Mar; 34(3): 339–347.

96 Gammage MD, Lieberman RA, Yee R, Manolis AS, Compton SJ, Khazen C, et al. Multi-center clinical experience with a lumenless, catheter-delivered, bipolar, permanent pacemaker lead: implant safety and electrical performance. *Pacing Clin Electrophysiol.* 2006 Aug; 29(8): 858–865.

97 Chakrabarti S, Morgan GJ, Kenny D, Walsh KP, Oslizlok P, Martin RP, et al. Initial experience of pacing with a lumenless lead system in patients with congenital heart disease. *Pacing Clin Electrophysiol.* 2009 Nov; 32(11): 1428–1433.

98 Daccarett M, Segerson NM, Bradley DJ, Etheridge SP, Freedman RA, Saarel EV. Bipolar lumenless lead performance in children and adults with congenital heart disease. *Congenit Heart Dis.* 2010 Mar-Apr; 5(2): 149–156.

99 Khan A, Zelin K, Karpawich PP. Performance of the lumenless 4.1-Fr diameter pacing lead implanted at alternative pacing sites in congenital heart: a chronic 5-year comparison. Pacing Clin Electrophysiol. 2010 Dec; 33(12): 1467–1474.

100 Bullock A, Finley J, Sharratt G, Ross D. Single lead VDD pacing in children with complete heart block. *Can J Cardiol.* 1998 Jan; 14(1): 58–62.

101 Horenstein MS, Karpawich PP, Tantengco MV. Single versus dual chamber pacing in the young: noninvasive comparative evaluation of cardiac function. *Pacing Clin Electrophysiol.* 2003 May; 26(5): 1208–1211.

102 Südkamp M, Schmid M, Geissler HJ, Emmel M, Gillor A, Mehlhorn U, Hekmat K. VDD-pacemaker in children: A long-term therapy? *Thorac Cardiovasc Surg.* 2005 Jun; 53(3): 158–161.

103 Seiden HS, Camuñas JL, Fishburger SB, Golinko RJ, Steinberg LG, Shagong U, Rossi AF. Use of single lead VDD pacing in children. *Pacing Clin Electrophysiol.* 1997 Aug; 20(8 Pt 1): 1967–1974.

104 Maginot KR, Mathewson JW, Bichell DP, Perry JC. Applications of pacing strategies in neonates and infants. *Progress in Ped Cardio.* 2000; 11: 65–75.

105 Agarwal R, Krishnan GS, Abraham S, Bhatt K, Sekar P, Kulkarni S, Cherian KM. Extrapleural intrathoracic implantation of permanent pacemaker in the pediatric age group. *Ann Thorac Surg.* 2007; 83: 1549–1552.

106 Villain E, Martelli H, Bonnet D, Iserin L, Butera G, Kachaner J. Characteristics and results of epicardial pacing in neonates and infants. *Pacing Clin Electrophysiol.* 2000; 23: 2052–2056.

107 Cherry J, Kaplan S, Demmler-Harrison G, Steinbach W. Infections related to prosthetic or artificial devices. In: *Feigin and Cherry's Textbook of Pediatric Infectious Diseases.* Philadelphia, PA: WB Saunders. 2009; 1(6): 1111–1200.

108 Silvetti MS, Drago F, Marcora S, Ravà L. Outcome of single-chamber, ventricular pacemakers with transvenous leads implanted in children. *Europace* 2007; 9: 894–899.

109 Dretzke J, Toff WD, Lip GYH, Raftery J, Fry-Smith A, Taylor RRS. Dual chamber versus single chamber ventricular pacemakers for sick sinus syndrome and atrioventricular block (review). *The Cochrane Library.* 2009; 1: 1–83.

110 Horenstein MS, Karpawich PP, Tantengco MVT. Single versus dual chamber pacing in the young: noninvasive comparative evaluation of cardiac function. *Pacing Clin Electrophysiol.* 2003; 26: 1208–1211.

111 Fishberger SB, Wernovsky G, Gentles TL, Gamble WJ, Gauvreau K, Burnett J, et al. Long-term outcome in patients with pacemakers following the Fontan operation. *Am J Cardiol.* 1996; 77: 887–889.

112 Kalin R, Stanton MS. Current clinical issues for MRI scanning of pacemaker and defibrillator patients. *Pacing Clin Electrophysiol.* 2005; 28: 326–328.

113 Kanal E, Borgstede JP, Barkovich AJ, Bell C, Bradley WG, Etheridge S, et al. American College of Radiology White Paper on MR Safety: 2004 Update and Revisions. *Amer J Radiol.* 2004; 182: 1111–1114.

114 Levine GN, Gomes AS, Arai AE, Bluemke DA, Flamm SF, Kanal EK, et al. Safety of magnetic resonance imaging in patients with cardiovascular devices: An American Heart Association scientific statement from the Committee on Diagnostic and Interventional Cardiac Catheterization, Council on Clinical Cardiology, and the Council on Cardiovascular Radiology and Intervention. *Circulation.* 2007; 116: 2878–2891.

115 Martin ET, Coman JA, Shellock FG, Pulling CC, Fair R, Jenkins K. Magnetic resonance imaging and cardiac pacemaker safety at 1.5-Tesla. *J Am Coll Cardiol.* 2004; 43: 1–10.

116 Gimbel JR. Magnetic resonance imaging of implantable cardiac rhythm devices at 3.0 Tesla. *Pacing and Clin Electrophysiol.* 2008; 31: 795–801.

117 Pulver AF, Puchalski MD, Bradley DJ, Minich LL, Su JT, Saarel EV, et al. Safety and imaging quality of MRI in pediatric and adult congenital heart disease patients with pacemakers. *Pacing Clin Electrophysiol.* 2009; 32: 450–456.

118 Cabrera ME, Hanisch DG, Cohen MH, Murtaugh R, Spector ML, Liebman J. Cardiopulmonary responses to exercise in children with activity sensing rate responsive ventricular pacemakers. *Pacing Clin Electrophysiol.* 1993; 16: 1386–1393.

119 Ragonese P, Guccione P, Drago F, Turchetta A, Galzolari A, Formigari R. Efficacy and safety of ventricular rate responsive pacing in children with complete atrioventricular block. *Pacing Clin Electrophysiol.* 1994; 17: 603–610.

120 Bauersfeld U, Nowak B, Molinari L, Malm T, Kampmann C, Schönbeck MH, Schüller H. Low-energy epicardial pacing in children: the benefit of autocapture. *Ann Thorac Surg.* 1999; 68: 1380–1383.

121 Tomaske M, Harpes P, Pretre R, Dodge-Khatami A, Bauersfeld U. Long-term experience with autocapture-controlled epicardial pacing in children. *Europace.* 2007; 9: 645–650.

122 Ellenbogen KA, Gold MR, Meyer TE, Lozano IF, Mittal S, Waggoner AD, et al. Primary results from the Smart-Delay determined AV optimization: a comparison to other AV delay methods used in cardiac resynchronization therapy (SMART-AV) trial: A randomized trial comparing empirical, echocardiography-guided, and algorithmic atrioventricular delay programming in cardiac resynchronization therapy. *Circulation.* 2010; 122: 2660–2668.

123 Kaltman JR, Ro PS, Zimmerman F, Moak JP, Epstein M, Zeltser IJ, et al. Managed ventricular pacing in pediatric patients and patients with congenital heart disease. *Am J Cardiol.* 2008; 102: 875–878.

124 Ammirati F, Colivicchi F, Toscano S, Pandozi C, Laudadio MT, De Seta F, Santini M. DDD pacing with rate drop response function versus DDI with rate hysteresis pacing for cardioinhibitory vasovagal syncope. *Pacing Clin Electrophysiol.* 1998; 21: 2178–2181.

125 Janko S, Hoffmann E. Atrial antitachycardia pacing: Do we still need to talk about it? (editorial). *Europace* 2009; 11: 977–979.

126 Kamp AN, LaPage MJ, Serwer G, Dick M, Bradley DJ. Anti-tachycardia pacemaker in congenital heart disease (abstract). *Presented at International Academy of Cardiology 16th World Congress on Heart Disease Annual Scientific Sessions* 2001.

127 Batra AS. Patient-activated antitachycardia pacing to terminate atrial tachycardias with 1:1 atrioventricular conduction in congenital heart disease. *Pediatr Cardiol.* 2008; 29: 851–854.

CHAPTER 4

Indications for implantable cardioverter defibrillator therapy, device, and lead selection

Mitchell I. Cohen[1] and Susan P. Etheridge[2]

[1]Co-Director Heart Center, Section Chief Cardiology, Phoenix Children's Hospital, Clinical Associate Professor of Child Health University of Arizona College of Medicine, Phoenix, AZ, USA

[2]Pediatric Electrophysiologist, Primary Children's Hospital, Professor of Pediatrics, University of Utah, Salt Lake City, UT, USA

Introduction

The indications for implantation of an implantable cardioverter-defibrillator (ICD) in the pediatric population and in adults with congenital heart disease (CHD) have expanded in the three decades since the introduction of this technology. The indications for device implantation in children often mirror those of adult patients although the technical issues surrounding implantation and late complications after implantation vary greatly. Furthermore, CHD patients represent a group without a comparable adult population. Application of ICD technology in all children is characterized by both unique anatomic and size considerations. The increasing complexity of ICD devices and leads with sophisticated discriminators, anti tachycardia protocols, and lead designs increases the potential for either ICD generator or lead failure and may necessitate removal/revision. The three largest ICD manufacturers (St. Jude Medical, St Paul, MN, Medtronic, Minneapolis, MN, and Guidant/Boston Scientific, Indianapolis, IN) have each had advisories related to their defibrillation systems. Given the impact lead failures, recalls and advisories have on patients it is critical that a thorough understanding of current leads and generators is well-grounded, pertinent decisions prior to implantation are made, and appropriate post-market surveillance is established.

This chapter addresses published guidelines regarding: (1) current indications for ICD implantation in children and young adults with CHD, and (2) novel ICD indications in the inheritable arrhythmias and structural and functional cardiac disease. Appropriate device and lead choices and programming strategies unique to these patients is also discussed. It is not feasible to address every clinical scenario and patient who may require an ICD. Although ICD implantation should be based primarily on a thoughtful assessment of arrhythmia risk using the patient's clinical history, hemodynamic status, ECG, and genetic information in

Cardiac Pacing and Defibrillation in Pediatric and Congenital Heart Disease, First Edition.
Edited by Maully Shah, Larry Rhodes and Jonathan Kaltman.
© 2017 John Wiley & Sons Ltd. Published 2017 by John Wiley & Sons Ltd.
Companion Website: www.wiley.com/go/shah/cardiac_pacing

decision-making, there are occasionally families in whom the previous tragic deaths make this, in part, an emotional decision. While we can and should counsel families using all the available data in the literature, each patient and family is unique and decisions concerning ICD implantation must be individualized and tailored to each patient (see Table 4.1). This chapter also provides a decision-making framework for choosing the most appropriate ICD generator and leads for a given patient. Issues regarding programming and troubleshooting are discussed elsewhere. Complications discussed in this chapter allow for a better understanding of the importance of device and lead choice.

ICD indications in patients with congenital heart disease (CHD)

The use of ICDs in children and adults with CHD is increasing. A greater number of patients with complex CHD are surviving to adulthood and arrhythmias must be considered intrinsic to the lives of these patients. Risk stratification, device choice, and programming are unique and differ from what is applied to a patient population with a normally formed heart. Arrhythmias are a main reason for hospitalization and are a frequent cause of morbidity and mortality in the CHD population.[1] Although arrhythmia management using catheter ablation in this population is possible, when compared to patients with structurally normal hearts, results are generally worse and occasionally the chamber of interest is inaccessible. Anti-arrhythmic agents are often poorly tolerated especially if hemodynamic compromise exists. In a multi-center series of pediatric ICD recipients, patients with CHD represented the largest subgroup.[2] CHD patients with the greatest risk of sudden death are those with l-transposition and d-transposition of the great arteries, Ebstein anomaly, aortic stenosis, single ventricle physiology, and tetralogy of Fallot (TOF).[1, 3] Despite the fairly frequent use of devices in CHD patients, algorithms for risk assessment for sudden death and indications for ICD implantation in the setting of CHD have not been established.

At present, patients with TOF constitute the largest subgroup of ICD recipients among CHD patients.[4, 5] With improved survival in patients with single ventricle physiology, in the future, these patients will likely constitute a greater proportion and one likely to be challenging to manage, especially from an implantation standpoint. In the analysis of indications for ICD implantation in the entire CHD population, one must extrapolate from patients with TOF where data are most robust and sudden death remains the most common cause of late mortality.[6–8] Sudden death prevention is a challenge that can be overcome with ICD implantation. In a recent multi-institutional analysis of adult TOF patients, 10% of the 556 patients had ICDs. Although ICD implantation for primary prevention remains controversial, in this series 59% were implanted for primary prevention[9] similar to the 52% of children with primary prevention device implantation reported in the Pediatric ICD Registry data.[2] Of note, 44% of the adult TOF patients with implantation for primary prevention had ventricular arrhythmias during study follow-up.

The CHD population is a heterogeneous group with a vast number of diagnoses, having had numerous different surgical procedures, in different eras, and at different ages. Previous reports outline the utility of invasive and noninvasive risk factors for sudden death in TOF.[6, 10] The QRS duration as a predictor of risk for clinical ventricular tachycardia (VT) has with stood the test of time and remains a valid indicator of risk.[9] It is not clear if this association is unique to the TOF population or can be extrapolated to others with CHD. There are some data that a more modest QRS duration prolongation of $>/= 140$ ms is associated with risk in patients with d-transposition after Mustard operation.[11] The number of cardiac surgeries and previous palliative shunts has been associated with inducible ventricular arrhythmias[10] and appropriate ICD shocks[12] in TOF patients, and these data may be applicable other CHD patients. Recommendations for ICD implantation in children and CHD patients were updated in 2012 (Table 4.1).[13] Recently, specific recommendations for ICD implantation in adults with CHD have also been published (Table 4.2).[14]

Table 4.1 *Recommendations for implantable cardioverter-defibrillators in pediatric patients and patients with congenital heart disease. Source: Epstein 2013. Reproduced with permission of Wolters Kluwer[13]*

Class I	Survivors of cardiac arrest after evaluation to define the cause of the event and to exclude any reversible causes
Class IIa	Reasonable for patients with CHD with recurrent syncope of undetermined origin in the presence of either ventricular dysfunction or inducible ventricular arrhythmias at EPS
Class IIb	May be considered for patients with recurrent syncope associated with complex CHD and advanced systemic ventricular dysfunction when thorough invasive and noninvasive investigations have failed to define a cause
Class III	Those who do not have a reasonable expectation of survival with an acceptable functional
1.	status for at least 1 year
2.	Incessant VT or VF
3.	Patients with significant psychiatric illnesses
4.	NYHA Class IV patients with drug-refractory congestive heart failure who are not
5.	candidates for cardiac transplantation or CRT-D Syncope of undetermined cause in a patient
6.	without inducible ventricular tachyarrhythmias and without structural heart disease VF or
7.	VT is amenable to surgical or catheter ablation (e.g., atrial arrhythmias associated with the Wolff-Parkinson-White syndrome, RV or LV outflow tract VT, idiopathic VT, or fascicular VT in the absence of structural heart disease Ventricular tachyarrhythmias due to a completely reversible disorder in the absence of structural heart disease

Notes: Class I – indicated, Class IIa – probably indicated, Class IIb – may be considered. AV– atrioventricular, CHD – congenital heart disease, CRT – cardiac resynchronization therapy, EPS – electrophysiology study, EF – ejection fraction, NYHA – New York Heart Association, LV – left ventricle, RV – right ventricle, VT – ventricular tachycardia, VF – ventricular fibrillation

As in other patient populations, ICD implantation in a survivor of a cardiac arrest is a Class I indication.[13, 14] In patients with documented or inducible VT, recommended therapies include catheter ablation or surgical resection. If unsuccessful, ICD implantation is recommended. Even after successful ablation of a single VT focus, one must be vigilant for the appearance of other tachycardia substrates that could cause sudden death. Unexplained syncope is very concerning and assessment should include a hemodynamic and electrophysiology evaluation. In patients with syncope in the setting of decreased systemic ventricular function without a reversible cause, ICD implantation should be considered (IIa level of evidence B).

Other factors that should be considered when deciding about ICD implantation in a patient with CHD include, ventricular diastolic dysfunction,[9] extensive fibrosis on MRI, inducible,[15] extensive fibrosis on MRI, inducible VT, a history of long-term palliative shunts, and older age at repair as a surrogate of long standing hemodynamic pressure or volume overload or long-standing cyanosis. Left ventricular diastolic function assessed using noninvasive measures has been independently associated with mortality and ventricular arrhythmias in TOF, sickle cell disease,[16] renal failure,[17] and others. As this population ages and develops co-morbidities such as diabetes, hypercholesterolemia, and hypertension, these also must factor into the ICD decision process.

This population is not uniform and therefore decisions about ICD implantation should be taken using a patient-by-patient approach. Occasionally clear indications for ICD implantation are present including: any survivor of a cardiac arrest, documented ventricular fibrillation (VF), hemodynamically unstable VT not able to be addressed by ablation, and syncope or VT in the setting of

Table 4.2 *Recommendations for ICD therapy in adults with CHD. Source: Khairy 2014. Reproduced with permission of Elsevier[14]*

Class I	Survivors of cardiac arrest
1.	due to VF or hemodynamically unstable VT after evaluation to define the cause of the event and
2.	exclude any completely reversible etiology
3.	Patients with sustained VT who have undergone hemodynamic and electrophysiologic evaluation
	Systemic LV EF ≤35%, biventricular physiology, and NYHA class II or III symptoms
Class IIa	Reasonable in selected adults with TOF and multiple risk factors for SCD, such as LV systolic or
	diastolic dysfunction, nonsustained VT, QRS duration ≥180 ms, extensive right ventricular scarring,
	or inducible sustained VT at EPS
Class IIb	Single or systemic RV EF <35%, particularly in the presence of additional risk factors such as
1.	complex ventricular arrhythmias, unexplained syncope, NYHA functional class II or III symptoms,
2.	QRS duration ≥140 ms, or severe systemic AV valve regurgitation
3.	Systemic ventricular EF <35% in the absence of overt symptoms (NYHA class I) or other known risk
4.	factors
5.	Syncope of unknown origin with hemodynamically significant sustained ventricular tachycardia or
	fibrillation inducible at EPS
	Non-hospitalized adults with CHD awaiting heart transplantation
	Syncope and moderate or complex CHD in whom there is a high clinical suspicion of ventricular
	arrhythmia and in whom thorough investigations have failed to define a cause
Class III	Life expectancy with an acceptable functional status <1 year
1.	Incessant VT or VF
2.	Significant psychiatric illness that may be aggravated by ICD or preclude systematic follow-up
3.	Patients with drug-refractory NYHA class IV symptoms who are not candidates for cardiac
4.	transplantation or CRT.
5.	Advanced pulmonary vascular disease (Eisenmenger syndrome)
6.	Endocardial leads are generally avoided in adults with CHD and intracardiac shunts

Notes: Class I – indicated, Class IIa – probably indicated, Class IIb – may be considered. AV – atrioventricular, CHD – congenital heart disease, CRT – cardiac resynchronization therapy, EPS – electrophysiology study, EF – ejection fraction, NYHA – New York Heart Association, LV – left ventricle, RV – right ventricle, VT – ventricular tachycardia, VF – ventricular fibrillation

decreased systemic ventricular function (a patient in whom one might also consider CRT therapy).

ICD indications in hypertrophic cardiomyopathy (HCM)

HCM is a heritable disease that usually involves mutations in sarcomeric proteins although non-sarcomeric disease genes have been implicated.[18] The condition may be asymptomatic, while in some the first symptom is sudden death. Identification of risk factors and the implantation of an ICD in high risk patients is the standard of care. Risk factors for sudden death are derived from a number of registries and observational studies.

However, other than cardiac arrest, each of the risk factors has low positive predictive value.[19] The reported risk factors include aborted sudden death, spontaneous sustained or nonsustained VT, unexplained syncope, left ventricular thickness ≥ 30 mm, abnormal exercise blood pressure, and a family history of sudden death. Left ventricular thickness > 30 mm may need to be adjusted downward in small children as suggested by a recent pediatric series.[20] In a large systematic analysis of the literature supporting the international guidelines on the assessment of sudden death risk factors in HCM, all major risk factors were found associated with a risk of sudden death but age was an important factor modifying the predictive power of these risk factors.[21] Nonsustained VT proved to be a significant independent risk factor in young HCM patients. In another study, an abnormal blood pressure response was associated with increased risk only in patients under age 50.[22] Some studies have addressed the combination of risk factors. One study found that patients with two or more risk factors had an estimated sudden death risk of 4–5%.[23] Although sudden death can occur without significant left ventricular outflow tract obstruction, recent data suggest this may be emerging as a risk,[21] but its use as a risk factor may be limited by the fact that the gradient is dynamic and highly variable.[19]

In a pediatric series, factors predictive of arrhythmic events in univariate risk analysis included ventricular septal thickness, VT induction by programmed ventricular stimulation, age and presyncope/syncope.[20] In a multivariate analysis septal thickness, age, presyncope/syncope, and VT induction were not independently predictive of risk for an arrhythmic event. However, the 5-year event rate was 15% when age ≥ 13 years and septal thickness of ≥ 20 mm were combined, and 23% (95% CI: 3–39%) when VT induction and septal thickness ≥ 20 mm were combined. Of the risk factors that were considered in this pediatric cohort, septal thickness and inducible VT were the most significant univariate predictors of risk. More traditional risk factors identified in older patients (family history of sudden death, VT on Holter, and exercise-induced hypotension) were not predictive of events in patients under 21 years of age. Similarly, in another pediatric high risk HCM cohort, appropriate ICD therapy occurred in 43 of 224 patients (19%) over a mean of 4.3 ± 3.3 years and extreme left ventricular hypertrophy was most frequently associated with appropriate interventions.[24]

Based on the 2011 guidelines, the placement of an ICD in the setting of HCM is recommended for patients with a prior documented cardiac arrest, VF, or hemodynamically significant VT (Class I, level of evidence B).[19] The same guidelines state that it is reasonable (Class IIa) to recommend an ICD in patients with HCM and a family history of sudden death in a first-degree relative, a maximum left ventricular wall dimension ≥ 30 mm, or recent unexplained syncope (all level of evidence C). Specific Class IIa recommendations related to children are included in this document and state that it is reasonable to recommend an ICD for children with unexplained syncope, massive left ventricular hypertrophy, or a family history of sudden death. They do caution that one must take into account the relatively high complication rate of long-term ICD implantation in children.[19] The Class IIb indications where an ICD is of uncertain benefit include those with nonsustained VT and those with an abnormal blood pressure response to exercise. Class III (potentially harmful) recommendations for ICD implantation continues to include routine management without an indication of risk and a strategy to allow the patient to participate in competitive sports.

ICD indications in patients with long QT syndrome (LQTS)

The LQTS represents a complex group of disorders characterized by syncope, "seizures" and sudden death due to mutations that interfere with cardiac ion channel function. Although there are 16 recognized types, the majority of patients have LQTS 1, 2, or 3. Data concerning risk stratification focus on these three types of LQTS and most patients in these series have LQT1 or LQT2.[14, 15, 25, 26] Data concerning risk in the less common types of LQTS are unavailable. The indications for ICD implantation in pediatric patients with LQTS are similar to indications in adults, although size considerations may impact these decisions. Occasionally, in a high-risk neonate in whom an ICD is warranted, pacing may be helpful until the patient achieves a size where an ICD is feasible. In this population, if feasible a dual chamber device that allows for antibradycardia pacing and AV synchrony is preferable. At present most would agree that ICD implantation is indicated in LQTS patients who survive a cardiac arrest with consideration for the possibility that beta-blocker noncompliance and/or the use of medications known to prolong repolarization may have precipitated the event. In other situations, it is less clear and debate exists. The renewed interest in the left cervical sympathetic denervation (LCSD) has proven effective in high-risk LQTS patients and may obviate the need for an ICD in some.[27, 28] Patients compliant with appropriate dose beta-blockers in whom syncope or ventricular arrhythmias persist, and those with symptoms and profound (>550 ms) QTc prolongation[29] are considered high risk and ICD implantation is recommended.[30]

LQT3 patients represent a management dilemma. They represent <10% of the population studied even from the large International LQTS Registry. Thus one must use caution when interpreting these data due to the small number of LQT3 patients represented.[15, 16, 26, 31] LQT3 patients have fewer events but a higher percentage of lethal events.[31] There are data to suggest that beta-blockers may be less effective in LQT3 compared to LQT1 and LQT2.[32] Nonetheless, at present, beta-blockers (in particular propranolol) should be considered first line therapy in LQT3 until further data are available that their use increases risk. LQT3 patients have been shown to be at higher risk in the setting of slow heart rates and events often occur with sleep or rest.[32] Thus events are often not witnessed and therefore unavailable for bystander CPR. Other therapy considerations include LCSD, a procedure that blunts adrenaline effect without reducing heart rate[33] and pacing that allows for the safe use of beta-blockers in patients with bradycardia or sinus pauses. The recognition that LQT3 patients are part of a larger and overlapping group of entities, the sodium channelopathies, adds to the complexity of management. The overlap, within a family and even within isolated patients, of LQT3, sinus and AV node dysfunction, Brugada syndrome, conduction system disease and even functional cardiac disease makes treatment choices difficult. Medications that might obviate the need for an ICD in a high risk LQT3 patient, like sodium channel blocking agents, have been shown to shorten the QTc but the response to this therapy may be mutation-specific.[34-36] Although, the use of sodium channel blocking agents has been incorporated into clinical guidelines, use should be guided by mutation-specific data when available and caution taken where these data are not available. and caution taken where these data are not available.

Primary prevention ICD implantation in LQTS should focus on those at high risk. Most agree this group includes patients with syncope and ventricular arrhythmias despite beta-blocker therapy. Intolerance to beta-blocker therapy is often listed as an indication for ICD implantation. Beta-blocker intolerance can be mitigated by starting the medication at a low dose and increasing gradually. Children usually tolerate beta-blockers. Profound QTc prolongation (>550 ms) may be a primary prevention indication in some, although not in LQT1 patients who are highly protected by beta-blockers.[17, 18] Other high-riskpatients are infants with functional 2:1 AV block, those with Jervell Lange-Nielsen and Timothy syndrome (TS, LQT8). TS is a rare and unique type of LQTS that affects multiple organ systems and has a high incidence of sudden death due to profound QT prolongation and resultant ventricular arrhythmias. TS patients reported in the literature are highly-affected individuals who present early in life with severe cardiac manifestations. As the disease is becoming more widely recognized, we will likely identify less severely affected patients in whom the clinical course is less profound. At present, mortality in TS is thought to be very high and the response to beta-blocker therapy incomplete. ICD implantationis indicated if feasible with additional consideration for an LCSD in patients with a high burden of ventricular arrhythmias or severe repolarization abnormalities.[38]

Because of the disease diversity, decisions about ICD implantation in LQTS patients must be made with a patient-centered approach. As genetic data are increasingly available in LQTS patients, the location of the mutations and the degree of ion channel dysfunction caused by the mutations are emerging as risk factors influencing the clinical course of this disorder and may factor into decisions about ICD implantation.[39]

ICD implantation in catecholaminergic polymorphic ventricular tachycardia (CPVT)

CPVT is a genetic disease resulting in arrhythmias and sudden death in the setting of a structurally normal heart. The resting ECG is normal in these patients who experience stress-induced supraventricular or ventricular arrhythmias. The classic ventricular arrhythmia is bidirectional or polymorphic VT.[19, 20, 40, 41] In 2001, Priori et al. identified that the autosomal dominant and most common form of CPVT was caused by mutations in the cardiac ryanodine receptor 2 gene (RyR2) which encodes the calcium-releasing channel of the sarcoplasmic reticulum.[42] Later, the calsequestrin 2 gene (CASQ2) was linked to the rare autosomal recessive form of CPVT.[43, 44] CPVT pathogenesis is linked to both calcium homeostasis and catecholamines.[21]

In a series of over 100 CPVT patients, the 8-year cardiac fatal and near-fatal event rates were 32 and 13%, respectively, with most events occurring between the ages of 13–26 years.[46] The mainstays of therapy are beta-blockers, recommended in all patients. However, these medications may offer only incomplete protection from sudden death thus the search for additional therapeutic strategies is on-going.[21] Furthermore, patients must understand that missing a single dose of the medication has been associated with the development of arrhythmias.[46]

Although the ICD was once thought the only consideration for additional therapy, recent data suggest other potential choices. After recognition that flecainide can prevent arrhythmias in a mouse CPVT model,[22] flecainide was shown to reduce exercise-induced ventricular arrhythmias in CPVT patients and may offer adjunct therapy in patients with an ICD and continued ventricular arrhythmias despite beta-blocker therapy.[48] There is evidence of an emerging role of calmodulin kinase II pathway as a transducer of adrenergic nervous system signal to the intracellular calcium handling system.[45] Inhibition of this effect may provide adjunct therapy in patients with arrhythmias despite beta-blockers. Using a mouse model of CPVT, researchers found cardiac calcium-calmodulin-dependent protein kinase inhibition was effective in suppressing arrhythmias induced by epinephrine and caffeine. Further research is needed to bring this approach into clinical practice.

ICD management in CPVT is problematic as the burden of arrhythmia is high and even a modest increase in adrenaline output can result in VT and trigger an ICD discharge. Furthermore, ICDs are not 100% effective.[49] Frequently, episodes of polymorphic VT or bidirectional VT are not successfully terminated by the ICD and may result in an ICD storm that may trigger more arrhythmias due to associated catecholamine surges. A recent study showed that only one-third of appropriate shocks were effective in terminating sustained ventricular arrhythmias and shocks delivered to initiating triggered arrhythmias nearly always failed.[50, 51] Programming considerations should include the detection and redetection durations to be maximized in view of the tendency for self-terminating arrhythmias, and the detection rates aimed at VF rather than the bidirectional or polymorphic VT.

A LCSD may represent an antifibrillatory intervention in those not fully protected by beta-blockers or in those with frequent ICD shocks.[52] Pediatric electrophysiologists who manage these patients remain concerned for fatalities even in those with ICDs. Inappropriate shocks or appropriate shocks that occur without loss of consciousness cause fear and pain, and result in increased catecholamines and a resultant increase in arrhythmias, more ICD shocks, and potential for an arrhythmic storm.[52] Risk stratification for CPVT is still not possible based on the small number of patients identified.[13] Beta-blockers are effective with ICDs recommended for patients who have an episode of VF, those with syncope secondary to ventricular arrhythmias and without another cause, poorly tolerated VT and sustained VT despite beta-blockers. In such patients an ICD is commonly used and a reasonable choice.[13]

ICD implantation in Brugada syndrome (BrS)

BrS is a rare channelopathy with an even more rare phenotypic expression in children. Inherited in an autosomal dominant pattern, genetic testing is positive in only 25–30% of patients with phenotypic disease. Most gene positive patients have a mutation in the sodium channel, SCN5A. Other rarerBrS associated mutations have been identified. All genetic defects identified to date lead to either a loss-of-function of the sodium channel or L-type calcium channel or a gain-in-function in the potassium channel, I_{to}. In BrS patients, arrhythmias usually occur at rest, often at night. Presymptomatic diagnosis is difficult

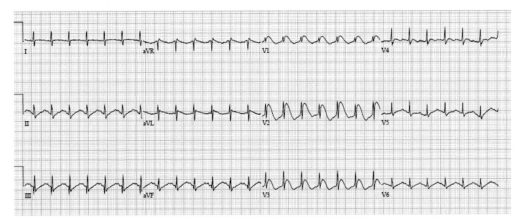

Figure 4.1 *Twelve lead ECG showing ST elevation (coved) in leads V1–V3 in a child with Brugada Syndrome during high grade fever.*

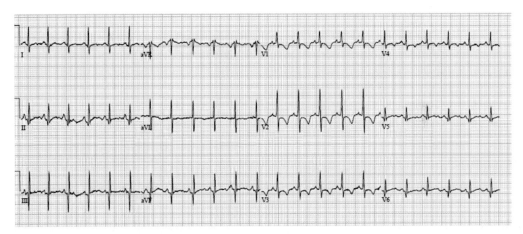

Figure 4.2 *Twelve lead ECG showing disappearance of ST segment elevation followed by appearance of T wave inversion in leads V1-V3 in the same child depicted in Figure 4.1 after resolution of fever.*

and there is potential overlap with the other sodium channelopathies.

The ECG changes typical of BrS may be spontaneous and persistent or may vary over days or even hours. Some patients require medications or fever to provoke the typical ECG changes (Figure 4.1) and the ECG changes resolve once the patient is afebrile (Figure 4.2). The type 1 BrS ECG pattern characteristically includes coved ST segment elevation followed by T wave inversion in the right precordial leads. This is a newly recognized condition and thus the electrophysiologic profile has yet to be fully established.

Therapeutic options are limited and although some data suggest quinidine may have efficacy,[53] there are insufficient data to recommend this as first-line treatment. Epicardial catheter ablation over the anterior right ventricular outflow tract has been shown to normalize the ECG pattern and prevent VF and may someday be an alternative or adjunct therapy.[54] Presently, ICDs are the only reliable treatment to prevent sudden death. High risk patients require an ICD. Defining high risk, while imperative, is a challenge. There is general agreement that patients with aborted sudden death or syncope are at high risk and should receive an ICD.[55] However, most sudden death victims have no recorded premorbid symptoms. Asymptomatic patients with spontaneous type 1 ECG patterns appear to be at higher risk.[23, 24, 55, 56] Although electrophysiological testing to induce sustained polymorphic VT/VF has been used to aid risk stratification,[57] meta-analyses have failed to find an association between inducibility and risk.[58] In asymptomatic patients, electrophysiology testing may have a useful negative predictive value.[59] There is on-going debate about the utility of programmed electrical stimulation in the identification of high-risk asymptomatic patients.[60, 61] In the most recent consensus report, an electrophysiology study was recommended for patients with a spontaneous type 1 ECG or a provoked type 1 ECG and a family history of sudden death.[55] This approach has come under question as it involves a large number of electrophysiology studies with their associated risk and expense and it may ultimately expose asymptomatic individuals to unnecessary ICD-related complications.[62] Those in favor argue that asymptomatic patients with a coved type ECG, either spontaneous or after provocation by a class I anti-arrhythmic agent, and a positive electrophysiology study should undergo ICD placement.[60] Others emphasize the large number of variables that impact the outcome of the electrophysiology study. They note that while some variables, such as cycle length, location, and amplitude of the impulse used, can be controlled, others, such as the level of anesthesia, concomitant medications, and time of day, cannot and may be quite relevant in the BrS patient.[61] This is a population where the amount of ST elevation in the right precordial leads can vary spontaneously over a matter of hours and the degree of elevation is associated with the arrhythmogenic substrate thus timing of the study should correspond with the maximal amount of ST change, an unpredictable and untenable goal.

The role of fever in BrS patients has been recognized as a precipitating factor for ventricular arrhythmias in adults[23] and children.[53] It has been shown that mutations responsible for BrS alter the temperature sensitivity of the fast activation of the sodium channel[63] but the exact mechanism by which fever triggers the arrhythmias remains in question. Parents of children with known or suspected BrS should be vigilant about fever control and some advocate ECG monitoring in the setting of fever.[53] In children where the diagnosis remains in question, we recommend an ECG be performed during fever to optimize the chances of capturing an ECG with the typical BrS pattern.

Risk stratification in BrS is a challenge. Ethnicity and gender factor into risk assessment with males of South East Asian origin at higher risk.[55] Late potentials on signal-averaged ECG are more common in symptomatic patients but not an independent risk factor. QRS fragmentation appears to predict patients at risk of syncope due to VF.[64] The presence of an SCN5A mutation was also strongly associated with a fragmented QRS. Using an isolated canine right ventricular tissue model of BrS, researchers have demonstrated that activation delay in the epicardium could reproduce similar fragmented QRS in the transmural ECG and was a possible mechanism for the clinical observations. The role of genetic testing in risk stratification is unknown as few patients have a mutation identified. A recent study has suggested earlier and more frequent VF in symptomatic BrS patients with SCN5A mutations compared with those without.[65] The severity of the biophysical consequence resulting from an SCN5A mutation appears to influence phenotype and possibly risk, with increased syncope and longer PR and QRS durations in patients with mutations leading to protein truncation compared with missense mutations.[66] As additional mutations are identified and functionally characterized, genetic data will impact the characterization of risk. Like many newly recognized conditions, we are presently identifying only patients with the most profound forms of the disease. As our phenotypic characterization, genetic diagnosis and screening improve we will better understand this BrS and its true risk.

ICD indications in arrhythmogenic right ventricular dysplasia/cardiomyopathy (ARVD/C)

ARVD/C is a unique inherited condition that links structural and electrophysiological cardiac disease. As a disease of the myocyte junction, ARVD/C results from mutations in proteins of the gap junction that are important in cell-to-cell electrical and physical coupling. ARVC/D affects the structural and electrical integrity of the myocardium usually, but not always, limited to the right ventricle. Cardiac cells lose cell-to-cell adhesion, become separated, die, and are replaced by fat or fibrotic material. This results in electrical disturbance characterized by ventricular ectopy and tachycardia, and a risk of sudden death and right ventricular dysfunction.[67, 68] In ARVD/C events are often precipitated by stress. In affected patients, disease progression is often nonlinear with periods of quiescence followed by abrupt worsening possibly instigated by exercise or infection.

One of the most important and most difficult decisions in these patients is whether to implant an ICD. ICD therapy is recommended as secondary prevention after cardiac arrest and in the setting of sustained VT or VF. There is a great deal more uncertainty about the approach for the patient in whom the ICD would be implanted for primary prevention. A recent evaluation of 84 young adults (age 32+/− 12 years) with ARVD/C reported a considerable number of appropriate ICD interventions in patients with devices implanted as primary prevention.[69] Inducibility at electrophysiology study, nonsustained VT, proband status, and Holter evidence of > 1000 PVCs in 24 hours were significant predictors of appropriate ICD therapy and the presence of multiple risk factors incrementally increased the likelihood of appropriate ICD therapy. Nearly one-half of the study patients had appropriate ICD therapy in the 5 years of follow-up. However, if one or no risk factors were identified, patients did not experience appropriate device intervention and were at low risk. In a European study of 106 ARVD/C patients with ICDs who did not have a history of VT or VF, 24% had an appropriate ICD therapy, 16% with an appropriate ICD shock in a 58-month study period.[70] In this study, syncope was the sole predictor of appropriate ICD therapy. These and previous studies suggest that ICD therapy in ARVD/C has a role in primary prevention in patients with defined risk factors.[25, 26, 71, 72]

ICD code

In 1981, the North American Society of Pacing and Electrophysiology and the British Pacing Group using nomenclature from the 1974 International Commission for Heart Disease, extended the code to account for new technology.

I	II	II	IV
Shock Chamber	Antitachy cardia-pacing chamber	Tachycardia Detection	Antibrady cardia-pacing chamber
O = None A = Atrium V = Ventricle D = Dual (A+V)	O = None A = Atrium V = Ventricle D = Dual (A+V)	E= Electrogram H= Hemodynamic	O = None A = Atrium V = Ventricle D = Dual (A+V)

The Short Form of the NASPE/BPEG Defibrillator (NBD) Code: ICD-S = ICD with shock capability only, ICD-B = ICD with **b**radycardia pacing as well as shock, **ICD-T** = ICD with **t**achycardia (and bradycardia) pacing as well as shock.[27]

ICD generator selection

Three fundamental questions arise once the decision has been made that a patient requires an ICD. (1) Should the patient receive a single or dual chamber ICD system? (2) Should the system be implanted via a transvenous or epicardial route? (3) What are the most appropriate ICD generator and specific lead(s) for a particular patient? The specifics of a particular device and lead selection are often based on experiential physician preference. Prior to deciding on a single or dual chamber system a number of considerations should be thoroughly reviewed. Highly important is whether there is a clinical need for atrial pacing, akin to other conditions whereby atrial or AV sequential anti-bradycardia pacing is warranted. It is critical that an exhaustive search for atrial arrhythmias be undertaken to optimally program atrial non-tracking modes and consider utilization of dual-chamber detection enhancements to minimize the morbidity associated with inappropriate ICD shocks. Unfortunately, the basis for upgrading to a dual chamber ICD is often not grounded in large multi-center prospective randomized trials but rather predicated on small retrospective studies, case–control studies, and extrapolation from adult studies that generally exclude adults with CHD. Prior to the decision to implant an ICD it is paramount that the implanting physician understands the cardiac pathophysiology, potential venous constraints, residual intracardiac shunts, and potential deleterious effects of right ventricular (RV) apical pacing.

Dual-chamber or single-chamber device

Physicians tasked with selecting an ICD generator must first address the question of whether an atrial lead is required. The addition of an atrial lead in children provides theoretical advantages, though clinical superiority has not been conclusively shown in a prospective trial. The use of a dual chamber ICD is widely accepted in patients with a clinical need for antibradycardia pacing. As a consideration for patients with supraventricular tachycardia (SVT) who may benefit from dual chamber detection enhancements, the argument however is slightly more contentious. The addition of an atrial lead increases the complexity of the procedure, may cause venous obstruction, complicates future lead extractions, and supports the concept that "the more hardware that is implanted the more things can go wrong." Data from 60,000 ICD implantations in the National Cardiovascular Data Registry ICD Registry demonstrated a higher peri-procedural complication rate for dual-chamber devices. Complications included lead dislodgement, pneumothorax, infection, and mortality.[74] However, it is equally important that if an atrial lead is required that the lead be placed at the initial operation to avoid potential reoperations and associated risks. Substrates for which dual-chamber defibrillators may be considered are highlighted below.

Bradycardia pacing

Patients with standard clinical indications for bradycardia pacing should undergo implantation of an atrial lead. Sinus node dysfunction (SND), either predominant junctional rhythm with loss of AV synchrony, or chronotropic incompetence are relatively common following the Fontan operation,[28, 29, 75, 76] atrial baffling procedures,[30, 77] and/or TOF.[78] Furthermore, the incidence of SND increases over time with certain anatomical substrates. In such cases where an ICD lead is needed and a high-suspicion exists that SND may develop, an atrial lead may be warranted.[79–81] In the setting of complete AV block following cardiac surgery or in rare cases of spontaneous AV block

associated with AV discordance,[82] patients will in all likelihood already have a DDD pacemaker in-situ. Continuation of AV synchrony should be maintained if the device needs to be upgraded to a defibrillator.

Maintenance of AV synchrony with AAIR pacing in adults with isolated SND has been shown to reduce the incidence of atrial fibrillation,[83, 84] and is superior to DDDR pacing in preserving left ventricular function.[31] However, in the absence of SND, dual chamber pacing for bradycardia secondary to AV block offers no clear advantage and may be more deleterious.[86] The concept that DDDR pacing in patients with ICDs was associated with poorer outcomes was first exhibited in the DAVID Trial (Dual Chamber and Implantable VVI Defibrillator Trial) that randomized adults undergoing ICD implantation without a need for anti-bradycardia pacing to either DDDR with a lower rate of 70 bpm or back-up VVI at 40 bpm.[87] Dual-chamber pacing was associated with poorer quality of life, increased heart-failure hospitalizations, all-cause mortality and no reduction in the incidence of inappropriate ICD shocks. The poorer outcomes in the dual-chamber group were attributed to an increased frequency of RV apical pacing and dyssynchrony, rather than to the device itself. A follow-up study, DAVID II, randomized patients with impaired ventricular function to AAI 70 bpm versus VVI 40 bpm with no significant difference in event-free survival or quality of life.[88] The results of these two studies challenged conventional wisdom regarding the benefits of dual-chamber ICDs and if extrapolated to children, support the concept that unless there is a clinical indication for atrial pacing, no clear advantage exists over a ventricular mode that minimizes ventricular pacing. This trial pre-dated current Medtronic dual chamber defibrillators that have an AAI(R) to DDD(R) mode, otherwise called Managed Ventricular Pacing mode.

Minimizing ventricular pacing in children and young adults, who will likely require life-long therapy, is reasonable considering the deleterious effects of chronic RV pacing. Knowledge of the maximum allowable AV interval is important and device specific and must be taken within the context of the PVARP so as to optimize upper-rate behavior (Table 4.3). The implanter must be familiar with

Table 4.3 Features and related parameters in current defibrillators to minimize RV pacing (RV, right ventricular; AV, atrioventricular; PAV, paced AV delay; SAV, sensed AV delay)

Pacing Features	Medtronic Evera™ XT DR	Medtronic Protecta™ DR D334DRG	St. Jude Current DR™ +DR CD2211	Boston Scientific Energen™	Boston Scientific Punctua™
Mode-based RV Pacing Reduction	Managed Ventricular Pacing	Managed Ventricular Pacing	None	RHYTHMIQ	None
AV-based RV Pacing Reduction	None	None	VIP	AV Search+	AV Search+
Max PAV (msec)	350	350	450	400	400
Max SAV (msec)	350	350	425	400	400
Maximum Tracking Rate (bpm)	175	175	150	185	185
Rate Response Sensor	Accelerometer	Accelerometer	Accelerometer	Accelerometer	Accelerometer
Maximum Sensor Rate (bpm)	175	175	150	185	185

the other features in current defibrillators that minimize RV pacing. Single-chamber hysteresis allows the sensed intrinsic rate to decrease to a value below the programmed lower rate before pacing resumes. Hysteresis provides the ability to maintain the patient's own heart rhythm as long as possible, while pacing at a faster rate if the intrinsic rhythm falls below the hysteresis rate.

In dual-chamber ICDs, AV Search Hysteresis (AVSH) reduces the percentage of ventricular pacing and mitigates the negative effects of chronic RV apical pacing. The Intrinsic RV Study (Inhibition of Unnecessary RV Pacing with AV Search Hysteresis in ICDs) randomized patients with NYHA III/IV and dual chamber ICDs to a DDDR AVSH 60–130 or VVI back-up pacing at 40 bpm (Vitality AVT; Guidant; Indianapolis, Indiana) and found non-inferiority for the endpoint of all cause-mortality and heart failure hospitalization between the two modes. [89] Managed ventricular pacing (MVP® *beginning with Medtronic Intrinsic models*; Medtronic Minneapolis, Minnesota) is an atrial-based pacing mode that prioritizes AV conduction with AAI(R) pacing while providing the safety of dual-chamber pacing if there is transient loss of AV conduction.[90]

Atrial pacing for chronotropic incompetence in the individual with a concomitant ICD necessitates an understanding of important differences between a pacemaker and an ICD. Unlike dual chamber pacemakers where upper sensing/tracking rates can achieve heart rates of 210 bpm, the same situation does not apply with defibrillators. Additionally, upper rate limits are also dependent on the ascribed VT detection zone. Some device companies do not allow bradycardia pacing to cross into a VT detection zone. This may be a consideration when placing an ICD in a patient with slow VT where bradycardia pacing is required. Early single-chamber ICDs (Guidant 1783, 1788, 1790; Medtronic 7223; St. Jude Medical V186, V180) allowed maximum pacing rates of only 90–120 bpm. More recent maximum pacing rates for single and dual-chamber ICDs approach 150 bpm. Currently rate-response sensors for bradycardia pacing in all the major device companies are based on accelerometers although differences exist on upper rate limit behaviors.

Resynchronization therapy

Patients with ventricular dysfunction secondary to ischemic or non-ischemic causes who have concomitant inter/intraventricular dyssynchrony may benefit from cardiac resynchronization therapy (CRT) (see Chapter 5) but also defibrillator therapy as part of primary prevention. Furthermore, there is an increasing subset of adults with repaired/palliated CHD who are at risk for sudden cardiac death[3] and also have dyssynchrony from post-surgical bundle-branch block[91] who may benefit from combined CRT and ICD therapies. Many of the general practicalities regarding dual-chamber ICDs, such as ICD lead selection can be expanded to the CRT-D cohort.

Unique conditions

Specific conditions exist whereby a dual-chamber ICD is preferable to a single chamber system. Patients with ICDs in the setting of HCM may develop atrial arrhythmias necessitating anti-arrhythmic therapy, antitachycardia pacing, or atrial preference pacing to minimize the atrial arrhythmia burden. Currently, only Medtronic dual-chamber ICDs offer ambulatory atrial burst and/or ramp termination therapies; however, both St. Jude (AF Suppression) and Medtronic (Atrial Preference Pacing, Atrial Rate Stabilization, and Post-Mode Switch Overdrive Pacing) utilize some form of atrial intervention pacing to prevent arrhythmia initiation.

Upwards of 30–50% of patients with HCM may develop left ventricular outflow tract obstruction.[92] Dual chamber pacing may be considered as adjuvant therapy in those patients who do not respond to medical therapy or are not ideal candidates for a septal myomectomy. Although variable in its response (ranges 10–90% echocardiographic or clinical response), some patients paced DDD or VDD with a short AV interval will have a pre-excited ventricular pattern that increases end-systolic volume and reduces LV outflow tract obstruction.[93–95] It is critical when programming the DDD-ICD, that the AV delay is set to pre-excite the apical RV without spontaneous His-Purkinje conduction while avoiding so short an AV interval that left atrial pressures critically rise.[96]

Patients with LQTS and symptomatic bradycardia secondary to beta-blockers may benefit from

AAI pacing and if an ICD is required both an atrial and ventricular lead should be implanted. While increased adrenergic tone may initiate ventricular arrhythmias in patients with LQTS, a significant number of arrhythmic events may be related to a short-long-short form of pause dependency.[97] Pause-preceded torsade de pointes tends to be genotype specific, more common with LQT2 than LQT1,[98] and in that contingent atrial pacing with rate-smoothing algorithms should be considered.[99] Patients with LQT3 who have associated bradycardia-related cardiac events should have an atrial lead at the time of ICD implantation. Despite continuous atrial pacing and beta-blocker therapy, 24% of high-risk LQTS patients may have sudden aborted sudden death and a dual-chambered ICD is likely more efficacious than medical or pacing therapy.[100] Our experience in patients with LQTS and a higher than expected ventricular arrhythmia burden may benefit from dual-chambered ICD with AAI pacing at rates 70–80 bpm so as to "push" beta-blocker therapy as high as tolerated to mitigate against VT/VF episodes.

Atrial arrhythmias

Prior to ICD implantation a detailed review of the patient's past medical history should search for atrial arrhythmias. Similarly, the implanting physician should have a reasonable knowledge as to which structural heart defects (i.e., Fontan; TOF), channelopathic conditions (SQTS), or myopathies have a high likelihood of developing atrial arrhythmias. The goal of the ICD manufacturer should be a device with 100% sensitivity in VF recognition with detection enhancements to achieve specificity approaching 100% with a low incidence of inappropriate ICD therapies. While discussed in greater detail in the section on "Lead Selection," a basic understanding of inappropriate therapies is needed so as to select the most optimal device. Supraventricular tachycardias account for 15–21% of inappropriate ICD shocks in children.[101–103] Sinus tachycardia attributable to either non-compliance with anti-arrhythmic therapy or a VF detection zone inadvertently programmed below the maximal achievable sinus rate is responsible for 10–42% of inappropriate ICD shocks.[101, 102]

Inappropriate ICD discharges have major adverse psychological effects on patients including depression and anxiety.[32, 33, 104, 105] Therefore, it is critical that the device algorithms successfully discriminate between true, shockable rhythms and false positives. The algorithms depend on whether there is just a single ventricular lead or if there is both an atrial and ventricular lead. While rate-based detection is accurate for VF, sinus tachycardia or SVT extending into a VT zone may result in false positive detection and inappropriate shocks. Single chamber discriminators allow determination of the tachycardia mechanism based on onset and/or regularity. Sudden-onset discriminates VT from sinus tachycardia by withholding therapy from tachycardias that "warm-up." While effective for rejecting sinus tachycardia, it fails for sudden-onset VT originating below the VT zone and VT that starts during SVT.[34] Stability discriminates VT from atrial fibrillation, which tends to have an irregular RR pattern. Manufacturers have different algorithms for both onset and stability. The third single chamber discriminator, morphology, distinguishes SVT from VT based on a pre-determined ventricular electrograms (VEGM) template. Morphology is predicated on a successful sinus template match and the VT being noticeably different from the baseline template. Aberrant SVT or template misalignments may render morphologic enhancement inferior (see Chapter 1 for details).

Dual-chamber defibrillators utilize information regarding atrial activity relative to ventricular activity to ascertain the mechanism of the tachycardia. While the device companies have slightly different algorithms they all tend to utilize the ratio of number of ventricular eletrograms relative to the number of atrial electrograms. In patients with either SVT or VT and a 1:1 relationship, the chamber of origin (short PP or short RR) may serve as a means to discriminate between the two.[35, 36] Unfortunately data regarding the benefits of dual-chamber devices compared to single chamber devices are conflicting.[33, 37–39, 105, 109–111] In the Detect Trial (Dual-Chamber Versus Single-Chamber Detection Enhancements of Implantable Rhythm Diagnosis Study- powered for inappropriate detection, not therapy) dual chamber ICDs had a significantly lower incidence of inappropriate detection than single chamber devices, except in the case of sinus tachycardia where no benefit was proven.[109] In a retrospective multi-center trial of 168 pediatric and young adults, there was no significant difference in the incidence of inappropriate ICD therapies between patients with single chamber and dual chamber devices (Single ICD: 7/252; Dual ICD 28/116).[112] In fact, in patients with myopathies the incidence of inappropriate ICD shocks was greater in those with dual-chamber devices than single chamber devices. Newer ICD models such as Medtronic Protecta™ family of ICDs and beyond have married features previously unique to either single or dual chamber defibrillators. Pattern based algorithms (atrial andventricular relationships) in conjunction with morphology recognition are now available and may reduce inappropriate SVT detection and therapies though this has not been formally shown in children. Unless, there are compelling data for bradycardia pacing or atrial anti-tachycardia pacing, strong consideration should be given to single-chamber devices as the benefit with dual-chamber devices solely for detection enhancements to reduce inappropriate ICD therapies is limited in children.

Size and longevity

ICD generator size is often a major concern for the pediatric patient. Even when placed in a sub-pectoral location, cosmetic concerns are a reality for the patient and need to be addressed before surgery. As a general rule, larger devices have greater battery capacity and longevity, often placing the pediatric implanter in a quandary as a smaller device is often preferred but at the expense of longevity. Dual-chamber devices are larger, especially the header, compared to single-chamber devices, often subjugating the electrophysiologist to critically assess the need for a dual-chamber ICD prior to implant. Technological advances in the last decade have reduced the size of the device from 300cc to < 32cc. Projected longevity for different manufacturer's devices are often calculated using pacing at lower rates than may be required for a given pediatric patient and should be taken into consideration when speaking with a patient/family prior to surgery (Table 4.4). In addition, high impedance leads with small diameter electrodes

have less ventricular current drain and have been shown to extend battery life.[40, 41, 113, 114] Although much of the life expectancy of a device is related to "static current and house-keeping functions," projected battery longevity may be disparate from actual longevity and patients and their families should be aware of that prior to surgery and during follow-up.[42, 43, 115, 116] Poor thresholds and an increased percentage paced will further diminish battery longevity.

Maximum shock output

Successful defibrillation is a function of multiple factors including lead design (single vs dual-coil), generator position relative to the fibrillating myocardium, shock waveform, shock polarity, timing of the shock, and minimization of anti-arrhythmic drugs known to reduce DFTs. High DFTs may prompt consideration for an alternative defibrillation vector such as subcutaneous (SQ) coil or sub-axillary array.[44, 45, 117, 118] The DFT can be influenced by the shock polarity and reconfiguration from cathodal to anodal DFT testing should be considered. Device companies' ship polarities differently. Medtronic and St. Jude Medical ships anodal and Boston Scientific and Biotronic devices are set for cathodal testing and should be reversed before usage. From a clinical perspective, high-output devices (>35 J) should be considered in patients with marked LV thickness such as HCM and right subclavian implants where the vector of defibrillation is away from the left ventricle. The Medtronic Evera™ and Boston Scientific Energen™ and Punctua™ family of devices deliver 35 J. The St. Jude Fortify® family of ICDs delivers 36 J on the firstshock and 40 J on subsequent shocks. The St. Jude Ellipse™ ICD allows for 35 J delivered energy with a volume of 31 cc. Most devices allow a maximum of six shocks. The Medtronic Protecta®(and future devices) ICD allows ATP during charging and also allows ATP discrimination in the VF zone. In addition, current devices from Medtronic, St. Jude, and Boston Scientific allow a programmable SVC vector and a programmable active can.

Lead selection

Over the last two decades, the ICD lead has undergone significant design changes with improvements

Table 4.4 Defibrillator size and projected battery longevity (LRL, lower rate limit)

Single & Dual Chamber Device Attributes	Medtronic Evera™ XT DR DDBB1D4	Medtronic Evera™ XT VR DVBB1D4	Medtronic Protecta™ DR D334DRG	St. Jude Current VR™ +VR CD1211	Sr. Jude Current DR™ +DR CD2211	St. Jude Ellipse VR™ VR CD1311	St. Jude Ellipse DR™ DR CD2311	Boston Scientific (V) Energen™	Boston Scientific (D) Energen™
Volume (cc)	34	33	37 (41 DF-4)	41	41	30	31	31.5	31.5
Mass (gm)	78	77	68 (73 DF-4)	79	80	67	68	72	72
Dimensions (h x w x t; mm)	68 x 51 x 13	64 x 51 x 13	64 x 51 x 15 (DF-1) 66 x 51 x 15 (DF-4)	74 x 50 x 14	74 x 50 x 14	66 x 51 x 12	70 x 51 x12	7.45 x 6.2 x 0.99 (DF-1) 6.9 x 6.2 x 0.99 (DF-4)	7.45 x 6.2 x 0.99 (DF-1) 7.40 x 6.2 x 0.99 (DF-4)
Connector	DF4	DF4	IS-1/DF-1 or IS-1/DF-4	DF4	DF4	DF4	DF4	IS-1/DF-1 or IS-1/DF-4	IS-1/DF-1 or IS-1/DF-4
Projected Longevity (years)									
0% pacing, no shocks	9.7	11	8	8.4	8.2	11.1	10.4	11.8	111.2
50% pacing, no shocks	8.3	10.1	7	7.6	7	10.1	8.9	11.1	10
100% pacing, no shocks	7.3	9.3	6.2	7	6.1	9.4	7.7	10.6	9.1
0% pacing, 2 shocks/yr			7.1	7.1	6.6	9.9	9.3	11.3	10.7
50% pacing, 2 shocks/yr			6.3	6.6	6	9.1	8.1	107	9.7
100% pacing, 2 shocks/yr			5.7	6.2	5.5	8.5	7.1	10.1	8.8

(Medtronic) Longevity estimates assume LRL o 60 bpm with a lead impedance of 500 ohms, 2.5V/0.4 msec

(St. Jude) Longevity estimates assume LRL at 60 bpm with lead impedances at 500 ohms

(BSI) Longevity estimates assume LRL of 60 bpm, pacing impedances of 500 ohm for both leads, 2.0V @ 0.5ms for both leads, pacing % the same for both A and V outputs, pacing % the same for both A and V leads, and remote monitoring.

in sensing qualities and defibrillation. However, despite the increasing sophistication, ICD leads have a finite life and the greater complexity compared to a pacemaker lead increases the propensity for early lead failures. Premature adverse failure of the pacing/sensing electrode, shocking coils, or both have come under tremendous public scrutiny.

More than three decades ago, epicardial patches and epicardial sensing leads ushered in a new era in the treatment of patients with potentially life-threatening arrhythmias. Epicardial ICD systems necessitated implantation via either a thoracotomy or a sternotomy and were marred by a significant surgical mortality and high rate of lead-malfunction. The ingenuity of this early technology, however, laid the foundation for successful defibrillation with endocardial leads. While novel non-endocardial leads may continue to be required or preferred in a subset of children and young adults, endocardial leads account for the majority of pediatric implants. The ICD lead in the pediatric population is subjected to significantly more stress than in adults both from activity level and somatic growth, both of which may increase tension on the lead. Dual coil ICD leads may be particularly problematic in children and may increase the complexity of future lead extractions.[119]

Many techniques employed in endocardial pacemaker lead implantations are applicable to an ICD lead implant. However, the ICD lead is unique and should have a combination of excellent sensing, capable of bradycardia and anti-tachycardia pacing, and serve as a component in the shocking vector. Endocardial ICD leads are not "all the same" and different ICD lead designs may be of particular benefit for the patient (Table 4.5). Implanting physicians also typically have personal preferences. The following sections subdivide endocardial leads based on specific features.

Lead survival

ICD lead and conductor failure in children and young adults with CHD has ranged from 5–20% over a 5-year period after implantation, noticeably higher than adult ICD lead failure.[2, 46–48, 120, 121] This likely reflects a combination of potential rapid somatic growth and increased activity in a younger population. Conclusive data regarding specific

ICD lead failure in adult studies have shown the average failure rate for Medtronic Sprint Quattro Secure® (0.55%/year) and Guidant Endotak® (0.42%/year) are all relatively comparable and noticeably less than the hazard lead failure rate for the Medtronic Sprint Fidelis® ICD lead failure rate (3.75%/year).[122] and the St. Jude Riata® ICD Lead (0.7–2.8%/year).[123, 124] Similarly, ICD lead perforation results appear to be relatively comparable across manufacturer lines (0.0–0.51%/year).[125, 126] While no lead has gone unscathed, the failure rate of the Medtronic Sprint Fidelis® ICD lead accelerated in the first few years after implant and has been shown to be more problematic in a younger pediatric cohort.[48–50, 121, 122, 127] A recent multi-institutional pediatric study showed a 9.2% yearly failure rate for the Medtronic Sprint Fidelis lead highlighting the biophysical differences between pediatric and adult patients.[128] Designs such as the Medtronic Sprint Fidelis lead appear to confer as significant risk for lead failure, potentially even more important that the intrinsic diameter.[129] Management issues regarding failed leads are discussed in later chapters, but undoubtedly careful scrutiny of any ICD lead should be paramount with early failure detection algorithms and quality measures crucial for prompt recognition of lead failure to avoid adverse events, most commonly inappropriate ICD therapies. Unfortunately, because most failed leads are not extracted or significant damage occurs at extraction, it is often difficult to give an accurate account of the cause of lead failure. Other factors that impact ICD lead survival include the different fixation mechanisms, lead insulation types, lead diameter, adequacy of slack, and the anchoring sleeves tie-downs.

True bipolar versus integrated bipolar lead

Currently most pediatric electrophysiologists utilize a true bipolar lead with active fixation and a tip-ring inter-electrode spacing 12–15 mm. The ring electrode may or may not be in contact with the endocardium and the coil to an "active" can is the most common vector for defibrillation. Additional leads containing defibrillation elements may be considered. Integrated bipolar leads use a distal tip electrode for pacing and sensing, a distal coil for pacing/sensing and defibrillation in conjunction with a proximal coil for defibrillation.

Table 4.5 *Characteristics of ICD leads (Fr, French)*

	Medtronic Sprint Quattro Secure® 6947	Medtronic Sprint Quattro Secure® 6935	St. Jude Durata® 7120-22Q	St. Jude Durata® 7120-22,7130-31	St. Jude Optisure TM LDA 220Q-210-230Q	Boston Scientific Endotak Reliance® G0184-0187	Boston Scientific Endotak Reliance® SG 0180-0183
General							
Insulation	Silicone w/poly overlay	Silicone w/poly overlay	Optim	Optim	Silicone with Optim overlay	Silicone	Silicone
Connector	IS-1/DF-1	IS-1/DF-1	DF-4	IS-1/DF-1	DF-4	IS-1/DF-1	IS-1/DF-1
Electrode Configuration	Dual Coil	Single Coil	Dual Coil (7120/21Q); Single Coil (7122Q)	Dual Coil (7120/21); Single Coil (7122)	Dual Coil (LDA 220Q/230Q); Single Coil (210Q)	Dual Coil	Single Coil
Polarity	True Bipolar	True Bipolar	True Bipolar	True Bipolar (712x); Integrated Bipolar (713x)	True Bipolar	Integrated Bipolar	Integrated Bipolar
Lead Body	8.2Fr	8.2Fr	6.8Fr	6.8Fr	7.6Fr	8.2Fr	8.2Fr
Introducer (Fr)	9Fr	9Fr	7Fr	7Fr	8Fr	9Fr	9Fr
Pacing Details							
Tip-Ring spacing (mm)	8	8	11	11	11		
Tip-Cathode Surface Area (sq.mm)	5.7	5.7	6	6	6	2	5.7
Ring-Anode Surface Area (sq.mm)	25.2	25.2	17	17	17		
High Voltage							
Coil-treatment	Silicone backfill	Silicone backfill	Silicone backfill	Silicone backfill	Silicone backfill	ePTFE	ePTFE
Tip-RV Coil Spacing (mm)	12	12	17	17	17	12	12
Tip-SVC Spacing (cm)	18		17 (71x0); 21 (71x1)	17 (71x0); 21 (71x1)	17 (LDA 220)	18	
Electrode Surface Area RV (sq.mm)	614	614	367	367	367	450	450
Electrode Surface Area RV (sq.mm)	860		588	588	638	660	

True bipolar leads have the most optimal sensing and the shorter tip-to-defibrillation coil distance in integrated bipolar leads may support better defibrillation success. However, the main disadvantage of integrated leads relates to the susceptibility to oversense diaphragmatic myopotential and atrial EGM oversensing which can be particularly problematic in children with smaller hearts.

Dual versus single coil ICD lead

Dual coil ICD leads have a distal coil in the body of the RV and a proximal coil near the SVC-right atrial (RA) junction, but depending on the size of the patient can also be closer to the innominate vein (Figure 4.3A). In typical single coil configurations, the ICD is active as the anodal component with the RV coil as the cathode (Figure 4.3B). While the vast majority of current ICD configurations are set with an active can, the shock vector can be noninvasively programmed in a reverse fashion; a feature which may be useful if the first few shocks fail. Older ICD devices may have an SVC coil that can only be removed from the shock vector by opening the pocket and plugging the SVC port. In a dual coil system, both the can and the proximal coil can serve as a combined anodal configuration or the proximal coil may itself be a single anode with the "can-off" feature applied. The principal advantage of a dual coil system is the theoreticalreduction in the DFT. The disadvantages of dual coil systems are the potential for fracture

within the un-insulated proximal coil and the greater difficulty in extracting the leads.

Children and young adults appear to have a higher incidence of ICD related complications compared to adults.[51] In addition, the proximal coil may become distorted secondary to tension from the RV tip transmitted longitudinally by forces from rapid somatic growth. Because the proximal coil is not insulated it is susceptible to fibrous in-growth, which may complicate future attempts at venous entry and may increase the complexity of lead extractions. Cooper et al. observed proximal coil distortion in 13% of pediatric leads at the time of lead extraction questioning the need to consider dual coils in growing children.[119]

Novel leads to consider for alternative configurations

The decision to implant a lead in an alternative site is less often related to the size of the device than the adequacy of the venous system. Given the need for probable life-long pacing/defibrillation, the implanting physician must adjudicate adequacy of the venous system to accommodate one to three leads and consider issues related to lead revision/extractions in the future. Alternative site defibrillation has been well reported in the pediatric literature. There are a number of non-transvenous configurations that may achieve acceptable defibrillation. A transvenous ICD lead may be placed on the epicardium, and an SVC coil or transvenous ICD lead may be placed

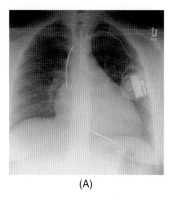
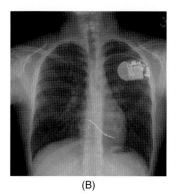

(A)   (B)

Figure 4.3 *(A) AP chest radiograph. Patient with HCM after myomectomy with a single chamber dual-coil ICD. The proximal coil is at the SVC-RA junction and is part of the defibrillation vector. (B) AP chest radiograph. Patient with LQTS and a single chamber ICD; there is a single coil lead with an adequate loop left in the RA to accommodate somatic growth.*

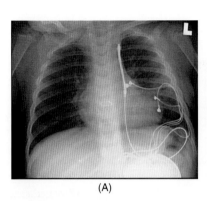
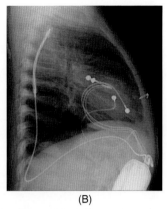

(A)   (B)

Figure 4.4 *Chest X-ray PA view (A) and lateral view (B) showing novel configuration with dual-chamber ICD with epicardial (Medtronic 4968® bipolar epicardial leads) and a subcutaneous array coil.*

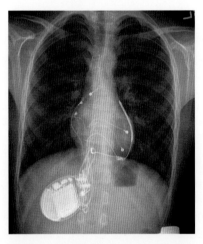

Figure 4.5 *Chest X-ray (PA view) showing ICD placement in a patient with a single left ventricle, ventricular tachycardia, complete heart block, s/p Fontan palliation. A Bipolar steroid-eluting lead is positioned on the left ventricular surface. A steroid-eluting bipolar lead is placed on the right atrial appendage. An old atrial lead has been cut with its distal end attached to the atrium. An SVC shocking coil was placed in the pericardial surface along the left ventricle. This was secured to the pericardium with interrupted sutures of 2–0 silk and the pacing leads and shocking coil were connected to the ICD generator which was implanted in a right sub-rectus abdominal pocket. (Source: Dr. Maully Shah, Division of Cardiology, The Children's Hospital of Philadelphia, U.S.A. Reproduced with courtesy of Dr. Maully Shah.)*

subcutaneously, in the pericardium or pleura (Figure 4.4A,B, Figure 4.5). Typically, a Medtronic 4968® epicardial bipolar pace/sense lead is used for the R wave sensing. An alternative bipolar epicardial lead includes the Great batch Medical

Myopore® Sutureless, Screw-In bipolar epicardial lead (Great batch Medical; Clarence NY, USA). Unipolar leads should generally be avoided given the potential for double-counting and inappropriate ICD shocks. Subcutaneous coil leads are single coil leads designed to be placed in the subcutaneous region, have no pacing or sensing capacity, and are inserted into the RV (HXB) port. The ICD coil portion of a standard ICD lead is smaller than the subcutaneous coil and theoretically is easier to insert, develops less scar tissue adhesions, and may have less coil outside of the desired shock vector. In these leads the pace/sense pin connector is "capped" and the high-voltage shocking component is used.

These non-traditional epicardial/pericardial ICD leads have a shorter life expectancy than typical endocardial ICD systems.[134] In a review of three pediatric and young adult studies with ICDs, involving 45 patients (mean age at ICD implant approximately 11.9 years) with a follow-up of 2.5 years, lead system revisions were required in ~25% of patients.[135–137] While appropriate ICD shocks were successful in 29% of subjects, inappropriate ICD shocks occurred in 20% within a very short follow-up. Newer advancements in lead design may allow this technology to be used as a bridge to an endocardial system in certain patients. There will continue to be a subset of patients with venous occlusion, significant right-to-left shunts, or cardiac baffles limiting vascular access to the heart that necessitate the pediatric ICD implanter to maintain a full repertoire of ICD configurations.

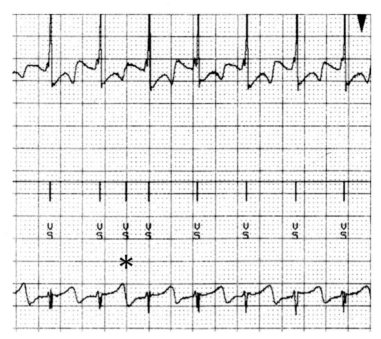

Figure 4.6 *Sinus tachycardia with intermittent "double-counting." Top channel: Far-field (Can/HVB); Middle channel: Marker; Bottom channel: Near-field (Vtip/Vring). * T wave larger than R wave resulting in T-wave oversensing. This patient had numerous inappropriate ICD shocks from T wave oversensing. The Medtronic ICD was exchanged for a St. Jude Medical ICD with extension of the decay delay and a higher threshold start resolved T wave oversensing.*

V sensing and refractory (unique to devices)

Each of the ICD manufacturers utilize a unique algorithm automatically adjusting the sensitivity following a sensed R wave to assure appropriate VF recognition while minimizing cardiac or extracardiac signals during regular rhythm. While T wave oversensing can often be resolved with adjustments in the programmed sensitivity there are different ICD manufacturer algorithms that may necessitate consideration for a particular device to reduce T wave oversensing and any potential inappropriate ICD therapies.

Following sensed ventricular events

Medtronic ICDs reset the sensing threshold to 8–10 times the programmed sensitivity, up to a maximum of 75% of the sensed R wave. The sensitivity then decays exponentially from the end of the (sense) blanking period with a time constant of 450 ms until it reaches the programmed (maximum) sensitivity. At the nominal sensitivity of 0.3 mV,

there is little difference between the sensitivity curves after large and small spontaneous R waves. If the R wave is large, the entire auto-adjusting sensitivity curve can be altered substantially by changing the programmed value of maximum sensitivity. In our experience T-wave oversensing and inappropriate ICD shocks are more commonly observed in electrical conditions (i.e., LQTS) than in congenital heart defects or cardiomyopathic conditions (Figure 4.6).

St. Jude Medical ICDs have a threshold start that begins at 62.5% of the measured R wave for values between 3–6 mV. If the R wave amplitude is > 6 mV or < 3 mV, the threshold start is set to 62.5% of these values. The threshold-start-decay delay, however, is programmable over a range of 50–100%. The sensing threshold remains constant at a decay delay of 60 ms. Both the threshold start percent and decay delay are programmable.

Guidant ICDs set the starting threshold to 75% of the sensed R wave with a half-time of 200 ms to a minimum value that depends on the dynamic range of the sensing amplifier.

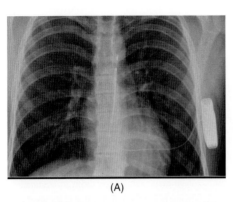 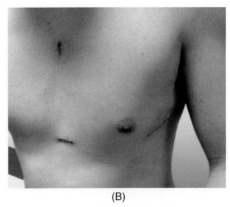

(A)   (B)

Figure 4.7 *(A) Chest X-ray of a patient with hypertrophic cardiomyopathy with an S-ICD showing the left lateral position of the pulse generator and parasternal location of the coil flanked by the distal and proximal electrodes. (B) View of the patient's chest after implantation of the subcutaneous ICD showing a left lateral incision for ICD generator placement and small superior vertical and inferior horizontal incisions at the sternum for securing the subcutaneously tunneled lead. (Source: Dr. Maully Shah, Division of Cardiology, The Children's Hospital of Philadelphia, U.S.A. Reproduced with courtesy of Dr. Maully Shah.)*

T wave oversensing may be predicted by exercise testing to assess for any rate-related changes, including diminution in the QRS complex or augmentation of the T wave.[138] In situations where the T waves > R waves, programming changes alone typically cannot resolve double counting and the patient will often need a new ICD or pace/sense lead. In situations where there is intermittent T wave oversensing whereby the R wave diminishes and the T waves get larger, programming changes may be of some benefit. In patients with LQTS, T waves may extend beyond a typical refractory pattern resulting indouble-counting. In these situations, it has been our preference to consider a St. Jude Medical device with changes in the decay delay and/or threshold start to extend the periods whereby potential physiologic changes may alter the QT interval. The current Medtronic family of ICDs in conjunction with a true bipolar lead allows RV sensing to occur between the RVtip-RVring electrode (bipolar) or between the RVtip-RVcoil electrodes. Adjusting these sensing configurations may reduce T-wave oversensing.

Subcutaneous ICD

A novel ICD configuration is the recently FDA approved totally subcutaneous device (S-ICD, Cameron Health/Boston Scientific Inc.). The subcutaneous pulse generator and electrode are placed in the extrathoracic space and no part of the system is exposed to most of the risks associated with an intravascular lead placement (Figure 4.7A,B). The three available sensing vectors utilize two sensing electrodes at either end of the coil electrode and the generator. The limitations include the inability of the device to provide ATP and advanced diagnostics as well as concerns about inappropriate shocks and device erosion. The current S-ICD model is thinner (59.5 cc) than the prototype and has remote patient monitoring capability. Initial results regarding safety and efficacy are promising. Although there are few published data regarding its sensing capabilities and efficacy in children, data from small studies is encouraging is a selective patient population.[139–141]

Conclusions

ICD implantation in children is complex and encompasses numerous structural and electrical conditions in a population often with complex anatomy, a need for somatic growth, and an active lifestyle. While there are guidelines to help in deciding the appropriate ICD candidate, decisions must be made using a patient-by-patient approach. Some adult recommendations are applicable to children. But, patients with CHD represent our largest device population and the group with whom there is no comparable adult population. The length of device therapy needed and the risks associated with the device also make the decision to implant a device in a child more difficult. Therefore, we must continue to study our ICD patients, preferably in a multi-centered and prospective manner and define for ourselves the appropriate ICD indications.

ICD generator and lead selection should clearly assess the clinical indications for an ICD but also the patient's underlying anatomy, venous drainage, body habitus, baseline rhythm, chronotropic competence, AV nodal function, history of atrial arrhythmias, and proclivity for new or different atrial and/or ventricular arrhythmias. Careful selection of the ICD and leads should take into consideration the specific clinical patient paradigms and the comfort level of the implanting physician with particular ICD systems.

References

1 Baumgartner H, Bonhoeffer P, De Groot NM, et al. ESC Guidelines for the management of grown-up congenital heart disease (new version 2010). *Eur Heart J* 2010;31:2915–2957.

2 Berul CI, Van Hare GF, Kertesz NJ, et al. Results of a multicenter retrospective implantable cardioverter-defibrillator registry of pediatric and congenital heart disease patients. *J Am Coll Cardiol* 2008;51:1685–1691.

3 Oechslin EN, Harrison DA, Connelly MS, Webb GD, Siu SC. Mode of death in adults with congenital heart disease. *Am J Cardiol* 2000;86:1111–1116.

4 Dore A, Santagata P, Dubuc M, Mercier LA. Implantable cardioverter defibrillators in adults with congenital heart disease: a single center experience. *Pacing Clin Electrophysiol* 2004;27:47–51.

5 Yap SC, Roos-Hesselink JW, Hoendermis ES, et al. Outcome of implantable cardioverter defibrillators in adults with congenital heart disease: a multi-centre study. *Eur Heart J* 2007;28:1854–1861.

6 Gatzoulis MA, Balaji S, Webber SA, et al. Risk factors for arrhythmia and sudden cardiac death late after repair of tetralogy of Fallot: a multicentre study. *Lancet* 2000;356:975–981.

7 Nollert G, Fischlein T, Bouterwek S, Bohmer C, Klinner W, Reichart B. Long-term survival in patients with repair of tetralogy of Fallot:36-year follow-up of 490 survivors of the first year after surgical repair. *J Am Coll Cardiol* 1997;30:1374–1383.

8 Silka MJ, Hardy BG, Menashe VD, Morris CD. A population-based prospective evaluation of risk of sudden cardiac death after operation for common congenital heart defects. *J Am Coll Cardiol* 1998;32:245–251.

9 Khairy P, Aboulhosn J, Gurvitz MZ, et al. Arrhythmia burden in adults with surgically repaired tetralogy of Fallot: a multi-institutional study. *Circulation* 2010;122:868–875.

10 Khairy P, Landzberg MJ, Gatzoulis MA, et al. Value of programmed ventricular stimulation after tetralogy of fallot repair: a multicenter study. *Circulation* 2004;109:1994–2000.

11 Schwerzmann M, Salehian O, Harris L, et al. Ventricular arrhythmias and sudden death in adults after a Mustard operation for transposition of the great arteries. *Eur Heart J* 2009;30:1873–1879.

12 Khairy P, Harris L, Landzberg MJ, et al. Implantable cardioverter-defibrillators in tetralogy of Fallot. *Circulation* 2008; 117: 363–370.

13 Epstein AE, DiMarco JP, Ellenbogen KA, Estes NA 3rd,, Freedman RA, Gettes LS, et al. and American College of Cardiology Foundation;American Heart Association Task Force on Practice Guidelines; Heart Rhythm Society. 2012 ACCF/AHA/HRS focused update incorporated into the ACCF/AHA/HRS 2008 guidelines for device-based therapy of cardiac rhythm abnormalities: a report of the American College of Cardiology Foundation/American Heart Association Task Force on Practice Guidelines and the Heart Rhythm Society. *J Am Coll Cardiol.* 2013 Jan 22;61(3):e6–75.

14 Khairy P, Van Hare GF, Balaji S, Berul CI, Cecchin F, Cohen MI, et al. PACES/HRS expert consensus statement on the recognition and management of arrhythmias in adult congenital heart disease: developed in partnership between the Pediatric and Congenital Electrophysiology Society (PACES) and the Heart Rhythm Society (HRS). Endorsed by the governing bodies of PACES, HRS, the American College of Cardiology (ACC), the American Heart Association (AHA), the European Heart Rhythm Association (EHRA), the Canadian Heart Rhythm Society (CHRS), and the International Society for Adult Congenital Heart Disease (ISACHD). *Heart Rhythm.* 2014 Oct;11(10):e102–165.

15 Khairy P, Landzberg MJ. Adult congenital heart disease: toward prospective risk assessment of a multisystemic condition. *Circulation* 2008;117:2311–2312.

16 Sachdev V, Machado RF, Shizukuda Y, et al. Diastolic dysfunction is an independent risk factor for death in patients with sickle cell disease. *J Am Coll Cardiol* 2007;49:472–479.

17 Zaslavsky LM, Pinotti AF, Gross JL. Diastolic dysfunction and mortality in diabetic patients on hemodialysis:

a 4.25-year controlled prospective study. *J Diabetes Complications* 2005;19:194–200.

18 Ackerman MJ, Priori SG, Willems S, et al. HRS/EHRA expert consensus statement on the state of genetic testing for the channelopathies and cardiomyopathies this document was developed as a partnership between the Heart Rhythm Society (HRS) and the European Heart Rhythm Association (EHRA). *Heart Rhythm* 2011;8:1308–1339.

19 Gersh BJ, Maron BJ, Bonow RO, et al. 2011 ACCF/AHA Guideline for the Diagnosis and Treatment of Hypertrophic Cardiomyopathy: Executive Summary: A Report of the American College of Cardiology Foundation/American Heart Association Task Force on Practice Guidelines. Circulation, 2011.

20 Moak JP, Leifer ES, Tripodi D, Mohiddin SA, Fananapazir L. Long-term follow-up of children and adolescents diagnosed with hypertrophic cardiomyopathy: risk factors for adverse arrhythmic events. *Pediatr Cardiol* 2011;32:1096–1105.

21 Christiaans I, van Engelen K, van Langen IM, et al. Risk stratification for sudden cardiac death in hypertrophic cardiomyopathy: systematic review of clinical risk markers. *Europace* 2010;12:313–321.

22 Olivotto I, Maron BJ, Montereggi A, Mazzuoli F, Dolara A, Cecchi F. Prognostic value of systemic blood pressure response during exercise in a community-based patient population with hypertrophic cardiomyopathy. *J Am Coll Cardiol* 1999;33:2044–2051.

23 Elliott PM, Poloniecki J, Dickie S, et al. Sudden death in hypertrophic cardiomyopathy: identification of high risk patients. *J Am Coll Cardiol* 2000;36:2212–2218.

24 Maron BJ, Spirito P, Ackerman MJ, Casey SA, Semsarian C, Estes NA 3rd, et al. Prevention of sudden cardiac death with implantable cardioverter-defibrillators in children and adolescents with hypertrophic cardiomyopathy. *J Am Coll Cardiol.* 2013 Apr 9;61(14):1527–1535.

25 Goldenberg I, Moss AJ, Zareba W, et al. Clinical course and risk stratification of patients affected with the Jervell and Lange–Nielsen syndrome. *J Cardiovasc Electrophysiol* 2006;17:1161–1168.

26 Priori SG, Schwartz PJ, Napolitano C, et al. Risk stratification in the long-QT syndrome. *N Engl J Med* 2003;348:1866–1874.

27 Collura CA, Johnson JN, Moir C, Ackerman MJ. Left cardiac sympathetic denervation for the treatment of long QT syndrome and catecholaminergic polymorphic ventricular tachycardia using video-assisted thoracic surgery. *Heart Rhythm* 2009;6:752–759.

28 Schwartz PJ, Priori SG, Cerrone M, et al. Left cardiac sympathetic denervation in the management of

high-risk patients affected by the long-QT syndrome. *Circulation* 2004;109:1826–1833.

29 Schwartz PJ, Spazzolini C, Crotti L. All LQT3 patients need an ICD: true or false? *Heart Rhythm* 2009;6:113–120.

30 Zareba W, Moss AJ, Daubert JP, Hall WJ, Robinson JL, Andrews M. Implantable cardioverter defibrillator in high-risk long QT syndrome patients. *J Cardiovasc Electrophysiol* 2003;14:337–341.

31 Zareba W, Moss AJ, Schwartz PJ, et al. Influence of genotype on the clinical course of the long-QT syndrome. International Long-QT Syndrome Registry Research Group. *N Engl J Med* 1998;339:960–965.

32 Schwartz PJ, Priori SG, Spazzolini C, et al. Genotype-phenotype correlation in the long-QT syndrome: gene-specific triggers for life-threatening arrhythmias. *Circulation* 2001;103:89–95.

33 Schwartz PJ, Stone HL. Effects of unilateral stellectomy upon cardiac performance during exercise in dogs. *Circ Res* 1979;44:637–645.

34 Ruan Y, Liu N, Bloise R, Napolitano C, Priori SG. Gating properties of SCN5A mutations and the response to mexiletine in long-QT syndrome type 3 patients. *Circulation* 2007;116:1137–1144.

35 Ruan Y, Denegri M, Liu N, et al. Trafficking defects and gating abnormalities of a novel SCN5A mutation question gene-specific therapy in long QT syndrome type 3. *Circ Res* 2010;106:1374–1383.

36 Fabritz L, Damke D, Emmerich M, et al. Autonomic modulation and antiarrhythmic therapy in a model of long QT syndrome type 3. *Cardiovasc Res* 2010;87:60–72.

37 Etheridge SP, Sanatani S, Cohen MI, Albaro CA, Saarel EV, Bradley DJ. Long QT syndrome in children in the era of implantable defibrillators. *J Am Coll Cardiol* 2007;50:1335–1340.

38 Etheridge SP, Bowles NE, Arrington CB, et al. Somatic mosaicism contributes to phenotypic variation in Timothy syndrome. *Am J Med Genet A* 2011;155A:2578–2583.

39 Moss AJ, Shimizu W, Wilde AA, et al. Clinical aspects of type-1 long-QT syndrome by location, coding type, and biophysical function of mutations involving the KCNQ1 gene. *Circulation* 2007;115:2481–2489.

40 Reid DS, Tynan M, Braidwood L, Fitzgerald GR. Bidirectional tachycardia in a child. A study using His bundle electrography. *Br Heart J* 1975;37:339–344.

41 Leenhardt A, Glaser E, Burguera M, Nurnberg M, Maison-Blanche P, Coumel P. Short-coupled variant of torsade de pointes. A new electrocardiographic entity in the spectrum of idiopathic ventricular tachyarrhythmias. *Circulation* 1994;89:206–215.

42 Priori SG, Napolitano C, Tiso N, et al. Mutations in the cardiac ryanodine receptor gene (hRyR2) underlie catecholaminergic polymorphic ventricular tachycardia. *Circulation* 2001;103:196–200.

43 Postma AV, Denjoy I, Hoorntje TM, et al. Absence of calsequestrin 2 causes severe forms of catecholaminergic polymorphic ventricular tachycardia. *Circ Res* 2002;91:e21–26.

44 Lahat H, Pras E, Olender T, et al. A missense mutation in a highly conserved region of CASQ2 is associated with autosomal recessive catecholamine-induced polymorphic ventricular tachycardia in Bedouin families from Israel. *Am J Hum Genet* 2001;69:1378–1384.

45 Napolitano C, Liu N, Priori SG. Role of calmodulin kinase in catecholaminergic polymorphic ventricular tachycardia. *Heart Rhythm* 2011;8:1601–1605.

46 Hayashi M, Denjoy I, Extramiana F, et al. Incidence and risk factors of arrhythmic events in catecholaminergic polymorphic ventricular tachycardia. *Circulation* 2009;119:2426–2434.

47 Watanabe H, Chopra N, Laver D, et al. Flecainide prevents catecholaminergic polymorphic ventricular tachycardia in mice and humans. *Nat Med* 2009;15:380–383.

48 van der Werf C, Kannankeril PJ, Sacher F, et al. Flecainide therapy reduces exercise-induced ventricular arrhythmias in patients with catecholaminergic polymorphic ventricular tachycardia. *J Am Coll Cardiol* 2011;57:2244–2254.

49 Mohamed U, Gollob MH, Gow RM, Krahn AD. Sudden cardiac death despite an implantable cardioverter-defibrillator in a young female with catecholaminergic ventricular tachycardia. *Heart Rhythm* 2006;3:1486–1489.

50 Miyake CY, Webster G, Czosek RJ, Kantoch MJ, Dubin AM, Avasarala K, Atallah J. Efficacy of implantable cardioverter defibrillators in young patients with catecholaminergic polymorphic ventricular tachycardia: success depends on substrate. *Circ Arrhythm Electrophysiol.* 2013 Jun;6(3)

51 Roses-Noguer F, Jarman JW, Clague JR, Till J.Outcomes of defibrillator therapy in catecholaminergic polymorphic ventricular tachycardia. *Heart Rhythm.* 2014 Jan;11(1):58–66.

52 Wilde AA, Bhuiyan ZA, Crotti L, et al. Left cardiac sympathetic denervation for catecholaminergic polymorphic ventricular tachycardia. *N Engl J Med* 2008;358:2024–2029.

53 Probst V, Denjoy I, Meregalli PG, et al. Clinical aspects and prognosis of Brugada syndrome in children. *Circulation* 2007;115:2042–2048.

54 Nademanee K, Veerakul G, Chandanamattha P, et al. Prevention of ventricular fibrillation episodes in Brugada syndrome by catheter ablation over the anterior right ventricular outflow tract epicardium. *Circulation* 2011;123:1270–1279.

55 Antzelevitch C, Brugada P, Borggrefe M, et al. Brugada syndrome: report of the second consensus conference: endorsed by the Heart Rhythm Society and the European Heart Rhythm Association. *Circulation* 2005;111:659–670.

56 Priori SG, Napolitano C, Gasparini M, et al. Natural history of Brugada syndrome:insights for risk stratification and management. *Circulation* 2002;105:1342–1347.

57 Brugada J, Brugada R, Brugada P. Determinants of sudden cardiac death in individuals with the electrocardiographic pattern of Brugada syndrome and no previous cardiac arrest. *Circulation* 2003;108:3092–3096.

58 Bastiaenen R, Behr ER. Sudden death and ion channel disease: pathophysiology and implications for management. *Heart* 2011;97:1365–1372.

59 Paul M, Gerss J, Schulze-Bahr E, et al. Role of programmed ventricular stimulation in patients with Brugada syndrome: a meta-analysis of worldwide published data. *Eur Heart J* 2007;28:2126–2133.

60 Brugada J, Brugada R, Brugada P. Electrophysiologic testing predicts events in Brugada syndrome patients. *Heart Rhythm* 2011;8:1595–1597.

61 Wilde AA, Viskin S. EP testing does not predict cardiac events in Brugada syndrome. *Heart Rhythm* 2011;8:1598–1600.

62 Probst V, Veltmann C, Eckardt L, et al. Long-term prognosis of patients diagnosed with Brugada syndrome: Results from the FINGER Brugada Syndrome Registry. *Circulation* 2010;121:635–643.

63 Dumaine R, Towbin JA, Brugada P, et al. Ionic mechanisms responsible for the electrocardiographic phenotype of the Brugada syndrome are temperature dependent. *Circ Res* 1999; 85: 803–809.

64 Morita H, Kusano KF, Miura D, et al. Fragmented QRS as a marker of conduction abnormality and a predictor of prognosis of Brugada syndrome. *Circulation* 2008; 118: 1697–1704.

65 Nishii N, Ogawa M, Morita H, et al. SCN5A mutation is associated with early and frequent recurrence of ventricular fibrillation in patients with Brugada syndrome. *Circ J* 2010;74:2572–2578.

66 Meregalli PG, Tan HL, Probst V, et al. Type of SCN5A mutation determines clinical severity and degree of conduction slowing in loss-of-function sodium channelopathies. *Heart Rhythm* 2009;6:341–348.

67 Marcus FI, Fontaine GH, Guiraudon G, et al. Right ventricular dysplasia: a report of 24 adult cases. *Circulation* 1982;65:384–398.

68 Thiene G, Nava A, Corrado D, Rossi L, Pennelli N. Right ventricular cardiomyopathy and sudden death in young people. *N Engl J Med* 1988;318:129–133.

69 Bhonsale A, James CA, Tichnell C, et al. Incidence and predictors of implantable cardioverter-defibrillator therapy in patients with arrhythmogenic right ventricular dysplasia/cardiomyopathy undergoing implantable cardioverter-defibrillator implantation for primary prevention. *J Am Coll Cardiol* 2011;58:1485–1496.

70 Corrado D, Calkins H, Link MS, et al. Prophylactic implantable defibrillator in patients with arrhythmogenic right ventricular cardiomyopathy/dysplasia and no prior ventricular fibrillation or sustained ventricular tachycardia. *Circulation* 2010;122:1144–1152.

71 Hodgkinson KA, Parfrey PS, Bassett AS, et al. The impact of implantable cardioverter-defibrillator therapy on survival in autosomal-dominant arrhythmogenic right ventricular cardiomyopathy (ARVD5). *J Am Coll Cardiol* 2005; 45: 400–408.

72 Piccini JP, Dalal D, Roguin A, et al. Predictors of appropriate implantable defibrillator therapies in patients with arrhythmogenic right ventricular dysplasia. *Heart Rhythm* 2005; 2: 1188–1194.

73 Bernstein AD, Camm AJ, Fisher JD, et al. North American Society of Pacing and Electrophysiology policy statement. The NASPE/BPEG defibrillator code. *Pacing Clin Electrophysiol* 1993; 16: 1776–1780.

74 Dewland TA, Pellegrini CN, Wang Y, Marcus GM, Keung E, Varosy PD. Dual-chamber implantable cardioverter-defibrillator selection is associated with increased complication rates and mortality among patients enrolled in the NCDR implantable cardioverter-defibrillator registry. *J Am Coll Cardiol* 2011; 58: 1007–1013.

75 Cohen MI, Rhodes LA. Sinus node dysfunction and atrial tachycardia after the Fontan procedure: The scope of the problem. *Semin Thorac Cardiovasc Surg Pediatr Card Surg Annu* 1998; 1: 41–52.

76 Cohen MI, Wernovsky G, Vetter VL, et al. Sinus node function after a systematically staged Fontan procedure. *Circulation* 1998; 98: II352–1358;discussion II8–I19.

77 Beerman LB, Neches WH, Fricker FJ, et al. Arrhythmias in transposition of the great arteries after the Mustard operation. *Am J Cardiol* 1983; 51: 1530–1534.

78 Roos-Hesselink J, Perlroth MG, McGhie J, Spitaels S. Atrial arrhythmias in adults after repair of tetralogy of Fallot. Correlations with clinical, exercise, and echocardiographic findings. *Circulation* 1995; 91: 2214–2219.

79 Helbing WA, Hansen B, Ottenkamp J, et al. Long-term results of atrial correction for transposition of the great arteries. Comparison of Mustard and Senning operations. *J Thorac Cardiovasc Surg* 1994; 108: 363–372.

80 Janousek J, Paul T, Luhmer I, Wilken M, Hruda J, Kallfelz HC. Atrial baffle procedures for complete transposition of the great arteries: natural course of sinus node dysfunction and risk factors for dysrhythmias and sudden death. *Z Kardiol* 1994; 83: 933–938.

81 Meijboom F, Szatmari A, Deckers JW, et al. Long-term follow-up (10 to 17 years) after Mustard repair for transposition of the great arteries. *J Thorac Cardiovasc Surg* 1996; 111: 1158–1168.

82 Huhta JC, Maloney JD, Ritter DG, Ilstrup DM, Feldt RH. Complete atrioventricular block in patients with atrioventricular discordance. *Circulation* 1983; 67: 1374–1377.

83 Lamas GA, Lee KL, Sweeney MO, et al. Ventricular pacing or dual-chamber pacing for sinus-node dysfunction. *N Engl J Med* 2002; 346: 1854–1862.

84 Nielsen JC, Kristensen L, Andersen HR, Mortensen PT, Pedersen OL, Pedersen AK. A randomized comparison of atrial and dual-chamber pacing in 177 consecutive patients with sick sinus syndrome: echocardiographic and clinical outcome. *J Am Coll Cardiol* 2003; 42: 614–623.

85 Albertsen AE, Nielsen JC. Selecting the appropriate pacing mode for patients with sick sinus syndrome: evidence from randomized clinical trials. *Card Electrophysiol Rev* 2003; 7: 406–410.

86 Toff WD, Skehan JD, De Bono DP, Camm AJ. The United Kingdom Pacing and Cardiovascular Events (UKPACE) trial. United Kingdom Pacing and Cardiovascular Events. *Heart* 1997; 78: 221–223.

87 Wilkoff BL, Cook JR, Epstein AE, et al. Dual-chamber pacing or ventricular backup pacing in patients with an implantable defibrillator: the Dual Chamber and VVI Implantable Defibrillator (DAVID) Trial. *JAMA* 2002; 288: 3115–3123.

88 Wilkoff BL, Kudenchuk PJ, Buxton AE, et al. The DAVID (Dual Chamber and VVI Implantable Defibrillator) II trial. *J Am Coll Cardiol* 2009; 53: 872–880.

89 Olshansky B, Day JD, Moore S, et al. Is dual-chamber programming inferior to single-chamber programming in an implantable cardioverter-defibrillator? Results of the INTRINSIC RV (Inhibition of Unnecessary RV Pacing With AVSH in ICDs) study. *Circulation* 2007; 115: 9–16.

90 Sweeney MO, Ellenbogen KA, Miller EH, Sherfesee L, Sheldon T, Whellan D. The Managed Ventricular pacing versus VVI 40 Pacing (MVP) Trial: clinical background, rationale, design, and implementation. *J Cardiovasc Electrophysiol* 2006; 17: 1295–1298.

91 Janousek J, Gebauer RA, Abdul-Khaliq H, et al. Cardiac resynchronisation therapy in paediatric and congenital

heart disease: differential effects in various anatomical and functional substrates. *Heart* 2009; 95: 1165–1171.

92 Nishimura RA, Holmes DR, Jr., Clinical practice. Hypertrophic obstructive cardiomyopathy. *N Engl J Med* 2004; 350: 1320–1327.

93 Jeanrenaud X, Goy JJ, Kappenberger L. Effects of dual-chamber pacing in hypertrophic obstructive cardiomyopathy. *Lancet* 1992; 339: 1318–1323.

94 Nishimura RA, Trusty JM, Hayes DL, et al. Dual-chamber pacing for hypertrophic cardiomyopathy: a randomized, double-blind, crossover trial. *J Am Coll Cardiol* 1997; 29: 435–441.

95 Maron BJ, Nishimura RA, McKenna WJ, Rakowski H, Josephson ME, Kieval RS. Assessment of permanent dual-chamber pacing as a treatment for drug-refractory symptomatic patients with obstructive hypertrophic cardiomyopathy. A randomized, double-blind, crossover study (M-PATHY). *Circulation* 1999; 99: 2927–2933.

96 Betocchi S, Losi MA, Piscione F, et al. Effects of dual-chamber pacing in hypertrophic cardiomyopathy on left ventricular outflow tract obstruction and on diastolic function. *Am J Cardiol* 1996; 77: 498–502.

97 Viskin S, Glikson M, Fish R, Glick A, Copperman Y, Saxon LA. Rate smoothing with cardiac pacing for preventing torsade de pointes. *Am J Cardiol* 2000; 86: 111K–115K.

98 Tan HL, Bardai A, Shimizu W, et al. Genotype-specific onset of arrhythmias in congenital long-QT syndrome: possible therapy implications. *Circulation* 2006; 114: 2096–2103.

99 Viskin S, Fish R, Roth A, Copperman Y. Prevention of torsade de pointes in the congenital long QT syndrome: use of a pause prevention pacing algorithm. *Heart* 1998; 79: 417–419.

100 Dorostkar PC, Eldar M, Belhassen B, Scheinman MM. Long-term follow-up of patients with long-QT syndrome treated with beta-blockers and continuous pacing. *Circulation* 1999; 100: 2431–2436.

101 Alexander ME, Cecchin F, Walsh EP, Triedman JK, Bevilacqua LM, Berul CI. Implications of implantable cardioverter defibrillator therapy in congenital heart disease and pediatrics. *J Cardiovasc Electrophysiol* 2004; 15: 72–76.

102 Korte T, Koditz H, Niehaus M, Paul T, Tebbenjohanns J. High incidence of appropriate and inappropriate ICD therapies in children and adolescents with implantable cardioverter defibrillator. *Pacing Clin Electrophysiol* 2004; 27: 924–932.

103 Love BA, Barrett KS, Alexander ME, et al. Supraventricular arrhythmias in children and young adults with implantable cardioverter defibrillators. *J Cardiovasc Electrophysiol* 2001; 12: 1097–1101.

104 DeMaso DR, Lauretti A, Spieth L, et al. Psychosocial factors and quality of life in children and adolescents with implantable cardioverter-defibrillators. *Am J Cardiol* 2004; 93: 582–587.

105 Deisenhofer I, Kolb C, Ndrepepa G, et al. Do current dual chamber cardioverter defibrillators have advantages over conventional single chamber cardioverter defibrillators in reducing inappropriate therapies? A randomized, prospective study. *J Cardiovasc Electrophysiol* 2001; 12: 134–142.

106 Swerdlow CD. Supraventricular tachycardia-ventricular tachycardia discrimination algorithms in implantable cardioverter defibrillators: state-of-the-art review. *J Cardiovasc Electrophysiol* 2001; 12: 606–612.

107 Nair M, Saoudi N, Kroiss D, Letac B. Automatic arrhythmia identification using analysis of the atrioventricular association. Application to a new generation of implantable defibrillators. Participating Centers of the Automatic Recognition of Arrhythmia Study Group. *Circulation* 1997; 95: 967–973.

108 Wilkoff BL, Kuhlkamp V, Volosin K, et al. Critical analysis of dual-chamber implantable cardioverter-defibrillator arrhythmia detection: results and technical considerations. *Circulation* 2001; 103: 381–386.

109 Friedman PA, McClelland RL, Bamlet WR, et al. Dual-chamber versus single-chamber detection enhancements for implantable defibrillator rhythm diagnosis: the detect supraventricular tachycardia study. *Circulation* 2006; 113: 2871–2879.

110 Kouakam C, Kacet S, Hazard JR, et al. Performance of a dual-chamber implantable defibrillator algorithm for discrimination of ventricular from supraventricular tachycardia. *Europace* 2004; 6: 32–42.

111 Theuns DA, Klootwijk AP, Goedhart DM, Jordaens LJ. Prevention of inappropriate therapy in implantable cardioverter-defibrillators: results of a prospective, randomized study of tachyarrhythmia detection algorithms. *J Am Coll Cardiol* 2004; 44: 2362–2367.

112 Lawrence D, Von Bergen N, Law IH, et al. Inappropriate ICD discharges in single-chamber versus dual-chamber devices in the pediatric and young adult population. *J Cardiovasc Electrophysiol* 2009; 20: 287–290.

113 Scherer M, Ezziddin K, Klesius A, et al. Extension of generator longevity by use of high impedance ventricular leads. *Pacing Clin Electrophysiol* 2001; 24: 206–211.

114 Berger T, Roithinger FX, Antretter H, Hangler H, Pachinger O, Hintringer F. The influence of high versus normal impedance ventricular leads on pacemaker generator longevity. *Pacing Clin Electrophysiol* 2003; 26: 2116–2120.

115 Shepard RK, Ellenbogen KA. Leads and longevity: how long will your pacemaker last? *Europace* 2009; 11: 142–143.

116 Etsadashvili K, Hintringer F, Stuhlinger M, et al. Long-term results of high vs. normal impedance ventricular leads on actual (Real-Life) pacemaker generator longevity. *Europace* 2009; 11: 200–205.

117 Kuhlkamp V, Khalighi K, Dornberger V, Ziemer G. Single-incision and single-element array electrode to lower the defibrillation threshold. *Ann Thorac Surg* 1997; 64: 1177–1179.

118 Kall JG, Kopp D, Lonchyna V, et al. Implantation of a subcutaneous lead array in combination with a transvenous defibrillation electrode via a single infra-clavicular incision. *Pacing Clin Electrophysiol* 1995; 18: 482–485.

119 Cooper JM, Stephenson EA, Berul CI, Walsh EP, Epstein LM. Implantable cardioverter defibrillator lead complications and laser extraction in children and young adults with congenital heart disease:implications for implantation and management. *J Cardiovasc Electrophysiol* 2003; 14: 344–349.

120 Stefanelli CB, Bradley DJ, Leroy S, Dick M, 2nd,, Serwer GA, Fischbach PS. Implantable cardioverter defibrillator therapy for life-threatening arrhythmias in young patients. *J Interv Card Electrophysiol* 2002; 6: 235–244.

121 Bonney WJ, Spotnitz HM, Liberman L, et al. Survival of transvenous ICD leads in young patients. *Pacing Clin Electrophysiol* 2010; 33: 186–191.

122 Hauser RG, Hayes DL. Increasing hazard of Sprint Fidelis implantable cardioverter-defibrillator lead failure. *Heart Rhythm* 2009; 6: 605–610.

123 Rordorf R, Poggio L, Savastano S, et al. Failure of implantable cardioverter-defibrillator leads: a matter of lead size? *Heart Rhythm* 2013; 10: 184–190.

124 Parkash R, Exner D, Champagne J, et al. Failure rate of the Riata lead under advisory: a report from the CHRS Device Committee. *Heart Rhythm* 2013; 10: 692–695.

125 Epstein AE, Baker JH, 2nd,, Beau SL, Deering TF, Greenberg SM, Goldman DS. Performance of the St. Jude Medical Riata leads. *Heart Rhythm* 2009; 6: 204–209.

126 Turakhia M, Prasad M, Olgin J, et al. Rates and severity of perforation from implantable cardioverter-defibrillator leads: a 4-year study. *J Interv Card Electrophysiol* 2009; 24: 47–52.

127 Hauser RG, Maisel WH, Friedman PA, et al. Longevity of Sprint Fidelis implantable cardioverter-defibrillator leads and risk factors for failure:implications for patient management. *Circulation* 2011; 123: 358–363.

128 Atallah J, Erickson CC, Cecchin F, et al. Multi-institutional study of implantable defibrillator lead performance in children and young adults: results of the Pediatric Lead Extractability and Survival Evaluation (PLEASE) study. *Circulation* 2013; 127: 2393–2402.

129 Janson CM, Patel AR, Bonney WJ, Smoots K, Shah MJ. Implantable cardioverter-defibrillator lead failure in children and young adults: a matter of lead diameter or lead design? *J Am Coll Cardiol* 2014; 63: 133–140.

130 Link MS, Hill SL, Cliff DL, et al. Comparison of frequency of complications of implantable cardioverter-defibrillators in children versus adults. *Am J Cardiol* 1999; 83: 263–6, A5–6.

131 Dorwarth U, Frey B, Dugas M, et al. Transvenous defibrillation leads: high incidence of failure during long-term follow-up. *J Cardiovasc Electrophysiol* 2003; 14: 38–43.

132 Kitamura S, Satomi K, Kurita T, et al. Long-term follow-up of transvenous defibrillation leads: high incidence of fracture in coaxial polyurethane lead. *Circ J* 2006; 70: 273–277.

133 Hayes DL, Graham KJ, Irwin M, et al. Multicenter experience with a bipolar tined polyurethane ventricular lead. *Pacing Clin Electrophysiol* 1995; 18: 999–1004.

134 Radbill AE, Triedman JK, Berul CI, et al. System survival of nontransvenous implantable cardioverter-defibrillators compared to transvenous implantable cardioverter-defibrillators in pediatric and congenital heart disease patients. *Heart Rhythm* 2010; 7: 193–198.

135 Stephenson EA, Batra AS, Knilans TK, et al. A multi-center experience with novel implantable cardioverter defibrillator configurations in the pediatric and congenital heart disease population. *J Cardiovasc Electrophysiol* 2006; 17: 41–46.

136 Tomaske M, Pretre R, Rahn M, Bauersfeld U. Epicardial and pleural lead ICD systems in children and adolescents maintain functionality over 5 years. *Europace* 2008; 10: 1152–1156.

137 Cannon BC, Friedman RA, Fenrich AL, Fraser CD, McKenzie ED, Kertesz NJ. Innovative techniques for placement of implantable cardioverter-defibrillator leads in patients with limited venous access to the heart. *Pacing Clin Electrophysiol* 2006; 29: 181–187.

138 Cohen MI, Shaffer J, Pedersen S, Sims JJ, Papez A. Limited utility of exercise-stress testing to prevent T-wave oversensing in pediatric internal cardioverter defibrillator recipients. *Pacing Clin Electrophysiol* 2011; 34: 436–442.

139 Pettit SJ, McLean A, Colquhoun I, Connelly D, McLeod K.Clinical experience of subcutaneous and transvenous implantable cardioverter defibrillators in children and

teenagers.*Pacing Clin Electrophysiol*. 2013 Dec; 36(12): 1532–1538.

140 Weiss R, Knight BP, Gold MR, Leon AR, Herre JM, Hood M, et al. Safety and efficacy of a totally subcutaneous implantable-cardioverter defibrillator. *Circulation*. 2013 Aug 27; 128(9): 944–953.

141 Jarman JW1, Lascelles K, Wong T, Markides V, Clague JR, Till J.Clinical experience of entirely subcutaneous implantable cardioverter-defibrillators in children and adults: cause for caution. *Eur Heart J*. 2012 Jun; 33(11): 1351–1359.

CHAPTER 5

Hemodynamics of pacing and cardiac resynchronization therapy (CRT) for the failing left and right ventricle

Kara S. Motonaga[1] and Anne M. Dubin[2]

[1] Pediatric Electrophysiologist, Lucile Packard Children's Hospital, Clinical Assistant Professor, Stanford University, Palo Alto, CA, USA
[2] Professor of Pediatrics, Stanford University School of Medicine, Director, Pediatric Electrophysiology, Lucile Salter Packard Children's Hospital Heart Center, Palo Alto, CA, USA

Cardiac Resynchronization Therapy (CRT) has transformed the cardiac pacemaker into a powerful tool that improves function, decreases mortality, and increases quality of life in adult left ventricular heart failure patients. However, 30% of adult CRT patients are non-responders, prompting further evaluation of electro-mechanical coupling interactions in dyssynchrony and cardiac pacing to determine the optimal pacing sites and selection criteria for CRT.[1,2] CRT in the pediatric heart failure population is even more difficult to evaluate due to complex anatomical abnormalities including single ventricles of left or right ventricular morphologies, and the higher proportion of right bundle branch block and right ventricular failure. The heterogeneous pediatric population has led to various pacing strategies for CRT with the ultimate goal of normalizing electrical and mechanical activation to preserve electromechanical synchrony and maximize cardiac function.

Physiology of electrical and mechanical activation

Electrical activation during sinus rhythm

Electrical activation in sinus rhythm begins with the sinus node, located in the high right atrium (RA) near the junction of the superior vena cava (see Figure 5.1).[3] The sinus node's automaticity results in spontaneous depolarization at a regular rate influenced by extrinsic neurohormonal control and atrial stretch. The action potential spreads from myocyte to myocyte via gap junctions throughout the atria. The activation of the entire atria takes approximately 100 ms in the human heart.[4]

The impulse reaches the atrioventricular (AV) node, which electrically connects the atria and the ventricles in the normal heart (Figure 5.1).[3] The remaining parts of the atria and ventricles are separated by the fibrous mitral and tricuspid valve

Cardiac Pacing and Defibrillation in Pediatric and Congenital Heart Disease, First Edition.
Edited by Maully Shah, Larry Rhodes and Jonathan Kaltman.
© 2017 John Wiley & Sons Ltd. Published 2017 by John Wiley & Sons Ltd.
Companion Website: www.wiley.com/go/shah/cardiac_pacing

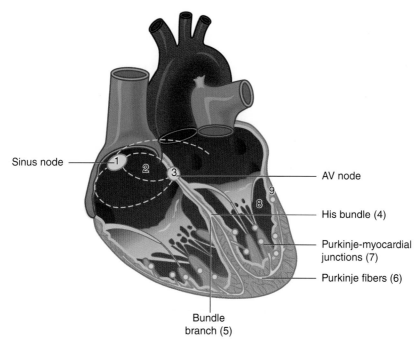

Sinus node

AV node

His bundle (4)

Purkinje-myocardial
junctions (7)

Purkinje fibers (6)

Bundle
branch (5)

Figure 5.1 *Illustration of the normal electrical conduction through the heart. The impulse originates in the sinus node (1) and spreads across the atrial wall (2) before reaching the AV node (3). The impulse is then conducted to the ventricles via the rapidly conducting His–Purkinje system that includes the His bundle (4), Bundle branches (5), and Purkinje fibers (6). The Purkinje fibers transfer the electrical impulse to the slowly conducting myocardium via the Purkinje-myocardial junctions in the endocardium (7), which is followed by slow conduction through the myocardium from endocardium to epicardium. (Source: Ellenbogen 2011. Reproduced with permission of Elsevier.)*

annulus. The AV node conducts electrical impulses slowly, taking approximately 80 ms for the impulse to travel from the atrial side to the ventricular side of the AV node, allowing time for optimal ventricular filling.

The electrical impulse travels from the AV node to the His–Purkinje system, consisting of the His bundle and the right and left bundle branches (Figure 5.1).[3] This specialized electrical tissue conducts impulses approximately four times faster (3–4 m/s) than the myocardium (0.3 to 1 m/s) due to a high concentration of gap junctions.[5–8] The right bundle branch (RBB) runs in the subendocardium along the right side of the interventricular septum and terminates in the Purkinje plexuses of the right ventricle (RV). The left bundle branch (LBB) initially was thought to divide into two fascicles called the anterior and posterior fascicles. Further studies demonstrated that the LBB network can have a third subdivision called the centroseptal

subdivision that supplies the midseptal area of the left ventricle (LV) and arises from either the anterior or posterior fascicles or both. The fascicles continue subendocardially in a network of Purkinje fibers that covers the lower third of the septum, free wall, and papillary muscles.[5,9] The rapidly conducting His bundle, as well as the right and left bundle branches, are electrically isolated from the slower conducting adjacent myocardium. They are electrically connected to the myocardium at discrete sites called Purkinje-myocardial junctions which are spatially inhomogenous with variable degrees of electromechanical coupling.[5,10]

Endocardial activation of the RV and LV starts low on the septum near the insertion of the anterior papillary muscle in the RV and the posteromedial papillary muscle in the LV at the myocardial breakthrough points of the Purkinje fibers (Figure 5.2 and Video clip 5.1). LV endocardial activation starts approximately 10 ms before the RV.[11] Activation of the normal myocardium occurs predominantly from apex to base and outflow tract as well as centrifugally from endocardium to epicardium.[11,12] This activation sequence has important ramifications to mechanical activation, as described later.

Total ventricular activation, studied in the isolated human heart by Durrer et al., lasts approximately 60–80 ms.[11] An *in vivo* study using three-dimensional electroanatomical mapping by Motonaga et al. demonstrated that right ventricular activation lasted approximately 56.2 ± 11.2 ms while left ventricular activation lasted approximately 48.9 ± 9.2 ms in normal pediatric hearts.[13] These short activation times illustrate the important role of the Purkinje fiber system with its unique rapid propagation properties and widespread ventricular distribution, which allows for a high degree of coordination between distant regions of the myocardium thereby maximizing myocardial synchrony.

Mechanical activation during sinus rhythm

Excitation-contraction (E-C) coupling allows electrical activation to translate to contraction in cardiac myocytes. The calcium ion plays a central role in this process as electrical depolarization leads to entry of calcium into the cell through voltage-dependent L-type calcium channels. This triggers a much larger release of calcium from the sarcoplasmic reticulum (calcium-induced calcium release), which catalyzes the binding of myosin and actin filaments leading to myocardial contraction (Figure 5.3).[14] After repolarization, calcium dissociates from the actin-myosin contractile apparatus leading to myocardial relaxation. The calcium is then taken up again by the sarcoplasmic reticulum via the sarcoplasmic reticular Ca^{2+} adenosine triphosphatase (SERCA) where it is stored until the next electrical depolarization. The sodium-calcium (Na^+/Ca^{2+}) exchanger maintains intracellular calcium homeostasis, usually by removing calcium from the cell. Although the intracellular calcium

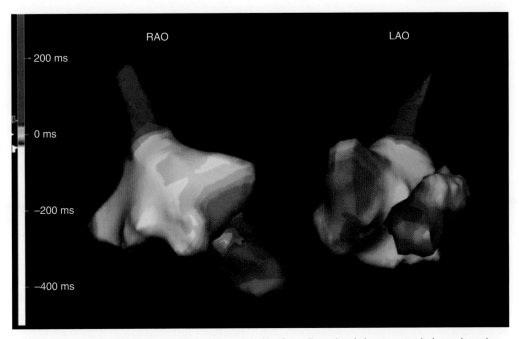

Figure 5.2 *Normal electrical activation pattern demonstrated by three-dimensional electroanatomical mapping using EnSite NavX Navigation & Visualization Technology (St. Jude Medical, St Paul, MN). The earliest electrical activation is seen midway down the ventricular septum (denoted by the white) with propagation of depolarization spreading to the apex and subsequently to the base and outflow tract (denoted by blue and purple). LAO = left anterior oblique; RAO = right anterior oblique. (Source: Motonaga 2012. Reproduced with permission of Elsevier.)*

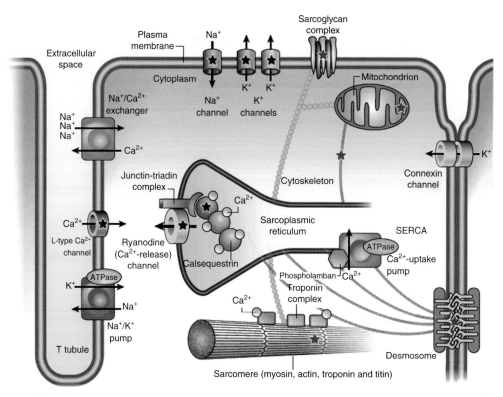

Figure 5.3 *Illustration of the excitation-contraction coupling process in the cardiac myocyte. Calcium enters the cell via L-type calcium channels which then triggers a much larger release of calcium from the sarcoplasmic reticulum through the ryanodine channel. This catalyzes the binding of myosin and actin filaments leading to myocardial contraction (calcium-induced calcium release). After repolarization, calcium dissociates from the actin-myosin contractile apparatus leading to myocardial relaxation. The calcium is then taken up again by the sarcoplasmic reticulum via the sarcoplasmic reticular Ca^{2+} adenosine triphosphatase (SERCA) where it is stored until the next electrical depolarization. The sodium-calcium (Na^+/Ca^{2+}) exchanger maintains intracellular calcium homeostasis, usually by removing calcium from the cell. (Source: Knollmann 2008. Reproduced with permission of Nature Publishing Group.)*

level rises rapidly after the upstroke of the action potential, there is about a 30 ms delay between the electrical depolarization and the development of contractile force.[15] This electromechanical delay dictates how tightly electrical activation and mechanical contraction can be coupled together and abnormalities in this timing can have negative hemodynamic consequences as described next.

Since atrial electrical activation precedes ventricular electrical activation and electrical depolarization and mechanical contraction are tightly coupled, it follows reason that atrial contraction precedes ventricular contraction. This antecedent atrial contraction is commonly referred to as the "atrial kick" and adds roughly 20% to the filling volume of the ventricles, which results in lengthening of the ventricular muscle cells and their sarcomeres. This lengthening allows for a greater contractile force, an effect known as the Frank–Starling relationship.[16]

The mechanical activation of the heart is also aided by the muscle fiber orientation within the ventricle. Francisco Torrent-Guasp demonstrated that the heart muscle can be unraveled into a continuous myocardial band that extends from the pulmonary artery to the aorta (Figure 5.4).[17,18] This band forms a basal loop in continuity with an apical loop consisting of a descending and an ascending segment in the left ventricular myocardial wall. The descending segment (subendocardium) forms a right-handed helix which

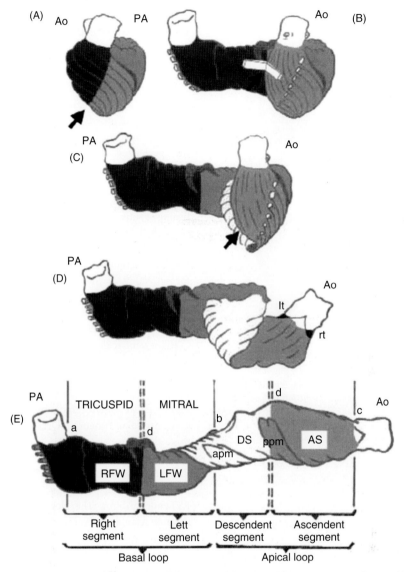

Figure 5.4 *Illustration of the myocardial band described by Torrent-Guasp and sequential stages of unwinding from A to E. The myocardial band extends between the pulmonary artery (PA) and the aorta (Ao) and can be divided into four segments (E): RV free wall (RFW, black), LV free wall (LFW, dark gray), descending segment (DS, white), and ascending segment (AS, light gray). These segments form a basal loop (from a to b, consisting of the RFW and LFW) and an apical loop (from b to c, consisting of the descending segment and the ascending segment). The cleavage plane that provides clues for unwinding the myocardial band are indicated by arrows. apm = Anterior papillary muscle; lt = left trigone of the aorta; ppm = posterior papillary muscle; rt = right trigone of the aorta. (Source: Torrent-Guasp 2001. Reproduced with permission of Elsevier.)*

transitions smoothly at the apex into a left-handed helix (subepicardium) as the ascending segment (Figure 5.5).[19]

Mechanical activation of the normal myocardium follows electrical activation in a predominantly apex to base and outflow tract progression as well as centrifugally from endocardium to epicardium. The oblique myocardial fiber orientation induces twisting around the long axis of the ventricle during contraction with the apex rotating in the

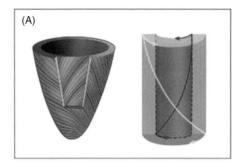

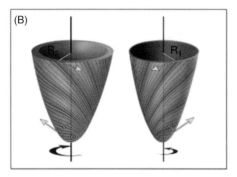

Figure 5.5 *Schematic diagram of the myofiber orientation. The image on the right side of panel B shows the right-handed helix (R1) that forms the descending loop (subendocardium). The image on the left side of panel B shows the left-handed helix (R2) that forms the ascending loop (epicardium). Each arm develops clockwise and counterclockwise motion resulting in the development of torsion as illustrated by the cylinder on the right side of panel A. (Source: Sengupta 2008. Reproduced with permission of Elsevier.)*

counterclockwise direction and the base rotating in the opposite clockwise direction (see Figure 5.5). The difference between the rotation of the base and apex of the LV relative to the long axis is referred to as ventricular torsion.

Torsion helps bring a uniform distribution of LV fiber stress and fiber shortening across the wall, contributing to an energy-efficient ejection with minimal endocardial strain and oxygen demand.[20] The normal heart rotates as a biventricular unit as the RV free wall also rotates with basal and apical rotation and torsion with the LV.[21] Disturbances in the electrical activation sequence and electromechanical coupling results in perturbation of the twist-torsion mechanics of ventricular contraction and thus decreased mechanical contraction and ventricular function.

Abnormal activation sequence during bundle branch block

A bundle branch block (right or left) can disturb the normal, physiologic, and synchronous sequence of electrical activation previously described. In such cases, the electrical impulse is conducted slowly through the surrounding working myocardium rather than rapidly through the specialized His–Purkinje conduction system. Electrical impulses from the normal myocardium are rarely able to reenter into parts of the rapid conduction system and therefore the sequence and timing of activation is governed by slow conduction through the myocardium, This can be up to four times slower than conduction through the normal Purkinje system.[5,12] As a result, the time required for activation of the entire ventricular muscle is at least twice as long as that during normal sinus rhythm. This manifests as prolongation of the QRS duration on surface ECG.

Right ventricular apex pacing induces an electrical activation sequence similar to the electrical activation sequence in left bundle branch block, making RV apex pacing an ideal model for studying the effects of left bundle branch block (LBBB) on ventricular function. Detailed studies of the three-dimensional spread of activation during ventricular pacing have been conducted since the 1960s on canine hearts.[12,22] In pacer-induced LBBB (RV apical pacing), activation starts at the RV endocardium. The electrical impulse breaks through a single site on the LV septum and travels gradually towards the distal LV free wall with the latest activation site generally being the LV inferoposterior wall.[11,23,24]

In a typical intrinsic LBBB, ventricular activation originates from the distal branching of the right bundle, and activation of the left endocardium starts with a significant delay (more than 50ms) due to the slow conduction throughout the interventricular septum. Within the left ventricle, the impulse propagates variably depending on the etiology of the underlying heart disease. High-resolution three-dimensional endocardial mapping techniques in patients with left bundle branch block have shown that LV activation patterns may differ among patients, largely due to the differences in the origin of the LBBB.[25,26]

Given the strong relationship between excitation and contraction in the myocardium, it is not surprising that depolarization from outside the normal conducting system alters the timing of electrical depolarization, and consequently, mechanical contraction.[22,27] Asynchronous electrical activation leads to asynchronous contraction. During bundle branch block, local contraction patterns differ not only in the onset of contraction but also, and more importantly, in the pattern of contraction. This disturbance in contraction patterns causes opposing regions of the ventricular wall to become out of phase. Energy generated by one region is dissipated in opposite regions leading to a decrease in energy efficiency and pump output. In summary, abnormal asynchronous electrical activation causes abnormal mechanical contraction patterns, inefficient and depressed pump function, and ultimately ventricular remodeling.[28–32]

Site specific hemodynamics of pacing

In pediatrics, the most common indication for a pacemaker is bradycardia due to complete heart block. While pacemakers may be necessary in these children to restore a normal heart rate, ventricular pacing results in abnormal electrical activation patterns, which in turn may cause electrical and mechanical dyssynchrony and ultimately impaired cardiac function. This has led to a number of studies evaluating the effects of pacing at various cardiac sites to find the most optimal pacing site that results in the most "normal" electromechanical activation.

RV apical pacing
The right ventricle (RV) has traditionally been the target of ventricular pacing as it is easily accessible both from the systemic venous system for transvenous leads, and via a sternotomy for epicardial pacemaker leads. This position has a relatively low dislodgement rate. Studies have shown, however, that RV apical pacing is associated with left ventricular (LV) dysfunction and pacemaker induced cardiomyopathy.[29,33–39]

In structurally normal hearts, RV apical pacing results in a left bundle branch block (LBBB) electrical activation pattern with the resultant issues

mentioned above. Early RV contraction increases RV pressure before the LV contracts leading to an abnormal early systolic pressure gradient between the two ventricles. As a result, the interventricular septum moves paradoxically and bulges into the LV in systole. Both animal and human studies suggest that chronic dyssynchronous contraction due to abnormal ventricular activation patterns from RV apical pacing are associated with abnormal regional myocardial perfusion and metabolism, resulting in structural changes and systolic and diastolic LV dysfunction. [40–45] RV apical pacing also leads to morphological and histological changes in the heart, which include myofiber size variation, fibrosis, fat deposition, and mitochondrial disorganization.[29,42,46,47]

Interestingly, although RV apical pacing results in abnormal electrical activation and ventricular dyssynchrony, it tends to be well tolerated in most children.[48,49] However, several studies have shown that RV apical pacing in children is associated with structural remodeling of the LV, leading to acute and chronic impairment of LV function and heart failure.[33,34,50] Cardiomyopathy with heart failure is reported in about 7% of pediatric patients, and impaired LV function in up to 13% of the chronically RV-paced pediatric patients after a decade of follow-up.[33,38,48,51]

RV septum pacing (His pacing)
Abnormal electrical activation and development of cardiomyopathy with RV apical pacing led to the search for alternative pacing sites that would lead to more normal electrical activation patterns. The His bundle emerged as a logical possibility for a pacing site that could result in more normal ventricular depolarization. The His bundle may be directly paced by lead insertion through the RV and placement of the lead high in the septum at the location of the His bundle. In patients without distal conduction abnormalities, His-bundle pacing should produce a normal physiological sequence of activation through the His–Purkinje system and therefore avoid the dyssynchronous electrical activation and detrimental effects of RV apical pacing.

Animal studies showed that QRS duration was shorter with pacing in the high ventricular septum than with RV apex pacing.[52–54] In the 1960s, Scherlag's group showed that His bundle pacing results in the same QRS duration and pressure development as sinus rhythm and atrial pacing and produces better hemodynamics than RV apex pacing.[55,56] Karpwich et al. demonstrated that the cellular and histological myocardial changes observed with RV apical pacing in canines do not occur when normal ventricular activation is maintained with RV septal pacing.[53]

Clinical studies in adults have reported the beneficial effects of successful His-bundle pacing in patients who had AV nodal ablation for atrial fibrillation with a significant improvement in NYHA functional class, exercise tolerance, quality of life, and interventricular mechanical delay compared to right ventricular apical pacing.[57–60] Zanon et al. showed that His bundle pacing preserves normal distribution of myocardial coronary blood flow and mechanics.[61]

Technical advances have improved the success rate of His-bundle pacing in adults, but implantation in this region is challenging. The His bundle lies deep within the RV septum, surrounded by an effective insulating tissue. In a study by Zanon et al., the time needed to successfully implant the pacing lead for His-pacing varied from 2–60 minutes and required approximately four attempts. Pacing thresholds were also significantly higher than with conventional RV apical pacing.[62] Therefore, while permanent pacing of the His bundle may be effective in preventing the dyssynchrony and negative effects of right ventricular apical pacing in adults, it is a complex method requiring longer implant times and higher acute pacing thresholds, making it a less feasible option in pediatrics. In addition, children with surgically induced AV block (the majority of pediatric patients requiring pacing) may have disease more distally in the conduction system which would still lead to abnormal ventricular activation and negative hemodynamic effects.

RVOT pacing

Pacing from the RVOT gained interest as an alternative pacing site secondary to the ease of accessibility during implantation. The development of active fixation electrodes allowed for stabilization and reduced the risk of dislocation.[63]

Studies in the literature often refer to this position as "high RV septal" or "RV outflow tract". It is important to be cautious when interpreting this data as there is some divergence in how RVOT pacing is defined. In some studies, "RVOT" may imply pacing at the high RV free wall in the RVOT. Studies have shown that QRS duration with pacing in this region remains wide and is not significantly different compared to RV apical pacing.[64–67]

Results of acute and long term effects of pacing from the RVOT have been inconsistent. Stambler et al. enrolled 103 patients in a randomized cross-over study and found that there were no significant differences observed between RVOT and RV apex pacing with respect to quality of life, New York Heart Association Classification (NYHA), 6-minute walk test, or LV ejection fraction.[68] In contrast, Giudici et al. showed in a nonrandomized study that RVOT pacing at the RV free wall resulted in improved cardiac output when compared to RV apical pacing.[64] Tse et al. randomized 24 patients with complete AV block and permanent ventricular pacing at the RV apex or at the right ventricular outflow tract. After 18 months of pacing, perfusion defects and regional wall motion abnormalities were less common and ejection fractions were higher in the high septal pacing group compared to the RV apical pacing group.[69]

LV apical pacing

Of late, the search for the ideal pacing site has focused on the left ventricle. Animal studies have shown that pacing in the LV septum and apex resulted in LV pump function close to that seen during normal sinus rhythm.[70,71] Mills et al. showed that LV apical and LV septal pacing in dogs with complete AV block resulted in only moderate electrical dyssynchrony and a minor redistribution of mechanical work and perfusion, with normal levels of contractility, relaxation, and myocardial efficiency after 4 months of pacing.[72]

In adult heart failure patients, single-site LV pacing induces a physiological apex to base sequence of activation, which results in synchronous electrical activation and contraction at the circumferential level of the LV.[70,73] This is supported by the observation of Gebauer et al. that LV apical pacing, compared with other sites, preserves septal to lateral LV synchrony and systolic function.[74] Indeed, several studies have shown that chronic LV apical pacing results in better LV function and mechanical synchrony when compared to RV pacing.[75]

Studies in children now support the superior performance of LV apical pacing over RV apical pacing with respect to hemodynamic function,[76] echocardiographic indices of dyssynchrony,[77] and reverse remodeling.[78] LV pacing has been shown to acutely increase pump function when compared with RV pacing in children undergoing cardiac surgery.[76,79]

In addition, children with LV dysfunction due to chronic RV pacing have shown functional improvement and reverse remodeling when they are transitioned to single site LV apical pacing.[78,80]

Unlike the RV apex, which can be easily and safely accessed via a transvenous approach, the LV apex is not as readily accessible. Transvenous LV apex pacing utilizing a transseptal approach has been reported in the adult literature, but it is not performed routinely because of the risk of embolization and stroke with a systemic lead.[81,82] In pediatric patients who required an epicardial pacing system, an epicardial left ventricular apical pacing lead can be easily placed via mini-sternotomy or mini-thoracotomy, making this site attractive and preferable.

Strategies to restore ventricular synchrony in adult heart failure

Restoring synchrony in the failing LV in adults

The concept of utilizing a pacemaker to restore ventricular synchrony and improve congestive heart failure (CHF) was first introduced in the early 1990s in adult patients.[83] One-third of adult patients with heart failure demonstrate a LBBB, with asynchronous ventricular contraction, and resultant poor hemodynamics. This substrate thus appeared an excellent target for pacing to synchronize the electrical activation of the ventricles, thereby restoring synchronous ventricular contraction. This initial pacing strategy, commonly referred to as Cardiac Resynchronization Therapy (CRT), involved simultaneously pacing from both the right and left ventricles (biventricular pacing) after a sensed or paced atrial event and an appropriate AV delay.

The initial CRT pacing systems were employed transvenously, with a lead in the RV apical region and a lead in a tributary of the coronary sinus, preferably on the lateral or posterolateral LV wall for left ventricular pacing (Figure 5.6).[2,84] As the use of CRT became more widespread, hybrid CRT pacing systems were utilized when the LV lead could not be successfully placed transvenously through the coronary sinus. In those cases, the right atrial and right ventricular leads were placed transvenously while the LV lead was placed

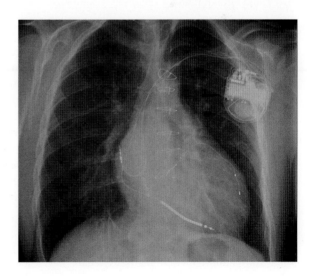

Figure 5.6 *Chest radiograph of a patient with a biventricular ICD system with transvenous right atrial, right ventricular, and left ventricular leads. The left ventricular lead is placed at the posterolateral LV wall via the coronary sinus.*

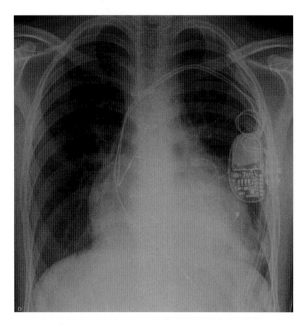

Figure 5.7 *Chest radiograph of a patient with a hybrid biventricular pacemaker system for resynchronization. The right atrial and right ventricular leads are placed transvenously while the left ventricular lead is placed epicardially via a left thoracotomy and tunneled up to the prepectoral pocket.*

epicardially through a median sternotomy or thoracotomy (Figure 5.7).

The beneficial effects of biventricular pacing for CRT in the management of adult congestive heart failure (CHF) has been validated in multiple prospective randomized trials.[1,2,84–94] The Multi-site Stimulation in Cardiomyopathy (MUSTIC) trial in 2001 was a prospective, single-blind, randomized crossover study in 48 patients in sinus rhythm with CHF due to severe left ventricular dysfunction (LVEF≤35%) and LBBB, NYHA Class III-IV, and QRS duration ≥120 ms.[84] It compared atrial synchronized biventricular (BiV) pacing to sinus rhythm with no pacing. CRT resulted in improvement in quality of life, 6-minute walk tests, and peak oxygen consumption, as well as a reduction in New York Heart Association (NYHA) classification.

These results were confirmed by the Multicenter InSync Randomized Clinical Evaluation (MIRA-CLE) trial, a prospective double-blind randomized controlled trial involving 453 adult patients with CHF, NYHA Class III, LV fraction ≤ 35%, and a QRS interval ≥130 ms randomly assigned to either a cardiac-resynchronization group with biventricular pacing (228 patients) or to a control group with no pacing (225 patients) for 6 months, while conventional therapy for heart failure was maintained.[2] The results confirmed the findings from the MUSTIC trial and showed that CRT led to improvements in NYHA classification, 6-minute walk tests, peak oxygen consumption, quality of life and a reduction in hospitalizations. In addition, this trial demonstrated that patients with CRT had reverse remodeling of the left ventricle as evidenced by reduced LV end-diastolic and end-systolic volumes, decreased LV mass, and improved LV ejection fraction. A number of large prospective adult trials have since reproduced these results demonstrating that, in the appropriate adult patient, CRT improves quality of life, decreases hospitalizations for worsening heart failure, results in reverse remodeling of the left ventricle, and can actually decrease mortality.[2,84,88,90]

A meta-analysis of multiple large randomized trials evaluating the effects of CRT in adult heart failure patients demonstrated that CRT alone, as compared with optimal medical therapy, significantly reduced all-cause mortality by 29% (Odds ratio 0.71, 95% confidence interval 0.57–0.88) and mortality due to progressive HF by 38% (Odds Ratio 0.62, 95% CI 0.45–0.84).[95] As a result, CRT has proven to be an important breakthrough in the treatment of adult heart failure.[96,97] In both European and North American guidelines, CRT is a Class I (level of evidence A) therapy for adult heart failure patients with an LV ejection fraction ≤35%, QRS duration ≥ 120 ms, and NYHA Class III-IV despite optimal medical therapy.[98-101]

A variety of cardiac and extracardiac processes are likely responsible for the long-term beneficial effects of CRT. Simultaneous biventricular pacing generates two activation wavefronts, one from each ventricle, which then merge.[73,102] As a result of this phenomenon, the time to maximum contraction in each ventricle is uniformly prolonged and thus restores a more coordinated contraction pattern. This results in a more homogenous distribution of regional loading conditions and myocardial strain.[103,104] Acute pacing studies demonstrated that improved ventricular synchrony leads to improved cardiac pump function as determined by LV dP/dt_{max}, pulse pressure, cardiac output, and ejection fraction.[102,105-108] Nelson et al. showed that restoring ventricular synchrony improves mechanical pump function while decreasing myocardial energy consumption. This suggests that CRT improves the efficiency of the cardiac pump.[109] The improved pump function reduces neurohumoral activation, evidenced by an increase in heart rate variability and a reduction in plasma brain natriuretic peptide (BNP) levels.[110] Furthermore, the improved contractility and pump efficiency at a smaller end-diastolic volume reduces mechanical ventricular stretch and may explain the beneficial reverse-remodeling effects of CRT.[103]

The preferred LV pacing site for CRT is often the latest-activated region, usually the basal part of the posterolateral LV wall.[26,111] Using extensive epicardial mapping and MRI strain analysis, Helm et al. demonstrated that, in dyssynchronous canine hearts, the area of latest electrical and mechanical activation closely matched the LV pacing site that caused the maximal LV dP/dt_{max} increase during biventricular CRT.[112] This region spans about 40% of the LV free wall, specifically the lateral wall. In addition, the optimal LV pacing site was the same regardless of whether RV pacing originated from the RV free wall or RV apex. Ansalone et al. investigated whether concordance of LV lead position and latest-activated region influences the outcome of CRT.[113] They found that the greatest effect on functional parameters was seen when the LV lead was in the latest-activated region.

Given the individual variations in etiology, severity, patterns of delayed ventricular activation, and location of scar regions in adult heart failure patients, it seems unlikely that the same pacing site will be optimal for every patient. Derval et al. investigated 11 LV pacing sites (10 endocardial LV sites, one coronary sinus site) in 35 non-ischemic dilated cardiomyopathy patients and failed to reveal a single optimal pacing site for all patients. This suggests that the optimal LV pacing site must be individualized for each patient.[114] This can be difficult to achieve when utilizing a transcoronary venous access, as LV sites are limited by underlying coronary venous anatomy.

Many strategies have been used to help identify the ideal LV pacing site, including, latest underlying LV electrogram, pressure volume loops, and mechanical indices.[107,115-119] The TARGET study, a randomized trial using echo guidance to determine optimal LV site for pacing in 220 patients undergoing CRT, found that 70% of patients with echo-guided LV leads placement had a greater than 15% reduction in LV end systolic volume at 6 months as compared to 55% of control patients.[115]

Alternative strategies for resynchronizing the failing LV in adults

Isolated left ventricular pacing has been proposed in adults to provide resynchronization in patients with LBBB and heart failure. Pacing at the LV lateral wall in a patient with LBBB creates an activation wavefront that moves in the opposite direction from the spontaneously occurring activation wavefront.[15,120] An appropriate AV interval can allow merging of the intrinsic activation originating from the right bundle with the wavefront created from the LV pacing lead. This merging wavefront leads to less electrical dyssynchrony when compared to left bundle branch block.[102]

Several studies evaluating acute hemodynamic effects of left ventricular versus biventricular pacing for resynchronization demonstrated similar or even greater benefits with left ventricular pacing alone.[105,106,109,121] In an acute hemodynamic study of 27 adult patients with a LBBB and severe heart failure due to dilated cardiomyopathy, pacing the lateral wall of the LV alone significantly improved systolic blood pressure and decreased pulmonary capillary wedge pressure compared to baseline. There was no significant difference in hemodynamic data between LV pacing alone and biventricular pacing. The QRS duration was shorter with LV pacing alone compared to baseline, but biventricular pacing resulted in a significantly shorter QRS duration when compared to LV pacing alone.[106]

A study by Blanc et al. evaluated the midterm effects of CRT using LV pacing only in 22 patients with LBBB and NYHA class III–IV.[122] The results demonstrated significant improvement in functional capacity, reverse remodeling with a decrease in LV dimensions, and increased left ventricular ejection fraction after one year. Other limited series of single-site LV pacing for CRT in adults with severe congestive heart failure have also demonstrated improved exercise tolerance and quality of life, [86] cardiac output, [109] LV resynchronization, [123] and improved LV function maintained at one year follow-up.[124]

A meta-analysis of five randomized controlled trials compared the effects of isolated left ventricular pacing to biventricular pacing for CRT in a combined total of 574 adult patients with heart failure and LBBB.[125] There were no statistically significant differences in improvement in clinical status (6-minute walk distance, quality of life, peak oxygen consumption, or NYHA class) between the two pacing methods. There was, however, a trend toward superiority of biventricular pacing over isolated left ventricular pacing for improvement in systolic function and reverse remodeling, although it did not reach statistical significance.

The clinical improvement seen in heart failure patients with isolated LV pacing may obviate right ventricular pacing entirely. This could increase the longevity of the device battery by up to 20% and simplify device implantation.[126] Despite these advantages, there are some limitations of isolated LV pacing in adult heart failure patients. CRT is indicated for adult patients with moderate to severe heart failure who are generally at high risk of sudden death and thus have indications for an implantable cardioverter-defibrillator (ICD) for primary prevention.[98] Current ICD systems require a right ventricular lead for tachyarrhythmia sensing and high-voltage therapies and therefore would require a biventricular system. In addition, while isolated left ventricular pacing for CRT does

result in clinical improvements for heart failure patients at midterm follow-up, there is insufficient evidence on whether it produces long-term improvement including decreased morbidity and mortality in adult patients with CHF.

Strategies to restore synchrony in pediatric and congenital heart disease

CRT has been successfully used in the treatment of ventricular failure in pediatric and congenital heart disease patients despite heterogeneity of anatomy and causes of electromechanical dyssynchrony. The strict application of the adult criteria for CRT to the pediatric population has many limitations. The substrate for CRT in the young is quite different from the substrate in the adult population where ischemic cardiomyopathy predominates.[127] In contrast to the adult population, the proportion of pediatric patients with the typical combination of systemic LV dysfunction and LBBB is low (9%).[127] RV dyssynchrony and a RBBB are much more common in children. The NYHA classification criteria were designed for adults, not children, and children remain clinically less symptomatic with a greater degree of cardiac dysfunction compared to adults. Estimation of ejection fraction in patients with complex anatomies is often difficult. In addition, the QRS duration varies with age such that there may be significant mechanical dyssynchrony despite a QRS duration <120 ms in a child. Taking into account these factors, CRT implantation guidelines have recently been published for adults with CHD (Table 5.1).[128]

Restoring synchrony in the failing LV

Between 45 and 77% of pediatric and congenital heart disease patients with CRT have ventricular dyssynchrony due to conventional single site pacing, usually in the right ventricle (see Video clips 5.2A and B).[127,129,130] A retrospective multicenter European study published by Janousek et al. in 2009 demonstrated major clinical improvement and LV reverse remodeling in pediatric and congenital heart disease patients with systemic left ventricles and RV pacing who were upgraded to BiV CRT (see Video clips 5.2C and D).[127] Correction of electrical dyssynchrony by CRT was highly

Table 5.1 *Recommendations for cardiac resynchronization therapy in adults with congenital heart disease*

Class I

1 Systemic LVEF ≤35%, sinus rhythm, complete LBBB with a QRS complex ≥150 ms (spontaneous or paced), and NYHA class II-IV (ambulatory) symptoms. (LOE:B)

Class IIa

1 Systemic LVEF ≤35%, sinus rhythm, complete LBBB with a QRS complex 120–149 ms (spontaneous or paced), and NYHA class II-IV (ambulatory) symptoms. (LOE:B)
2 Systemic RVEF ≤35%, right ventricular dilation, NYHA class II-IV (ambulatory) symptoms, and complete RBBB with a QRS complex ≥150 ms (spontaneous or paced). (LOE:C)
3 Systemic ventricular EF ≤35%, an intrinsically narrow QRS complex, and NYHA class I-IV (ambulatory) symptoms who are undergoing new or replacement device implantation with anticipated requirement for significant (>40%) ventricular pacing. Single-site pacing from the systemic ventricular apex/mid-lateral wall may be considered as an alternative. (LOE:C)
4 Single ventricle EF ≤35%, ventricular dilatation, NYHA class II-IV (ambulatory) symptoms, and a QRS complex ≥150 ms due to intraventricular conduction delay that produces a complete RBBB or LBBB morphology. (LOE:C)

Class IIb

1 Systemic ventricular EF >35%, an intrinsically narrow QRS complex, and NYHA class I-IV (ambulatory) symptoms who are undergoing new or replacement device implantation with anticipated requirement for significant (>40%) ventricular pacing. Single-site pacing from the systemic ventricular apex/mid-lateral wall may be considered as an alternative. (LOE:C)
2 Patients undergoing CHD surgery with an intrinsic or paced QRS duration ≥150 ms, complete bundle branch block morphology ipsilateral to the systemic ventricular (left or right), NYHA class I-IV (ambulatory) symptoms, and progressive systolic systemic ventricular dysfunction and/or dilatation or expectation of such development regardless of the ejection fraction value, especially if epicardial access is required to implement CRT. (LOE:B)
3 Systemic RV undergoing cardiac surgery for tricuspid valve regurgitation with an intrinsic or paced QRS duration ≥150 ms, complete RBBB, and NYHA class I-IV (ambulatory) symptoms, regardless of the degree of RV systolic dysfunction. (LOE:B)
4 CHD (e.g., tetralogy of Fallot) with severe subpulmonary right ventricular dilatation and dysfunction, complete RBBB with a QRS complex ≥150 ms, and NYHA class II-IV (ambulatory) symptoms. (LOE:C)
5 NYHA class IV symptoms, and severe systemic ventricular dysfunction in an attempt to delay or avert cardiac transplantation or mechanical support. (LOE:C)

Class III

1 CRT is not indicated in adults with CHD and a narrow QRS complex (<120 ms) (LOE:B)
2 CRT is not indicated in adults with CHD whose comorbidities and/or frailty limit survival with good functional capacity to less than 1 year. (LOE:C)

Notes: Class I – indicated, Class IIa – probably indicated, Class IIb – may be considered. AV- atrioventricular, CHD – congenital heart disease, CRT- cardiac resynchronization therapy, EPS- electrophysiology study, EF- ejection fraction, LBBB- Left bundle branch block, RBBB- right bundle branch block, NYHA- New York Heart Association, LV- left ventricle, RV- right ventricle, LOE-Level of Evidence.

successful in this patient subgroup, as shown by a significant decrease in QRS duration (Figure 5.8). Studies in adult patients with RV pacing induced ventricular dysfunction also demonstrated similar clinical improvement and LV reverse remodeling with upgrading to a BiV CRT system.[131,132]

Pediatric patients who develop cardiomyopathy associated with conventional RV pacing often require epicardial pacemaker systems due body size limitations. Upgrading to a biventricular device in these patients involves the addition of an epicardial LV lead (Figure 5.9). This can be placed through a

(A)   Conventional right ventricular pacing only

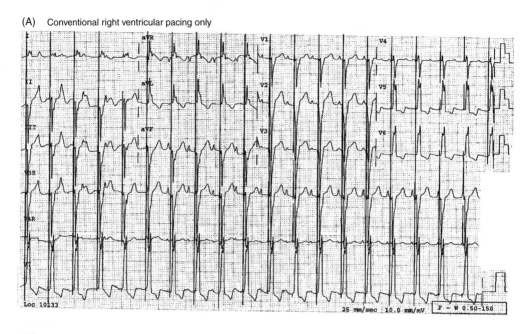

(B)   Biventricular pacing

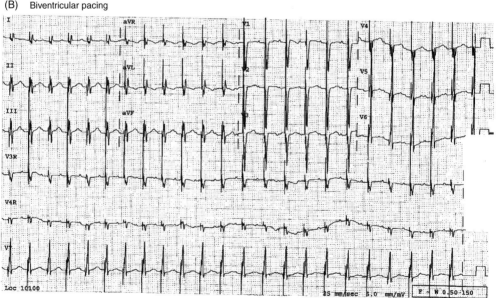

Figure 5.8 *Twelve-lead ECG of a patient with congenital complete heart block and pacing induced cardiomyopathy before and after CRT. The 12-lead ECG with conventional right ventricular apex pacing has a QRS of approximately 120 ms (A). After CRT with biventricular pacing, the QRS decreased to approximately 80 ms (B).*

mini-sternotomy, although scarring from previous surgeries or structural abnormalities in congenital heart disease may make it difficult to access the left ventricle from this approach. An alternative approach is to implant the epicardial LV lead via mini-thoracotomy. From this approach, the LV can be easily reached with excellent functional and cosmetic results (Figure 5.9).[133] The added LV lead can then be tunneled to the existing pacemaker pocket.

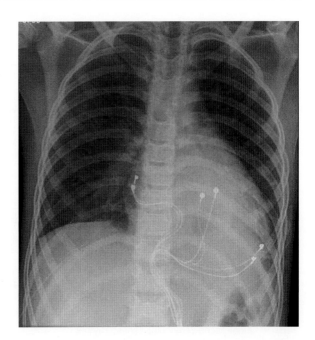

Figure 5.9 *Chest radiograph of a patient with an epicardial biventricular pacemaker system. The right atrial, right ventricular, and left ventricular leads were all placed via a midline sternotomy.*

Restoring synchrony in the failing V

More than 70% of CRT in the pediatric age group has been in the setting of congenital heart disease with 30–40% involving the RV.[129,130] The RV dysfunction and RV failure in congenital heart disease is often multifactorial in origin. It may be due to chronic pressure overload, volume overload, myocardial injury associated with cardiopulmonary bypass or surgical repair, or a combination of these factors. One model of the failing RV is seen in patients with repaired tetralogy of Fallot (TOF). These patients commonly have RBBB associated with ventricular septal defect (VSD) repair (Figure 5.10A). They develop right ventricular scar as well as RV pressure and/or volume overload secondary to pulmonary regurgitation and/or stenosis. These factors can converge to result in right-sided heart failure. Vogel et al. demonstrated abnormal regional wall motion in the RV free wall and interventricular septum using tissue Doppler imaging, suggesting a substrate for resynchronization.[134] Uebing et al. subsequently showed a delay in the onset of RV free wall contraction with correlation of severity of delay to duration of the surface QRS complex in these patients.[135]

It has been hypothesized that, similar to LV pacing in adults with LBBB, RV pacing in patients with RBBB creates an activation wavefront that moves in the opposite direction from the spontaneously occurring activation wavefront. An appropriate AV interval can allow merging of the intrinsic activation originating from the left bundle with the wavefront created from the RV pacing lead, resulting in less electrical dyssynchrony.

Initial studies in children focused on acute effects of RV pacing in patients with congenital heart disease and RBBB using temporary stimulation via epicardial pacing wires. Janousek et al. in 2001 showed that atrioventricular, intraventricular resynchronization, or a combination of both, increased systolic blood pressure in 14 post-operative patients with two ventricles and variable degrees of post-operative AV block and RBBB.[136] Resynchronization was achieved by atrial synchronous single site RV pacing in seven of these patients.

Zimmerman et al. examined the effect of multisite RV pacing in post-operative pediatric patients with RBBB after surgical repair.[137] Pacing electrodes were placed on the RV free wall, distal RVOT and diaphragmatic surface. By pacing through all three leads, simultaneous stimulation of the lateral RV free wall and RVOT was achieved. This resulted in a decrease in QRS duration, improved cardiac index, and increased systolic blood pressure.

(A)   Sinus rhythm

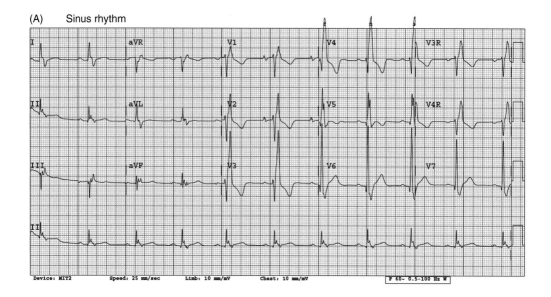

(B)   Atrial-paced ventricular-sensed rhythm

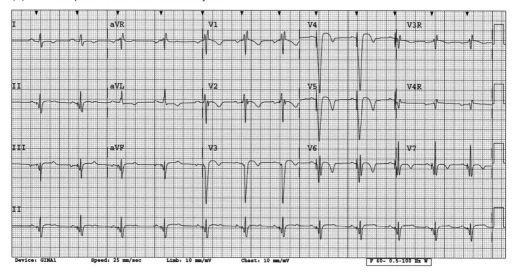

Figure 5.10 *12-lead ECG of a patient with Tetraology of Fallot in sinus rhythm with a right bundle branch block (A) and with single site right ventricular pacing for resynchronization (B). The QRS decreased from 190 ms to 120 ms with resynchronization.*

A third study by Dubin et al. evaluated the acute hemodynamic effects of transvenous single site RV pacing for resynchronization in seven patients with RBBB and RV dysfunction.[138] Transvenous pacing catheters were positioned in the RA and RV and three separate RV pacing sites (apex, outflow tract, and septum) were assessed. AV sequential pacing was performed with a PR interval that allowed for maximum fusion with the intrinsic activation wavefront. They found that AV sequential pacing in the RV decreased QRS duration and improved right ventricular dP/dt_{max} and cardiac output. The optimal RV site for pacing varied among patients and interestingly, the site that produced the narrowest QRS did not correlate with the one yielding the optimal RV function. There was, however, a strong relationship between degree of QRS improvement and increase in cardiac output. Stephenson et al. also found that RV pacing with optimization of the AV interval in patients with RBBB after Tetralogy of Fallot repair resulted in decreased QRS duration, potentially resynchronizing the RV in these patients.[139]

Thus, cardiac resynchronization therapy with chronic single site RV or biventricular stimulation has been proposed as a modality to improve right-sided heart failure. In 2008, Dubin et al. conducted a pilot prospective single-blinded crossover study in patients with TOF and right heart failure who already had a dual chamber ICD in place.[140] The patients were evaluated at baseline, after 3 months of CRT using atrial synchronous RV pacing with maximal fusion noted on EKG, and 3 months without pacing (Figure 5.10). Results demonstrated improved RV ejection fraction and quality of life in this patient population (see Video clips 5.3A and B).

Thambo et al. evaluated the immediate effects of single site RV versus biventricular stimulation in eight adult patients with TOF and RV dysfunction.[141] Single site RV stimulation resulted in improvement in RV dP/dt_{max} but a decrease in LV dP/dt_{max}. However, biventricular stimulation resulted in a decrease in QRS duration and improved contractility of both ventricles by invasive measures (LV and RV dP/dt_{max}) and by echocardiography. Interestingly, the patients in both the single site RV pacing and biventricular pacing groups had evidence of systemic LV dysfunction which may explain some of the differences seen between these finding by Thambo et al. and the previously discussed findings in the pilot study by Dubin et al. Thambo et al. also evaluated the effects of chronic biventricular CRT after 6 months in nine adult patients with TOF and RV dysfunction.[142] They found a significant improvement in exercise tolerance and NYHA functional class as well as improvement in synchrony in these patients.

Single site RV pacing has the advantage of being technically straightforward for implantation and widely applicable. While theoretically appealing, it may be difficult to maintain a stable degree of electrical fusion over a wide range of activities and heart rates with this approach, due to variations in intrinsic AV conduction. In addition, if there is a significantly prolonged baseline PR interval, this may prevent fusion between paced and physiologic activation due to limitations in the maximum programmable AV interval on current pacemaker devices. Biventricular stimulation enables a consistently homogenous ventricular activation when resynchronization with isolated RV pacing is not feasible or if concomitant LV dysfunction is present.

Patients with systemic RVs (congenitally corrected transposition of the great arteries and d-TGA patients s/p intra-atrial baffle repair) may also develop RV dysfunction. Over one-third of these patients develop moderate to severely depressed systemic RV function and impaired exercise tolerance.[143] Technical feasibility and hemodynamic benefits of CRT were formally assessed by Janousek et al. in eight patients with systemic right ventricles.[144] Six of the patients had conventional pacing systems with LV pacing induced-conduction delay and a QRS interval of 161 ± 21 ms. The RV leads were placed epicardially at the border between the basal and mid-ventricular free wall segments. Areas of late ventricular activation were targeted by measuring the latest activation time compared to intrinsic QRS during implantation. CRT was achieved by atrial synchronous simultaneous biventricular pacing. This strategy resulted in a decrease in QRS duration, reduction in interventricular mechanical delay, and modest improvements in RV function over a median of 17.4 months of follow-up.

A multicenter international study by Dubin et al. included 17 patients with systemic right ventricles.[129] These patients had a significant improvement in systemic right ventricular ejection fraction and a significant decrease in QRS duration. Thirteen of these patients had clinical improvement with a median follow-up duration of 4 months. However, these results were not supported by two studies with longer follow-up. Both Cecchin et al.[130] and Janousek et al.[127] found mixed results in patients with systemic RVs who had been resynchronized. Janousek's retrospective review of pediatric and congenital heart disease patients with CRT included 27 patients with systemic right ventricles who underwent biventricular CRT with a median follow-up duration of 7.3 months.[127] Interestingly, systemic RV patients had improvement in both EF and NYHA classification with resynchronization, but had a less pronounced response than patients with systemic LVs. A smaller benefit of CRT in a systemic RV may lie in the different RV architecture and decreased myocardial perfusion reserve as described in patients after atrial switch repair.[145,146]

Restoring synchrony in the failing single ventricle

The single ventricle patient undergoing palliative surgery remains at high risk for postoperative myocardial dysfunction. These patients may have inadequate myocardial protection, multiple scars, and a systemic right ventricle.[147,148] In fact, myocardial dysfunction remains the leading cause of death after both stage I Norwood palliation and the Fontan procedure.[147-149] The traditional management of a failing single ventricle patient after surgery is inotropic support that comes at a significant cost of increased myocardial oxygen consumption in the setting of adverse mechanical energetics. Thus, newer strategies to improve the function of the single ventricle are an important goal.

Multisite pacing CRT for the treatment of ventricular failure in single ventricle patients was first evaluated in two acute post-operative pacing studies. Zimmerman et al. initially evaluated the effects of acute multisite pacing in 14 single ventricle patients[137] while Bacha et al.[150] later evaluated the effects of acute multisite pacing in 26 post-operative patients with single ventricle anatomy. Three unipolar temporary epicardial pacing leads were placed as far apart from each other on the ventricle as possible on the right and left sided free wall and the third was placed in the midline near the apex (Figure 5.11). This allowed for simultaneous stimulation of the right and left lateral walls. Multisite ventricular pacing in both of these studies demonstrated an improvement in systolic blood pressure, cardiac index, and echocardiographic indices of synchrony. Both studies demonstrated narrowing of the QRS duration with multisite pacing despite normal baseline QRS durations.

The single center 5-year experience with multisite pacing in congenital heart disease published by Cecchin et al. included 13 patients with single

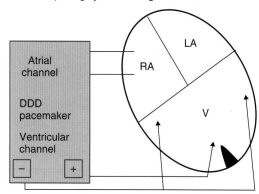

Multi-site pacing system in single ventricle

Figure 5.11 *Schema for multi-site pacing in ventricular failure in single ventricle patients. Two atrial and three ventricular tempoarary epicardial pacing leads are placed. The three ventricular pacing leads are positoned to produce an equidistant triangle with two leads as far apart as possible on the right- and left-sided free walls, and a third in the midline near the apex. The latter lead is connected to the positive port and other two leads to the negative port of the ventricular connector. RA: right atrium, LA: left atrium, V: ventricle, DDD: dual chamber pacing mode.*

ventricle physiology.[130] Eight of these patients had previous pacemakers due to complete heart block. Seven of these patients demonstrated an improvement in NYHA functional class and the median ejection fraction improved from 37 to 48% at acute follow-up. After 3–12 months of multisite pacing, the median ejection fraction was stable at 47%. Baseline median QRS in single ventricle patients was 129 ms, which shortened to 116 ms within 30 days of initiating CRT. Two of the 13 single ventricle patients were non-responders.

A retrospective multicenter European study published by Janousek et al. in 2009 included four patients with single ventricle physiology who underwent CRT with multisite pacing.[127] Three of the four patients had improvement in NYHA functional class over an average follow-up of 7.9 months while one patient was a non-responder with no change in clinical status.

In contrast, the international multicenter retrospective study published by Dubin et al. in 2005 included seven patients with single ventricle physiology.[129] These patients all received epicardial multisite pacing systems for CRT. There was no significant increase in ejection fraction or change in qualitative echo measurements, but there was a significant decrease in QRS duration. Clinical improvement was seen in only two of the seven patients.

The mixed response to CRT in single ventricle patients is a reflection of the complexity and heterogeneity of these patients. The structural abnormalities and associated morbidities make patient selection and optimal lead placement extremely challenging. Ultimately the role of CRT in improving outcomes in single ventricle patients will require a better understanding of electrical and mechanical interactions in this population.

Short and midterm outcomes of CRT in pediatric and congenital heart disease

At present, there are only two multicenter studies evaluating the effects of permanent CRT in pediatric and congenital heart disease patients. These studies both include a heterogeneous population of cardiac abnormalities including systemic left and right ventricles as well as single and two ventricle patients.

The first, published in 2005 by Dubin et al., included 103 patients from 22 international institutions.[129] The median duration of follow-up was 4 months with a range from 22 days to one year. CRT resulted in a statistically significant increase in the ejection fraction by 13% and a decrease in QRS duration by 40 ms. There did not appear to be any significant difference when comparing improvement in ejection fraction or QRS duration by type of heart disease. Of the 18 patients listed for transplantation at the time of CRT implantation, three improved and were removed from active listing, five underwent transplantation, and eight were still awaiting transplant. There were 11 non-responders (10.7%) to CRT, defined as those who either had no change or a decrease in their ejection fraction, a substantially lower non-response rate compared to the 30% seen in adult trials.[84] The only difference between responders and non-responders was the higher initial systemic ejection fraction in non-responders although the analysis did not include the type of heart disease as an independent variable.

The overall adverse event rate with CRT in Dubin's study was 29%, which is comparable to the experience with adults.[151] Overall mortality was 5% which is also comparable to the 5% mortality reported in the Multicenter Insync Randomized Clinical Evaluation (MIRACLE) trial.[152] Coronary sinus lead issues were found in 18% of all transvenous pacemakers placed, which accounted for 23% of the reported complications and were the single most common major complication. This is somewhat higher than the complication rate found in the MIRACLE trial in adults (12% for dissection, perforation, or lead dislodgement).[152] This may be related to anatomic issues found in the pediatric patient or patient with congenital heart disease. No differences in complication rates could be seen when comparing transvenous placement versus epicardial or mixed placement devices.

The second study, published by Janousek et al., included 109 patients from 17 European pediatric cardiology and cardiac surgery centers. The median duration of follow-up was 7.5 months.[127] CRT resulted in improvement in ejection fraction by 11.5%, decrease in QRS duration by 30 ms, and improvement in NYHA functional class. Of the 10 patients originally listed for heart transplantation, 4 were removed from the transplant list because of improvement in cardiac function with CRT. The presence of a systemic left ventricle was the strongest multivariable predictor of improvement in ventricular function with CRT. There were 15 non-responders (18.5%), substantially fewer than the 30% non-response rate seen in the adult literature. Two independent predictors of non-response were identified by multivariable analysis. Patients with idiopathic dilated cardiomyopathy responded poorly to CRT suggesting that CRT is ineffective in reversing the malignant course of this disease in pediatrics. A poor initial NYHA class also predicted non-responders, with the majority of non-responders being NYHA Class III or IV. The acute complication rate was 9.2% in this study but with CRT lead dislodgement accounting for only 1.8% of complications.

Although there are no large prospective and randomized trial data in pediatric and congenital heart disease, these retrospective studies show that CRT is similarly effective for managing dyssynchrony associated heart failure in this young heterogeneous population, as it is for treating adults with ischemic cardiomyopathy. At present, there are no long-term outcome studies of CRT in the pediatric and congenital heart disease population. Perera et al. recently presented the largest single-center retrospective study with the longest follow-up period thus far (67 patients with a mean follow-up of 2.75 years). Forty-eight patients (72%) received conventional pacing before upgrading to CRT. There was an overall increase in EF of 10%, a decrease in QRS duration by 27 ms, and a decrease in systemic ventricular end-diastolic volume by 39 mL. There were five deaths (7%), including two sudden deaths, and there was an overall increased incidence of ventricular tachyarrhythmias noted with CRT (10% before CRT versus 25% after CRT). It is disturbing that the incidence of ventricular arrhythmias doubled after CRT. Whether this is the natural history of the disease or some proarrhythmia effect secondary to heterogeneous depolarization caused by CRT is unclear.[153]

CRT offers significant benefit in specific pediatric patients. Appropriate patient identification is crucial in maximizing the effectiveness of this treatment modality. A recent single center retrospective study by Schiller et al. demonstrated that the currently recommended Class I criteria for CRT in adults were inadequate for the pediatric dilated cardiomyopathy population as none of the study subjects fulfilled the LBBB criteria for CRT.[154] Clearly, further work is required to delineate who will best benefit from CRT in this complex and heterogeneous group of patients and which diagnostic instruments will be the most useful in identifying CRT responders.[155]

Innovative tools such as noninvasive assessment of dyssynchrony by 3D echocardiography, 2D speckle-tracking strain analysis, electrocardiographic imaging (ECGI), as well as assessment of electrical dyssynchrony by 3D electroanatomical mapping can help localize optimal pacing sites for improved response to CRT.[112,156–162] Intra-cardiac mapping and ECGI enable a detailed analysis of electrical activation sequences far beyond that of the standard 12-lead ECG and can be used as a tool to better understand the relationship between electrical and mechanical dyssynchrony in complex congenital heart disease patients where patient selection criteria for CRT are less well defined.

Conclusions

Direct comparison of electrical activation patterns with parameters of mechanical dyssynchrony will be important in understanding the relationship between electromechanical interactions and hopefully, in optimizing pacing strategies for the most effective cardiac resynchronization therapy.

References

1 Young JB, Abraham WT, Smith AL, et al. Combined cardiac resynchronization and implantable cardioversion defibrillation in advanced chronic heart failure: the MIRACLE ICD Trial. *JAMA*. 2003; 289(20): 2685–2694.

2 Abraham WT, Fisher WG, Smith AL, et al. MIRACLE Study Group. Multicenter InSync Randomized Clinical Evaluation. Cardiac resynchronization in chronic heart failure. *N Engl J Med*. 2002; 346(24): 1845–1853.

3 Ellenbogen K, Wilkoff B, Kay G, et al. *Clinical Cardiac Pacing, Defibrillation, and Resynchronization Therapy*, 4th Edn. Philadelphia: Elsevier Saunders; 2011.

4 Smeets JLRM, Ben-Haim SA, Rodriguez L-M, et al. New method for nonfluoroscopic endocardial mapping in humans: accuracy assessment and first clinical results. *Circulation*. 1998; 97(24): 2426–2432.

5 Myerburg RJ, Nilsson K, Gelband H. Physiology of canine intraventricular conduction and endocardial excitation. *Circulation Research*. 1972; 30(2): 217–243.

6 Saffitz JE, Davis LM, Darrow BJ, et al. The molecular basis of anisotropy: role of gap junctions. *Journal of Cardiovascular Electrophysiology*. 1995; 6(6): 498–510.

7 Scher AM, Young AC, Malmghen AL, et al. Spread of electrical activity through the wall of the ventricle. *Circulation Research*. 1953; 1(6): 539–547.

8 Scher AM, Young AC, Malmgren AL, et al. Activation of the interventricular septum. *Circulation Research*. 1955; 3(1): 56–64.

9 Uhley HN, Rivkin L. Peripheral distribution of the canine A-V conduction system: Observations on gross morphology. *The American Journal of Cardiology*. 1960; 5(5): 688–691.

10 Berenfeld O, Jalife J. Purkinje-muscle reentry as a mechanism of polymorphic ventricular arrhythmias in a 3-dimensional model of the ventricles. *Circulation Research*. 1998; 82(10): 1063–1077.

11 Durrer D, Van Dam RT, Freud GE, et al. Total excitation of the isolated human heart. *Circulation*. 1970; 41(6): 899–912.

12 Spach M, Barr R. Analysis of ventricular activation and repolarization from intramural and epicardial potential distributions for ectopic beats in the intact dog. *Circulation Research*. 1975; 37(6): 830–843.

13 Motonaga KS, Miyake CY, Punn R, et al. Insights into dyssynchrony in hypoplastic left heart syndrome. *Heart Rhythm*. 2012; 9(12): 2010–2015.

14 Knollmann BC, Roden DM. A genetic framework for improving arrhythmia therapy. *Nature*. 2008; 451(7181): 929–936.

15 Prinzen FW, Augustijn CH, Allessie MA, et al. The time sequence of electrical and mechanical activation during spontaneous beating and ectopic stimulation. *Eur Heart J*. 1992; 13(4): 535–543.

16 Gi C. Load and length regulation of cardiac energetics. *Annu Rev Physiol*. 1990; 52: 505–522.

17 Torrent-Guasp F, Buckberg GD, Clemente C, et al. The structure and function of the helical heart and its buttress wrapping. I. The normal macroscopic structure of the heart. *Semin Thorac Cardiovasc Surg*. 2001; 13(4): 301–319.

18 Torrent-Guasp F, Ballester M, Buckberg GD, et al. Spatial orientation of the ventricular muscle band: physiologic contribution and surgical implications. *J Thorac Cardiovasc Surg*. 2001; 122(2): 389–392.

19 Sengupta PP, Tajik AJ, Chandrasekaran K, et al. Twist mechanics of the left ventricle: principles and application. *JACC Cardiovasc Imaging*. 2008; 1(3): 366–376.

20 Arts T, Veenstra PC, Reneman RS. Epicardial deformation and left ventricular wall mechanisms during ejection in the dog. *Am J Physiol*. 1982; 243(3): H379–390.

21 Haber I, Metaxas DN, Geva T, et al. Three-dimensional systolic kinematics of the right ventricle. *Am J Physiol Heart Circ Physiol*. 2005; 289(5): H1826–1833.

22 Lister JW, Klotz DH, Jomain SL, et al. Effect of pacemaker site on cardiac output and ventricular activation in dogs with complete heart block. *Am J Cardiol*. 1964; 14: 494–503.

23 Vassallo JA, Cassidy DM, Marchlinski FE, et al. Endocardial activation of left bundle branch block. *Circulation*. 1984; 69(5): 914–923.

24 Vassallo JA, Cassidy DM, Miller JM, et al. Left ventricular endocardial activation during right ventricular pacing: effect of underlying heart disease. *J Am Coll Cardiol*. 1986; 7(6): 1228–1233.

25 Auricchio A, Fantoni C, Regoli F, et al. Characterization of left ventricular activation in patients with heart failure and left bundle-branch block. *Circulation*. 2004; 109(9): 1133–1139.

26 Rodriguez LM, Timmermans C, Nabar A, et al. Variable patterns of septal activation in patients with left bundle branch block and heart failure. *J Cardiovasc Electrophysiol*. 2003; 14(2): 135–141.

27 Badke FR, Boinay P, Covell JW. Effects of ventricular pacing on regional left ventricular performance in the dog. *Am J Physiol*. 1980; 238(6): H858–H867.

28 Prinzen F, Vernooy K, Deboeck B, et al. Mechano-energetics of the asynchronous and resynchronized heart. *Heart Fail Rev*. 2011; 16(3): 215–224.

29 Karpawich PP, Rabah R, Haas JE. Altered cardiac histology following apical right ventricular pacing in patients with congenital atrioventricular block. *Pacing Clin Electrophysiol*. 1999; 22(9): 1372–1377.

30 Prinzen FW, Peschar M. Relation between the pacing induced sequence of activation and left ventricular pump function in animals. *Pacing and Clinical Electrophysiology*. 2002; 25(4): 484–498.

31 Vernooy K, Verbeek XA, Peschar M, et al. Left bundle branch block induces ventricular remodelling and functional septal hypoperfusion. *Eur Heart J*. 2005; 26(1): 91–98.

32 Vernooy K, Verbeek XaaM, Peschar M, et al. Relation between abnormal ventricular impulse conduction and heart failure. *Journal of Interventional Cardiology*. 2003; 16(6): 557–562.

33 Moak JP, Barron KS, Hougen TJ, et al. Congenital heart block: development of late-onset cardiomyopathy, a previously underappreciated sequela. *J Am Coll Cardiol*. 2001; 37(1): 238–242.

34 Tantengco MV, Thomas RL, Karpawich PP. Left ventricular dysfunction after long-term right ventricular apical pacing in the young. *J Am Coll Cardiol*. 2001; 37(8): 2093–2100.

35 Karpawich PP. Chronic right ventricular pacing and cardiac performance: the pediatric perspective. *Pacing Clin Electrophysiol*. 2004; 27(6 Pt 2): 844–849.

36 Thambo JB, Bordachar P, Garrigue S, et al. Detrimental ventricular remodeling in patients with congenital complete heart block and chronic right ventricular apical pacing. *Circulation*. 2004; 110(25): 3766–3772.

37 Janousek J, Tomek V, Chaloupecky V, et al. Dilated cardiomyopathy associated with dual-chamber pacing in infants: improvement through either left ventricular cardiac resynchronization or programming the pacemaker off allowing intrinsic normal conduction. *J Cardiovasc Electrophysiol*. 2004; 15(4): 470–474.

38 Kim JJ, Friedman RA, Eidem BW, et al. Ventricular function and long-term pacing in children with congenital complete atrioventricular block. *J Cardiovasc Electrophysiol*. 2007; 18(4): 373–377.

39 Manolis AS. The deleterious consequences of right ventricular apical pacing: time to seek alternate site pacing. *Pacing Clin Electrophysiol*. 2006; 29(3): 298–315.

40 Rosenqvist M, Isaaz K, Botvinick EH, et al. Relative importance of activation sequence compared to atrioventricular synchrony in left ventricular function. *Am J Cardiol*. 1991; 67(2): 148–156.

41 Prinzen FW, Van Oosterhout MF, Vanagt WY, et al. Optimization of ventricular function by improving

the activation sequence during ventricular pacing. *Pacing Clin Electrophysiol.* 1998; 21(11 Pt 2): 2256–2260.

42 Prinzen FW, Hunter WC, Wyman BT, et al. Mapping of regional myocardial strain and work during ventricular pacing: experimental study using magnetic resonance imaging tagging. *J Am Coll Cardiol.* 1999; 33(6): 1735–1742.

43 Nielsen JC, Bottcher M, Nielsen TT, et al. Regional myocardial blood flow in patients with sick sinus syndrome randomized to long-term single chamber atrial or dual chamber pacing—effect of pacing mode and rate. *J Am Coll Cardiol.* 2000; 35(6): 1453–1461.

44 Skalidis EI, Kochiadakis GE, Koukouraki SI, et al. Myocardial perfusion in patients with permanent ventricular pacing and normal coronary arteries. *J Am Coll Cardiol.* 2001; 37(1): 124–129.

45 Tse HF, Lau CP. Long-term effect of right ventricular pacing on myocardial perfusion and function. *J Am Coll Cardiol.* 1997; 29(4): 744–749.

46 Prinzen FW, Cheriex EC, Delhaas T, et al. Asymmetric thickness of the left ventricular wall resulting from asynchronous electric activation: a study in dogs with ventricular pacing and in patients with left bundle branch block. *Am Heart J.* 1995; 130(5): 1045–1053.

47 Karpawich PP, Justice CD, Cavitt DL, et al. Developmental sequelae of fixed-rate ventricular pacing in the immature canine heart: an electrophysiologic, hemodynamic, and histopathologic evaluation. *Am Heart J.* 1990; 119(5): 1077–1083.

48 Vatasescu R, Shalganov T, Paprika D, et al. Evolution of left ventricular function in paediatric patients with permanent right ventricular pacing for isolated congenital heart block: a medium term follow-up. *Europace.* 2007; 9(4): 228–232.

49 Shalganov TN, Paprika D, Vatasescu R, et al. Mid-term echocardiographic follow up of left ventricular function with permanent right ventricular pacing in pediatric patients with and without structural heart disease. *Cardiovasc Ultrasound.* 2007; 5: 13.

50 Karpawich PP, Mital S. Comparative left ventricular function following atrial, septal, and apical single chamber heart pacing in the young. *Pacing Clin Electrophysiol.* 1997; 20(8 Pt 1): 1983–1988.

51 Gebauer RA, Tomek V, Salameh A, et al. Predictors of left ventricular remodelling and failure in right ventricular pacing in the young. *Eur Heart J.* 2009; 30(9): 1097–1104.

52 Rosenqvist M, Bergfeldt L, Haga Y, et al. The effect of ventricular activation sequence on cardiac performance during pacing. *Pacing Clin Electrophysiol.* 1996; 19(9): 1279–1286.

53 Karpawich PP, Justice CD, Chang CH, et al. Septal ventricular pacing in the immature canine heart: a new perspective. *Am Heart J.* 1991; 121(3 Pt 1): 827–833.

54 Karpawich PP, Gates J, Stokes KB. Septal His-Purkinje ventricular pacing in canines: a new endocardial electrode approach. *Pacing Clin Electrophysiol.* 1992; 15(11 Pt 2): 2011–2015.

55 Kosowsky BD, Scherlag BJ, Damato AN. Re-evaluation of the atrial contribution to ventricular function: study using His bundle pacing. *Am J Cardiol.* 1968; 21(4): 518–524.

56 Scherlag BJ, Kosowsky BD, Damato AN. A technique for ventricular pacing from the His bundle of the intact heart. *J Appl Physiol.* 1967; 22(3): 584–587.

57 Deshmukh P, Casavant DA, Romanyshyn M, et al. Permanent, direct His-bundle pacing: a novel approach to cardiac pacing in patients with normal His–Purkinje activation. *Circulation.* 2000; 101(8): 869–877.

58 Deshmukh PM, Romanyshyn M. Direct His-bundle pacing: present and future. *Pacing Clin Electrophysiol.* 2004; 27(6 Pt 2): 862–870.

59 Mera F, Delurgio DB, Patterson RE, et al. A comparison of ventricular function during high right ventricular septal and apical pacing after His-bundle ablation for refractory atrial fibrillation. *Pacing and Clinical Electrophysiology.* 1999; 22(8): 1234–1239.

60 Occhetta E, Bortnik M, Magnani A, et al. Prevention of ventricular desynchronization by permanent para-Hisian pacing after atrioventricular node ablation in chronic atrial fibrillation: a crossover, blinded, randomized study versus apical right ventricular pacing. *J Am Coll Cardiol.* 2006; 47(10): 1938–1945.

61 Zanon F, Bacchiega E, Rampin L, et al. Direct His bundle pacing preserves coronary perfusion compared with right ventricular apical pacing: a prospective, cross-over mid-term study. *Europace.* 2008; 10(5): 580–587.

62 Zanon F, Baracca E, Aggio S, et al. A feasible approach for direct His-bundle pacing using a new steerable catheter to facilitate precise lead placement. *J Cardiovasc Electrophysiol.* 2006; 17(1): 29–33.

63 Barin ES, Jones SM, Ward DE, et al. The right ventricular outflow tract as an alternative permanent pacing site: long-term follow-up. *Pacing Clin Electrophysiol.* 1991; 14(1): 3–6.

64 Giudici MC, Thornburg GA, Buck DL, et al. Comparison of right ventricular outflow tract and apical lead permanent pacing on cardiac output. *Am J Cardiol.* 1997; 79(2): 209–212.

65 Victor F, Leclercq C, Mabo P, et al. Optimal right ventricular pacing site in chronically implanted patients: a prospective randomized crossover comparison of

apical and outflow tract pacing. *J Am Coll Cardiol.* 1999; 33(2): 311–316.

66 Buckingham TA, Candinas R, Schlapfer J, et al. Acute hemodynamic effects of atrioventricular pacing at differing sites in the right ventricle individually and simultaneously. *Pacing Clin Electrophysiol.* 1997; 20(4 Pt 1): 909–915.

67 Schwaab B, Frohlig G, Alexander C, et al. Influence of right ventricular stimulation site on left ventricular function in atrial synchronous ventricular pacing. *J Am Coll Cardiol.* 1999; 33(2): 317–323.

68 Stambler BS, Ellenbogen K, Zhang X, et al. Right ventricular outflow versus apical pacing in pacemaker patients with congestive heart failure and atrial fibrillation. *J Cardiovasc Electrophysiol.* 2003; 14(11): 1180–1186.

69 Tse HF, Yu C, Wong KK, et al. Functional abnormalities in patients with permanent right ventricular pacing: the effect of sites of electrical stimulation. *J Am Coll Cardiol.* 2002; 40(8): 1451–1458.

70 Peschar M, De Swart H, Michels KJ, et al. Left ventricular septal and apex pacing for optimal pump function in canine hearts. *J Am Coll Cardiol.* 2003; 41(7): 1218–1226.

71 Tyers GF. Comparison of the effect on cardiac function of single-site and simultaneous multiple-site ventricular stimulation after A-V block. *J Thorac Cardiovasc Surg.* 1970; 59(2): 211–217.

72 Mills R, Cornelussen R, Mulligan L, et al. Left ventricular septal and left ventricular apical pacing chronically maintain cardiac contractile coordination, pump function and efficiency. *Circ Arrhythm Electrophysiol.* 2009; 2(5): 571–579.

73 Wyman BT, Hunter WC, Prinzen FW, et al. Effects of single- and biventricular pacing on temporal and spatial dynamics of ventricular contraction. *Am J Physiol Heart Circ Physiol.* 2002; 282(1): H372–379.

74 Gebauer RA, Tomek V, Kubuš P, et al. Differential effects of the site of permanent epicardial pacing on left ventricular synchrony and function in the young: implications for lead placement. *Europace.* 2009; 11(12): 1654–1659.

75 Tomaske M, Breithardt OA, Bauersfeld U. Preserved cardiac synchrony and function with single-site left ventricular epicardial pacing during mid-term follow-up in paediatric patients. *Europace.* 2009; 11(9): 1168–1176.

76 Vanagt WY, Verbeek XA, Delhaas T, et al. The left ventricular apex is the optimal site for pediatric pacing: correlation with animal experience. *Pacing Clin Electrophysiol.* 2004; 27(6 Pt 2): 837–843.

77 Gebauer RA, Tomek V, Kubus P, et al. Differential effects of the site of permanent epicardial pacing on left ventricular synchrony and function in the young: implications for lead placement. *Europace.* 2009; 11(12): 1654–1659.

78 Vanagt WY, Prinzen FW, Delhaas T. Reversal of pacing-induced heart failure by left ventricular apical pacing. *N Engl J Med.* 2007; 357(25): 2637–2638.

79 Vanagt WY, Verbeek XA, Delhaas T, et al. Acute hemodynamic benefit of left ventricular apex pacing in children. *Ann Thorac Surg.* 2005; 79(3): 932–936.

80 Tomaske M, Breithardt OA, Balmer C, et al. Successful cardiac resynchronization with single-site left ventricular pacing in children. *Int J Cardiol.* 2009; 136(2): 136–143.

81 Pasquie JL, Massin F, Macia JC, et al. Long-term follow-up of biventricular pacing using a totally endocardial approach in patients with end-stage cardiac failure. *Pacing Clin Electrophysiol.* 2007; 30(1): S31–33.

82 Jais P, Takahashi A, Garrigue S, et al. Mid-term follow-up of endocardial biventricular pacing. *Pacing Clin Electrophysiol.* 2000; 23(11 Pt 2): 1744–1747.

83 Cazeau S, Ritter P, Bakdach S, et al. Four chamber pacing in dilated cardiomyopathy. *Pacing Clin Electrophysiol.* 1994; 17(11 Pt 2): 1974–1979.

84 Cazeau S, Leclercq C, Lavergne T, et al. Effects of multisite biventricular pacing in patients with heart failure and intraventricular conduction delay. *N Engl J Med.* 2001; 344(12): 873–880.

85 Auricchio A, Stellbrink C, Sack S, et al. Long-term clinical effect of hemodynamically optimized cardiac resynchronization therapy in patients with heart failure and ventricular conduction delay. *J Am Coll Cardiol.* 2002; 39(12): 2026–2033.

86 Auricchio A, Stellbrink C, Butter C, et al. Clinical efficacy of cardiac resynchronization therapy using left ventricular pacing in heart failure patients stratified by severity of ventricular conduction delay. *J Am Coll Cardiol.* 2003; 42(12): 2109–2116.

87 Higgins SL, Hummel JD, Niazi IK, et al. Cardiac resynchronization therapy for the treatment of heart failure in patients with intraventricular conduction delay and malignant ventricular tachyarrhythmias. *J Am Coll Cardiol.* 2003; 42(8): 1454–1459.

88 Bristow MR, Saxon LA, Boehmer J, et al. Cardiac-resynchronization therapy with or without an implantable defibrillator in advanced chronic heart failure. *N Engl J Med.* 2004; 350(21): 2140–2150.

89 Anand IS, Carson P, Galle E, et al. Cardiac resynchronization therapy reduces the risk of hospitalizations in patients with advanced heart failure: results from the Comparison of Medical Therapy, Pacing and Defibrillation in Heart Failure (COMPANION) trial. *Circulation.* 2009; 119(7): 969–977.

90 Cleland JG, Daubert JC, Erdmann E, et al. The effect of cardiac resynchronization on morbidity and mortality in heart failure. *N Engl J Med.* 2005; 352(15): 1539–1549.

91 Linde C, Abraham WT, Gold MR, et al. Randomized trial of cardiac resynchronization in mildly symptomatic heart failure patients and in asymptomatic patients with left ventricular dysfunction and previous heart failure symptoms. *J Am Coll Cardiol.* 2008; 52(23): 1834–1843.

92 Moss AJ, Hall WJ, Cannom DS, et al. Cardiac-resynchronization therapy for the prevention of heart-failure events. *N Engl J Med.* 2009; 361(14): 1329–1338.

93 Tang AS, Wells GA, Talajic M, et al. Cardiac-resynchronization therapy for mild-to-moderate heart failure. *N Engl J Med.* 2010; 363(25): 2385–2395.

94 Abraham WT, Young JB, Leon AR, et al. Effects of cardiac resynchronization on disease progression in patients with left ventricular systolic dysfunction, an indication for an implantable cardioverter-defibrillator, and mildly symptomatic chronic heart failure. *Circulation.* 2004; 110(18): 2864–2868.

95 Rivero-Ayerza M, Theuns DA, Garcia-Garcia HM, et al. Effects of cardiac resynchronization therapy on overall mortality and mode of death: a meta-analysis of randomized controlled trials. *Eur Heart J.* 2006; 27(22): 2682–2688.

96 Bertoldi EG, Polanczyk CA, Cunha V, et al. Mortality reduction of cardiac resynchronization and implantable cardioverter-defibrillator therapy in heart failure: an updated meta-analysis. Does recent evidence change the standard of care? *J Card Fail.* 2011; 17(10): 860–866.

97 Rossi A, Rossi G, Piacenti M, et al. The current role of cardiac resynchronization therapy in reducing mortality and hospitalization in heart failure patients: a meta-analysis from clinical trials. *Heart Vessels.* 2008; 23(4): 217–223.

98 Dickstein K, Vardas PE, Auricchio A, et al. 2010 Focused Update of ESC Guidelines on device therapy in heart failure: an update of the 2008 ESC Guidelines for the diagnosis and treatment of acute and chronic heart failure and the 2007 ESC Guidelines for cardiac and resynchronization therapy. Developed with the special contribution of the Heart Failure Association and the European Heart Rhythm Association. *Europace.* 2010; 12(11): 1526–1536.

99 Stevenson WG, Hernandez AF, Carson PE, et al. Indications for cardiac resynchronization therapy: 2011 Update from the Heart Failure Society of America Guideline Committee. *Journal of Cardiac Failure.* 2012; 18(2): 94–106.

100 McMurray JJ, Adamopoulos S, Anker SD, et al. ESC Guidelines for the diagnosis and treatment of acute and chronic heart failure 2012: The Task Force for the Diagnosis and Treatment of Acute and Chronic Heart Failure 2012 of the European Society of Cardiology. Developed in collaboration with the Heart Failure Association (HFA) of the ESC. *Eur Heart J.* 2012; 33(14): 1787–1847.

101 Tracy CM, Epstein AE, Darbar D, et al. 2012 ACCF/AHA/HRS focused update of the 2008 guidelines for device-based therapy of cardiac rhythm abnormalities: a report of the American College of Cardiology Foundation/American Heart Association Task Force on Practice Guidelines. *Circulation.* 2012; 126(14): 1784–1800.

102 Verbeek XA, Vernooy K, Peschar M, et al. Intraventricular resynchronization for optimal left ventricular function during pacing in experimental left bundle branch block. *J Am Coll Cardiol.* 2003; 42(3): 558–567.

103 Yu CM, Chau E, Sanderson JE, et al. Tissue Doppler echocardiographic evidence of reverse remodeling and improved synchronicity by simultaneously delaying regional contraction after biventricular pacing therapy in heart failure. *Circulation.* 2002; 105(4): 438–445.

104 Klimusina J, De Boeck BW, Leenders GE, et al. Redistribution of left ventricular strain by cardiac resynchronization therapy in heart failure patients. *Eur J Heart Fail.* 2011; 13(2): 186–194.

105 Auricchio A, Stellbrink C, Block M, et al. Effect of pacing chamber and atrioventricular delay on acute systolic function of paced patients with congestive heart failure. The Pacing Therapies for Congestive Heart Failure Study Group. The Guidant Congestive Heart Failure Research Group. *Circulation.* 1999; 99(23): 2993–3001.

106 Blanc JJ, Etienne Y, Gilard M, et al. Evaluation of different ventricular pacing sites in patients with severe heart failure: results of an acute hemodynamic study. *Circulation.* 1997; 96(10): 3273–3277.

107 Dekker AL, Phelps B, Dijkman B, et al. Epicardial left ventricular lead placement for cardiac resynchronization therapy: optimal pace site selection with pressure-volume loops. *J Thorac Cardiovasc Surg.* 2004; 127(6): 1641–1647.

108 Van Gelder BM, Bracke FA, Meijer A, et al. Effect of optimizing the VV interval on left ventricular contractility in cardiac resynchronization therapy. *Am J Cardiol.* 2004; 93(12): 1500–1503.

109 Nelson GS, Berger RD, Fetics BJ, et al. Left ventricular or biventricular pacing improves cardiac function at diminished energy cost in patients with

dilated cardiomyopathy and left bundle-branch block. *Circulation.* 2000; 102(25): 3053–3059.

110 Adamson PB, Kleckner KJ, Vanhout WL, et al. Cardiac resynchronization therapy improves heart rate variability in patients with symptomatic heart failure. *Circulation.* 2003; 108(3): 266–269.

111 Auricchio A, Abraham WT. Cardiac resynchronization therapy: current state of the art: cost versus benefit. *Circulation.* 2004; 109(3): 300–307.

112 Helm RH, Byrne M, Helm PA, et al. Three-dimensional mapping of optimal left ventricular pacing site for cardiac resynchronization. *Circulation.* 2007; 115(8): 953–961.

113 Ansalone G, Giannantoni P, Ricci R, et al. Doppler myocardial imaging to evaluate the effectiveness of pacing sites in patients receiving biventricular pacing. *J Am Coll Cardiol.* 2002; 39(3): 489–499.

114 Derval N, Steendijk P, Gula LJ, et al. Optimizing hemodynamics in heart failure patients by systematic screening of left ventricular pacing sites: the lateral left ventricular wall and the coronary sinus are rarely the best sites. *J Am Coll Cardiol.* 2010; 55(6): 566–575.

115 Khan FZ, Virdee MS, Palmer CR, et al. Targeted left ventricular lead placement to guide cardiac resynchronization therapy: the TARGET study: a randomized, controlled trial. *J Am Coll Cardiol.* 2012; 59(17): 1509–1518.

116 Polasek R, Kucera P, Nedbal P, et al. Local electrogram delay recorded from left ventricular lead at implant predicts response to cardiac resynchronization therapy: retrospective study with 1 year follow up. *BMC Cardiovasc Disord.* 2012; 12: 34.

117 Duckett SG, Ginks M, Shetty AK, et al. Invasive acute hemodynamic response to guide left ventricular lead implantation predicts chronic remodeling in patients undergoing cardiac resynchronization therapy. *J Am Coll Cardiol.* 2011; 58(11): 1128–1136.

118 Boogers MJ, Chen J, Van Bommel RJ, et al. Optimal left ventricular lead position assessed with phase analysis on gated myocardial perfusion SPECT. *Eur J Nucl Med Mol Imaging.* 2011; 38(2): 230–238.

119 Blendea D, Singh JP. Lead positioning strategies to enhance response to cardiac resynchronization therapy. *Heart Fail Rev.* 2011; 16(3): 291–303.

120 Wyman BT, Hunter WC, Prinzen FW, et al. Mapping propagation of mechanical activation in the paced heart with MRI tagging. *Am J Physiol.* 1999; 276(3 Pt 2): H881–891.

121 Bordachar P, Lafitte S, Reuter S, et al. Biventricular pacing and left ventricular pacing in heart failure: similar hemodynamic improvement despite marked electromechanical differences. *J Cardiovasc Electrophysiol.* 2004; 15(12): 1342–1347.

122 Blanc JJ, Bertault-Valls V, Fatemi M, et al. Midterm benefits of left univentricular pacing in patients with congestive heart failure. *Circulation.* 2004; 109(14): 1741–1744.

123 Turner MS, Bleasdale RA, Vinereanu D, et al. Electrical and mechanical components of dyssynchrony in heart failure patients with normal QRS duration and left bundle-branch block: impact of left and biventricular pacing. *Circulation.* 2004; 109(21): 2544–2549.

124 Gasparini M, Bocchiardo M, Lunati M, et al. Comparison of 1-year effects of left ventricular and biventricular pacing in patients with heart failure who have ventricular arrhythmias and left bundle-branch block: the Bi vs Left ventricular pacing: an International pilot Evaluation on heart failure patients with VEntricular arrhythmias (BELIEVE) multicenter prospective randomized pilot study. *Am Heart J.* 2006; 152(1): e1–7.

125 Liang Y, Pan W, Su Y, et al. Meta-analysis of randomized controlled trials comparing isolated left ventricular and biventricular pacing in patients with chronic heart failure. *Am J Cardiol.* 2011; 108(8): 1160–1165.

126 Boriani G, Kranig W, Donal E, et al. A randomized double-blind comparison of biventricular versus left ventricular stimulation for cardiac resynchronization therapy: the Biventricular versus Left Univentricular Pacing with ICD Back-up in Heart Failure Patients (B-LEFT HF) trial. *Am Heart J.* 2010; 159(6): 1052–1058.

127 Janoušek J, Gebauer RA, Abdul-Khaliq H, et al. Cardiac resynchronisation therapy in paediatric and congenital heart disease: differential effects in various anatomical and functional substrates. *Heart.* 2009; 95(14): 1165–1171.

128 Khairy P, Van Hare GF, Balaji S, et al. PACES/HRS Expert Consensus Statement on the Recognition and Management of Arrhythmias in Adult Congenital Heart Disease: developed in partnership between the Pediatric and Congenital Electrophysiology Society (PACES) and the Heart Rhythm Society (HRS). Endorsed by the governing bodies of PACES, HRS, the American College of Cardiology (ACC), the American Heart Association (AHA), the European Heart Rhythm Association (EHRA), the Canadian Heart Rhythm Society (CHRS), and the International Society for Adult Congenital Heart Disease (ISACHD). *Heart Rhythm.* 2014; 11(10): e102–165.

129 Dubin AM, Janousek J, Rhee E, et al. Resynchronization therapy in pediatric and congenital heart disease patients: an international multicenter study. *J Am Coll Cardiol.* 2005; 46(12): 2277–2283.

130 Cecchin F, Frangini PA, Brown DW, et al. Cardiac resynchronization therapy (and multisite pacing) in pediatrics and congenital heart disease: five years

experience in a single institution. *J Cardiovasc Electrophysiol.* 2009; 20(1): 58–65.

131 Valls-Bertault V, Fatemi M, Gilard M, et al. Assessment of upgrading to biventricular pacing in patients with right ventricular pacing and congestive heart failure after atrioventricular junctional ablation for chronic atrial fibrillation. *Europace.* 2004; 6(5): 438–443.

132 Leon AR, Greenberg JM, Kanuru N, et al. Cardiac resynchronization in patients with congestive heart failure and chronic atrial fibrillation: effect of upgrading to biventricular pacing after chronic right ventricular pacing. *J Am Coll Cardiol.* 2002; 39(8): 1258–1263.

133 Dodge-Khatami A, Kadner A, Dave H, et al. Left heart atrial and ventricular epicardial pacing through a left lateral thoracotomy in children: a safe approach with excellent functional and cosmetic results. *Eur J Cardiothorac Surg.* 2005; 28(4): 541–545.

134 Vogel M, Sponring J, Cullen S, et al. Regional wall motion and abnormalities of electrical depolarization and repolarization in patients after surgical repair of tetralogy of Fallot. *Circulation.* 2001; 103(12): 1669–1673.

135 Uebing A, Gibson DG, Babu-Narayan SV, et al. Right Ventricular mechanics and QRS duration in patients with repaired tetralogy of Fallot. *Circulation.* 2007; 116(14): 1532–1539.

136 Janousek J, Vojtovic P, Hucin B, et al. Resynchronization pacing is a useful adjunct to the management of acute heart failure after surgery for congenital heart defects. *Am J Cardiol.* 2001; 88(2): 145–152.

137 Zimmerman FJ, Starr JP, Koenig PR, et al. Acute hemodynamic benefit of multisite ventricular pacing after congenital heart surgery. *Ann Thorac Surg.* 2003; 75(6): 1775–1780.

138 Dubin AM, Feinstein JA, Reddy VM, et al. Electrical resynchronization: a novel therapy for the failing right ventricle. *Circulation.* 2003; 107(18): 2287–2289.

139 Stephenson EA, Cecchin F, Alexander ME, et al. Relation of right ventricular pacing in tetralogy of Fallot to electrical resynchronization. *The American Journal of Cardiology.* 2004; 93(11): 1449–1452.

140 Dubin AM, Hanisch D, Chin C, et al. A prospective pilot study of right ventricular resynchronization (Abstract). *Heart Rhythm.* 2008; 5(5): S42.

141 Thambo JB, Dos Santos P, De Guillebon M, et al. Biventricular stimulation improves right and left ventricular function after tetralogy of Fallot repair: acute animal and clinical studies. *Heart Rhythm.* 2010; 7(3): 344–350.

142 Thambo JB, De Guillebon M, Xhaet O, et al. Biventricular pacing in patients with Tetralogy of Fallot:

Non-invasive epicardial mapping and clinical impact. *Int J Cardiol.* 2011; 30: 30.

143 Khairy P, Landzberg MJ, Lambert J, et al. Long-term outcomes after the atrial switch for surgical correction of transposition: a meta-analysis comparing the Mustard and Senning procedures. *Cardiol Young.* 2004; 14(3): 284–292.

144 Janousek J, Tomek V, Chaloupecky VA, et al. Cardiac resynchronization therapy: a novel adjunct to the treatment and prevention of systemic right ventricular failure. *J Am Coll Cardiol.* 2004; 44(9): 1927–1931.

145 Lubiszewska B, Gosiewska E, Hoffman P, et al. Myocardial perfusion and function of the systemic right ventricle in patients after atrial switch procedure for complete transposition: long-term follow-up. *J Am Coll Cardiol.* 2000; 36(4): 1365–1370.

146 Millane T, Bernard EJ, Jaeggi E, et al. Role of ischemia and infarction in late right ventricular dysfunction after atrial repair of transposition of the great arteries. *J Am Coll Cardiol.* 2000; 35(6): 1661–1668.

147 Kiaffas MG, Van Praagh R, Hanioti C, et al. The modified Fontan procedure: morphometry and surgical implications. *Ann Thorac Surg.* 1999; 67(6): 1746–1753.

148 Altmann K, Printz BF, Solowiejczky DE, et al. Two-dimensional echocardiographic assessment of right ventricular function as a predictor of outcome in hypoplastic left heart syndrome. *Am J Cardiol.* 2000; 86(9): 964–968.

149 Daebritz SH, Nollert GD, Zurakowski D, et al. Results of Norwood stage I operation: comparison of hypoplastic left heart syndrome with other malformations. *J Thorac Cardiovasc Surg.* 2000; 119(2): 358–367.

150 Bacha EA, Zimmerman FJ, Mor-Avi V, et al. Ventricular resynchronization by multisite pacing improves myocardial performance in the postoperative single-ventricle patient. *Ann Thorac Surg.* 2004; 78(5): 1678–1683.

151 Bhatta L, Luck JC, Wolbrette DL, et al. Complications of biventricular pacing. *Curr Opin Cardiol.* 2004; 19(1): 31–35.

152 Abraham WT. Cardiac resynchronization therapy for heart failure: biventricular pacing and beyond. *Curr Opin Cardiol.* 2002; 17(4): 346–352.

153 Perera JL, Motonaga KS, Miyake CY, et al. Does pediatric CRT increase the risk of ventricular tachycardia? (Abstract). *Heart Rhythm.* 2013; 10(5): S210–211.

154 Schiller O, Dham N, Greene EA, et al. Pediatric dilated cardiomyopathy patients do not meet traditional cardiac resynchronization criteria. *J Cardiovasc Electrophysiol.* 2015; 26(8): 885–889.

155 Fishberger SB, Kanter RJ. Applying cardiac resynchronization criteria to pediatric patients: fitting a square peg into a round hole? *J Cardiovasc Electrophysiol.* 2015; 26(8): 890–892.

156 Van De Veire NR, Marsan NA, Schuijf JD, et al. Noninvasive imaging of cardiac venous anatomy with 64-slice multi-slice computed tomography and noninvasive assessment of left ventricular dyssynchrony by 3-dimensional tissue synchronization imaging in patients with heart failure scheduled for cardiac resynchronization therapy. *Am J Cardiol.* 2008; 101(7): 1023–1029.

157 Silva JN, Ghosh S, Bowman TM, et al. Cardiac resynchronization therapy in pediatric congenital heart disease: insights from noninvasive electrocardiographic imaging. *Heart Rhythm.* 2009; 6(8): 1178–1185.

158 Kiuchi K, Yoshida A, Fukuzawa K, et al. Identification of the right ventricular pacing site for cardiac resynchronization therapy (CRT) guided by electroanatomical mapping (CARTO). *Circ J.* 2007; 71(10): 1599–1605.

159 Kautzner J, Peichl P. Selecting CRT candidates: the value of intracardiac mapping. *Europace.* 2008; 10(3): iii106–109.

160 Ryu K, D'avila A, Heist EK, et al. Simultaneous electrical and mechanical mapping using 3D cardiac mapping system: novel approach for optimal cardiac resynchronization therapy. *J Cardiovasc Electrophysiol.* 2010; 21(2): 219–222.

161 Lambiase PD, Rinaldi A, Hauck J, et al. Non-contact left ventricular endocardial mapping in cardiac resynchronisation therapy. *Heart.* 2004; 90(1): 44–51.

162 Forsha D, Slorach C, Chen CK, et al. Classic-pattern dyssynchrony and electrical activation delays in pediatric dilated cardiomyopathy. *J Am Soc Echocardiogr.* 2014; 27(9): 956–964.

CHAPTER 6

Sensor driven pacing: Ideal characteristics in pediatrics

David Bradley[1] and Peter S. Fischbach[2]

[1] Director Pediatric Electrophysiology, C.S. Mott Children's Hospital, and Professor of Pediatrics, University of Michigan School of Medicine, Ann Arbor, MI, USA

[2] Pediatric Electrophysiologist, Children's Healthcare of Atlanta, Sibley Heart Center Cardiology, and Associate Professor of Pediatrics, Emory University School of Medicine, Atlanta, GA, USA

Introduction

In the intact healthy heart, the sinus node varies the heart rate to ensure adequate cardiac output to meet the metabolic needs of the body. This includes increasing the heart rate in times of physiologic demand and decreasing the heart rate during times of low energy requirements. The sinus node may become unable to meet these needs as a result of disease, pharmacologic alterations, or mechanical trauma such as following surgery for congenital heart disease. When the sinus node cannot adequately alter the heart rate to deliver appropriate blood flow to the peripheral tissues, symptoms such as fatigue, exercise intolerance, and syncope may result. While standard pacing will overcome limited cardiac output due to bradycardia induced by atrioventricular block, it does not address low cardiac output due to chronotropic incompetence of the sinus node.

The era of rate responsive pacing began in the late 1970s with the implantation of a pacemaker which responded to changes in a patient's serum pH.[1] Over the ensuing four decades, several different sensors have been advanced both experimentally and clinically. None have proven to mimic the complexity of the healthy sinus node.

The goal of the rate response sensor is to adjust the heart rate based on the metabolic needs of the individual. The basic system involves a sensor and electronics to calculate a graded and appropriate output rate from the measured input. Many sensors have been investigated and used clinically, as detailed in Table 6.1. Currently, the most commonly used sensor responds to device motion, a simple and reasonable correlate of the heart rate during common activities.

It has been demonstrated that chronotropic insufficiency is common following surgery for congenital heart disease (CHD) and is associated with an increased risk of mortality.[2] In individuals who have undergone surgical intervention for CHD, one in three fails to reach 80% of the maximum predicted heart rate two decades after surgery. This is a surprisingly high proportion when compared to patients with coronary artery disease (11%) and adults with congestive heart failure or dilated cardiomyopathy (25%).[3]

Cardiac Pacing and Defibrillation in Pediatric and Congenital Heart Disease, First Edition.
Edited by Maully Shah, Larry Rhodes and Jonathan Kaltman.
© 2017 John Wiley & Sons Ltd. Published 2017 by John Wiley & Sons Ltd.
Companion Website: www.wiley.com/go/shah/cardiac_pacing

Table 6.1 *Available and investigated sensor systems for rate responsive pacing*

	Vendor[a]	Required Hardware[b]	Disadvantages	Advantages
Myocardial conductance ("closed-loop stimulation")	B	V	Potential abnormal response to myocardial injury	Reliably reflective of autonomic nervous system activity emotional as well as exertional
Transthoracic impedance ("minute ventilation")	BS, S	pect	Resp. rate not directly related to HR during early exercise	Responsive to stresses of diverse types
Body movement, (accelerometer)	M, B, BS, SJ, V		Does not account for post-exertion "oxygen deficit," many non-exercise influences, poor response to isometric or low-impact exertion	Technically simple; rapid response; contained within generator;
Transvalvar impedance	Mc	A+V, endo	A and V endocardial leads needed	Preload independent; may also provide capture verification
blood pH	n/a	Ded endo	Delayed response, Long term sensor reliability questioned	Measurable physiologic variable
QT interval	n/a	V	Delayed response, undersensing of T wave common; inaccurate with drugs, ischemia	Good correlation to sympathetic tone regardless of type of exertion or emotion
MvO2	n/a	V, endo	Light sensor unstable long term; positive feedback with angina, ischemia; incompatible with CHD	Proportionality to metabolic demand
Peak endocardial acceleration ("PEA")	n/a	Ded V	Long term sensor reliability questioned;	rapid response to physiologic changes; CRT or A-V optimization
RV pressure (dP/dT)	n/a	Ded V	Long term sensor reliability questioned; artifacts from body position	rapid response to physiologic changes; CRT optimization
temperature	n/a	Ded endo	Central venous temperature increases slowly with exercise – slow response	Effective with isometric or dynamic exercise
Ventricular depolarization gradient	n/a	V	Certain leads incompatible	Closely coupled to contractility

[a]B = Biotronik (BIOTRONIK SE & Co.KG, Berlin, Germany); BS = Boston Scientific (Boston Scientific Inc., Natick, MA); ELA = ELA medical; Mc = Medico S.p.A; M = Medtronic; S = Sorin; SJ = St. Jude; V = Vitatron; CHD = congenital heart disease;
[b]A = atrial lead; Ded = dedicated lead model needed; V = ventricular lead

Basic physiology of exercise

With the initiation of exercise, the body makes several adaptations to deliver adequate blood flow to the peripheral muscles and vital organs. This provides fuel (oxygen and glucose) to the muscles and removes metabolic waste while also maintaining an appropriate body temperature. This balance of supply and demand occurs via a complex interaction of neural and neurohormonal factors. The result may be an increase in cardiac output of more than six-fold.[4]

Cardiac output is the product of heart rate and stroke volume. During exercise, increased preload resulting from enhanced venous return combined with increased sympathetic stimulation leads to increased contractility, decreased peripheral vascular resistance, and as a result, an increase of up to 150% in the stroke volume.[5] The increase in the stroke volume occurs primarily during the early portion of exercise and reaches a maximum by the midpoint between rest and maximal exercise. Heart rate tends to increase slightly prior to the onset of activity and increases rapidly after the initiation of exercise. The initial steep slope of heart rate acceleration is due to parasympathetic withdrawal while the continued heart rate acceleration results from sympathetic stimulation.[6] At the conclusion of exercise, ongoing metabolic activity of muscles and the need to clear accumulated lactate result in a gradual return to baseline heart rate.

Characteristics of an ideal rate-adaptive pacing system

The goal of rate responsive pacemakers – to recreate the complex function of the sinus node – has proven to be a difficult task. There are limited data in adult patients regarding the ability of rate responsive devices to mimic the output from the sinus node, and even less is known in pediatric patients and those with congenital heart disease. In pediatric patients with congenital heart block, using the Medtronic (Medtronic Inc., Minneapolis, MN) Kappa platform (accelerometer), it was demonstrated that even with the pacemaker programmed to its maximally responsive settings, the pacemakers were not able to recreate the same heart rate variability (including time spent at the upper heart rates) as an intact sinus node.[7]

Heart rate sensors can operate in either a "closed-loop" or "open-loop" fashion. In a closed loop system, the physiologic parameter being monitored effects a change in the heart rate. This change in the heart rate alters the physiologic parameter thereby creating a negative feedback loop. This system therefore should be fully "automatic" and not require any physician input. While this system seems ideal, the reality is that the normally

functioning sinus node has multiple inputs influencing the heart rate. The overwhelming majority of commercially available rate sensors today use an open-loop system in which the change in the heart rate does not feed back on the parameter being measured.

A normally functioning sinus node alters the heart rate in response to various physiologic stimuli. Upon exercise, the heart rate increases linearly in relation to the VO2. The heart rate response to other stimuli such as emotion or fever is more complex, however. It also remains unclear if reproducing the function of the normal sinus node is essential for all clinical conditions. The high level of function of many pediatric patients with nonphysiologic heart rates, such as unpaced school-aged children with congenital heart block, calls into question the necessity of the heart rate being tuned to metabolic need. Nonetheless, it is clear that in VVI paced patients increasing the ventricular rate achieves improvement in cardiac output more than by merely establishing AV synchrony.[8]

While it is known that chronotropic incompetence is a risk factor for increased mortality in adults with repaired congenital heart disease[2] limited information exists regarding the effect of rate responsive pacing on mortality and quality of life in this patient population. The relationship of cardiac output and heart rate is particularly complex in patients with single ventricle physiology following staged surgical palliation. This is important as the incidence of late sinus node dysfunction after the Fontan operation has been reported to range between 9 and 60%.[9] While chronotropic incompetence has been linked with more depressed ventricular function and worse NYHA heart failure status following surgery for CHD, it remains unclear whether this is a contributing factor.

Sensors

Sensor technology aims to approximate the normal changes in heart rate observed with physical activity and other physiologic perturbations, which may not involve body movement such as fever, stress, sleep, and emotion. Multiple approaches have been taken to address this complex physiology (Table 6.1).

A sensor system includes four components: (1) a parameter that correlates with heart rate changes in normal individuals; (2) a means of measuring that parameter accurately; (3) an algorithm that computes the appropriate heart rate from that measurement; and (4) the pacing system from which it is delivered.

A wide array of parameters has been identified as markers of changing metabolic need. While many have undergone clinical testing, only activity and respiration sensors have achieved broad clinical use. Reasons for this appear less evidence-based than due to manufacturing, regulatory, and logistical issues. For example, sensors of venous pH, intra-chamber pressure, and endocardial acceleration, which require dedicated (non-international standard, or IS-1) leads, have not had a lasting market presence. In contrast, the accelerometer, despite obvious shortcomings, is the most widely available rate response sensor.

Accelerometer
The accelerometer is a small component in the pulse generator. A common design is a small flexible arm with a weight at one end, secured to a piezoelectric crystal, which produces a current when the arm is flexed. The current fluctuations are counted by the device computer, and a rate is computed in proportion to the number of counts. Its rapid response to common activities and durability make the accelerometer a useful system. Sensitive to vibrations within the torso, however, this modality may inappropriately elevate rates in the presence of passive movement, such as riding in a car on an uneven road, or even in the presence of loud sounds, such as in a movie theater. Additionally, it may fail to respond physiologically during certain forms of low-impact exercise such as riding a bicycle or swimming. Notable also is its ineffectiveness for the non-ambulatory patient or infant, in whom it will inadequately vary heart rate.

Chest impedance or "minute ventilation"
Impedance, or resistance across the chest, to a small electrical current, falls with the filling of the lungs with air. Just as respiratory rate can be estimated on bedside monitors by this principle, it can be measured between a pectoral generator and intracardiac lead, allowing sensing of exertion regardless of the degree of body movement. The minute ventilation (MV), or respiratory rate, does not increase instantaneously with exercise, so MV sensors are included in a "blended" algorithm with another sensor type to achieve physiologic heart rates. Its utility in the presence of rapid respiratory rates seen in small patients is debated,[10] but probably acceptable.[11]

Myocardial conductance
One manufacturer, Biotronik (Biotronik SE & Co.KG, Berlin, Germany), currently produces devices with a sensor system based on a timed measurement of myocardial impedance that correlates closely with the sympathetic state of the heart. The instantaneous impedance measurement at the lead tip fluctuates in a pattern that differs significantly between times of low and elevated sympathetic tone. The slope of this change at a specific window after myocardial activation provides the measure from which physiological changes in heart rate are computed by this closed-loop system. Appropriate responses not only to exercise but also positional changes and mental stress can thereby be approximated.[12-15]

Practical considerations
The majority of pediatric patients will not require sensor driven pacing. Of those that do, available systems will be appropriate for most. One exception is the non-ambulatory child with a single lead system. The most commonly used motion sensors will be ineffective in this patient who may effectively be left with fixed rate pacing. Another may be the small patient in whom it is desired to limit the amount of hardware implanted. Finally, for those patients with chronic atrial arrhythmias, rate responsive ventricular pacing may be the most practical pacing mode. Ensuring appropriate heart rate variability in these patients is a challenge to which attentive device choice and programming will be required.

Conclusion
While there is clear evidence for the benefit of sensor driven rate response to approximate the

changes seen in heart rate under different physiologic conditions, comparisons between available systems for pediatric applications are few. Most children and young adults requiring rate responsive pacing experience acceptable performance provided by an accelerometer based system, which will be durable and sensitive. Knowledge of the available sensor types, along with the other features of the devices which accompany them, allows the clinician to make reasonable patient-specific device selection and programming.

References

1 Cammilli L, Alcidi L, Papeschi G, et al. Preliminary experience with the pH-triggered pacemaker. *Pacing and Clinical Electrophysiology: PACE.* 1978; 1(4): 448–457.

2 Diller G-P, Dimopoulos K, Okonko D, et al. Heart rate response during exercise predicts survival in adults with congenital heart disease. *Journal of the American College of Cardiology.* 2006; 48(6): 1250–1256.

3 Norozi K, Wessel A, Alpers V, et al. Chronotropic incompetence in adolescents and adults with congenital heart disease after cardiac surgery. *Journal of Cardiac Failure.* 2007; 13(4): 263–268.

4 Spina RJ, Ogawa T, Martin WH, et al. Exercise training prevents decline in stroke volume during exercise in young healthy subjects. *Journal of Applied Physiology (Bethesda, Md.: 1985).* 1992; 72(6): 2458–2462.

5 Bada AA, Svendsen JH, Secher NH, Saltin B, Mortensen SP. Peripheral vasodilation determines cardiac output in exercising humans: Insight from atrial pacing. *The Journal of Physiology.* 2012; 8: 2051–2060.

6 Robinson BF, Epstein SE, Beiser GD, Braunwald E. Control of heart rate by the autonomic nervous system. Studies in man on the interrelation between baroreceptor mechanisms and exercise. *Circ Res.* 1966; 19(2): 400–411.

7 Fischbach PS, Saarel EV, Condie C, DICK II M, Serwer GA. Sinus heart rate compared with sensor driven rate in young patients with pacemakers. *Heart Rhythm.* 2004; 1(1S): 693A.

8 Pehrsson SK. Influence of heart rate and atrioventricular synchronization on maximal work tolerance in patients treated with artificial pacemakers. *Acta Medica Scandinavica.* 1983; 214(4): 311–315.

9 Collins KK. The spectrum of long-term electrophysiologic abnormalities in patients with univentricular hearts. *Congenital Heart Disease.* 2009; 4(5): 310–317.

10 Padeletti L, Pieragnoli P, Di Biase L, et al. Is a dual-sensor pacemaker appropriate in patients with sino-atrial disease? Results from the DUSISLOG study. *Pacing and Clinical Electrophysiology: PACE.* 2006; 29(1): 34–40.

11 Cabrera ME, Portzline G, Aach S, et al. Can current minute ventilation rate adaptive pacemakers provide appropriate chronotropic response in pediatric patients? *Pacing and Clinical Electrophysiology.* 2002; 25(6): 907–914.

12 Drago F, Silvetti MS, de Santis A, et al. Closed loop stimulation improves ejection fraction in pediatric patients with pacemaker and ventricular dysfunction. *Pacing and Clinical Electrophysiology.* 2007; 30(1): 33–37.

13 Chandiramani S, Cohorn LC, Chandiramani S. Heart rate changes during acute mental stress with closed loop stimulation: report on two single-blinded, pacemaker studies. *Pacing and Clinical Electrophysiology: PACE.* 2007; 30(8): 976–984.

14 Christ T. Rate-adaptive pacing using intracardiac impedance shows no evidence for positive feedback during dobutamine stress test. *Europace.* 2002; 4(3): 311–315.

15 Palmisano P, Zaccaria M, Luzzi G, et al. Closed-loop cardiac pacing vs. conventional dual-chamber pacing with specialized sensing and pacing algorithms for syncope prevention in patients with refractory vasovagal syncope: results of a long-term follow-up. *Europace: European Pacing, Arrhythmias, and Cardiac Electrophysiology: Journal of the Working Groups on Cardiac Pacing, Arrhythmias, and Cardiac Cellular Electrophysiology of the European Society of Cardiology.* 2012; 18(7): 1038–1043.

CHAPTER 7

Implantable cardioverter-defibrillator testing in pediatric and congenital heart disease

Elizabeth A. Stephenson[1] and Charles I. Berul[2]

[1] Staff Cardiologist, The Hospital for Sick Children, Associate Professor of Pediatrics, The University of Toronto, Toronto, ON, Canada

[2] Electrophysiologist and Staff Cardiologist, The Hospital for Sick Children, Associate Professor of Pediatrics, The University of Toronto, Toronto, ON, Canada

Implantable cardioverter-defibrillators (ICDs) are effective interventions in preventing sudden death in pediatric and congenital heart disease patients.[1] Inherited cardiomyopathies and primary electrical diseases, such as the long QT syndrome, catecholaminergic polymorphic ventricular tachycardia, and Brugada syndrome, may place young people at high risk of malignant arrhythmias.[2, 3] Similarly, repaired congenital heart disease also carries a risk of ventricular arrhythmias, particularly in older children and adults. Implantable defibrillators are commonly used for secondary prevention, such as in patients resuscitated from cardiac arrest or those with documented ventricular arrhythmia. ICDs are placed for primary prevention in clinical scenarios that carry high risk of malignant arrhythmias, but prior to a life-threatening event. Once the decision has been made, and an ICD has been implanted, there are unique aspects to the testing of ICD function that differ from the testing of other implantable cardiac rhythm devices such as pacemakers. This chapter will focus on the initial evaluation of high energy output and ongoing assessment of the adequacy of programmed shock output.

Fibrillation and defibrillation

Ventricular fibrillation is an apparently chaotic rhythm that is frequently described as dependent on multiple eddy currents. Recent work has supported the theory that within this chaotic rhythm there exists a more organized underlying rhythm, described as a mother rotor, which drives the continuing fibrillation.[4, 5] Successful defibrillation requires creation of a voltage gradient large enough to disrupt the eddy currents and allow uniform depolarization.[6] Defibrillation threshold (DFT) testing began as a means to determine the likelihood of converting out of ventricular fibrillation. However, the threshold at which this gradient exists is well recognized to be dynamic, and thus is understood to be probabilistic in nature.[6] Histori-cally, the DFT was defined as the energy at which successful defibrillation was achieved 90% of the time; ICDs were then programmed with a margin of safety (at least 10 J) above that DFT to increase the likelihood of reliable defibrillation.

Defibrillation threshold testing and lowest energy tested

At the time ICDs were first introduced clini-cally, exacting defibrillation threshold testing was performed in the vast majority of patients. Ventric-ular fibrillation can be induced with a low-energy shock (typically 0.5–2 J) delivered on the vulnera-ble phase of the T wave (Figure 7.1a), programmed

ventricular extra-stimulation, or rapid cycle (50 Hz) stimulation. The implanted defibrilla-tor was then tasked with adequate sensing of low-amplitude signal during fibrillation, charging to a predetermined programmed energy, and deliv-ering a defibrillation shock to convert back into sinus rhythm (Figure 7.1b). DFT testing typically consisted of a multi-shock step-up or step-down algorithm until the margin between failed and successful shock was narrowed to identify the true defibrillation threshold. As the technology of ICDs improved, including biphasic waveforms, nonthoracotomy transvenous lead designs, and higher energy outputs, many practitioners con-verted to a "Lowest Energy Tested" (LET) strategy, to establish a safety margin (often 10 J) between

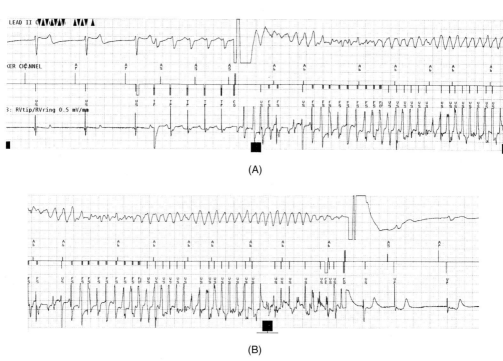

(A)

(B)

Figure 7.1 *(A) The printout from a defibrillation induction using a T wave shock delivered on the vulnerable timing of the T wave. These are three channel recordings, with the upper tracing representing the surface electrocardiogram, the middle is the marker channel from the defibrillator, and the lower channel is the intracardiac bipolar electrogram from the RV tip to RV ring. At the left of the image, the rhythm begins as atrial paced with intrinsic atrioventricular conduction. There are then five ventricular paced beats at a cycle length of 400 ms (150 bpm) followed by a low-energy T wave shock. The shock induces ventricular fibrillation, which is appropriately sensed by the ICD. (B) This is a continuation of the prior tracings, showing ventricular fibrillation while the ICD is sensing and charging, followed by successful defibrillation. There is occasional "drop-out" where not every beat of low amplitude fibrillation is detected. This is a typical example of a successful DFT.*

a successful defibrillation and the programmed high energy output. Typically, what is currently described as DFT testing is in fact actually LET testing, however, the terms are sometimes used nearly interchangeably.

In the early era of ICD implantation, DFTs were routinely performed at implant, prior to discharge, and on a regular ongoing basis (i.e., annually) as a monitoring technique for system functionality. Routine follow-up DFTs are now less common, due to the improved reliability of current transvenous systems utilizing biphasic waveforms and active can configurations. Recently the clinical practice of routine DFT or LET testing at the time of implantation has also come into question, as the possible adverse consequences of DFT testing and shocks are increasingly recognized.[7-9] Despite being used as a tool to increase the safety of an ICD system, DFTs are not without risk. Hemodynamic challenges, increased anesthetics, and possible myocardial injury from multiple high energy shocks can lead to complications from DFT testing. The risk of such testing will vary from patient to patient, and the clinical context must be taken into account when assessing the need for a DFT. However, there is a reported failure rate of defibrillation at routine energy levels 6–12% of the time, and thus completely eliminating DFT testing will inevitably leave a small proportion of patients with unrecognized high DFTs and inadequate energy outputs.[10, 11] Several recent studies in adult patients have revealed no difference in intermediate-term outcomes between those with and without DFT testing at time of ICD placement. Single shock threshold testing protocols have also been examined; in a study of 318 adults, ICD patients were randomized to a full DFT protocol versus a single 14 J shock. They found that the successful spontaneous conversion rate of ventricular fibrillation was similarly successful between the two groups, suggesting that the additional testing and multiple shocks provided no enhanced safety while increasing potential added risk.[12] One recent study compared the 2-year mortality and the frequency of ICD shocks, and found a similar rate between DFT and no-DFT groups.[13]

Common methods of determining DFT in pediatrics and CHD in the current era

Although some centers that implant ICDs in adults with structurally normal hearts are moving away from routine DFTs at implantation, DFT or LET assessment remains the norm at most pediatric and congenital heart disease ICD implantation centers. Variations in size, heterogeneous anatomy, can to coil configurations and myocardial hypertrophy potentially all lead to unpredictable vectors of defibrillation in this unique group of patients.[14] This may lead to unpredictability in DFT, and thus testing continues in most patients. In certain patients at particular high risk from DFT testing, such as those with restrictive cardiomyopathy or severe cardiac dysfunction, physicians may opt to omit DFT testing. This decision should be made on a case-by-case basis. The most common protocol for high output testing is two successful defibrillations at 10 J or more below the maximum output of the device, followed by programming of the device at maximum output. Alternatively, one successful defibrillation at 15–20 Js below the maximum output has also been shown to provide an adequate margin of safety when the first shock is then programmed at maximum output.[15] In a very recent pediatric study, a small group of patients were evaluated prospectively and found to have low DFTs and would all have been within the probabilistic margin of safety if the devices had simply been programmed at maximal output of at least 31 J.[16]

Upper limit of vulnerability

For centers that are opting to withhold routine DFT testing at implant, examining upper limit of vulnerability (ULV) may offer another way to evaluate expected efficacy of defibrillation. ULV utilizes the existence of a "vulnerable period" in the cardiac cycle, at the peak of the T wave; a lower energy shock delivered into that period will induce ventricular fibrillation (VF).[6] However, at increasing strengths of shocks delivered into the vulnerable period, there is a threshold at which VF

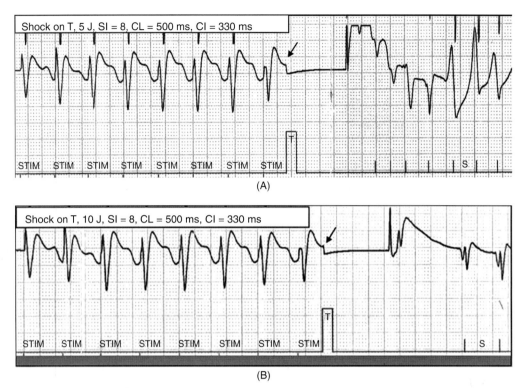

Figure 7.2 *(A) VF is induced with a 5 J T wave shock delivered during the vulnerable phase of the T-wave after a paced drive train of eight beats at a cycle length of 500 ms from the ICD lead in the right ventricular apex. The coupling interval for the induction shock is 330 ms. (B) In the same patient, VF can no longer be induced with a higher strength (10 J) T wave induction shock delivered at the same coupling interval, indicating the upper limit of vulnerability (ULV). J = Joules, S1 = number of intervals during paced drive train, CL = cycle length, CI = coupling interval measured from the stimulus to the vulnerable point in the T wave, arrow-delivery of T shock.*

will not be induced. The ULV is the weakest shock that, when delivered into the vulnerable period, will not induce VF (Figure 7.2A and B). This measurement has been shown to correlate with DFT, and can be used with far fewer inductions of VF. If one can establish an adequate safety margin with the ULV, it may not be necessary to induce VF.[17] Although this form of evaluating defibrillation efficacy has not been widely adopted in pediatric and congenital electrophysiology, it may have a role in minimizing VF in those patients at highest risk from standard DFT testing.

Equipment and personnel readiness for defibrillation testing at implant

Regardless of whether ICD implantation (with or without DFT testing) is being performed in the catheterization laboratory or the operating room, it essential that appropriate measures be in place to ensure patient safety. Although rare, complications of DFT testing do occur. In one large series of over 19,000 adults undergoing peri-implant DFTs, there were 3 deaths, 5 cerebrovascular events, and 27 episodes of prolonged resuscitation.[9] Not surprisingly, patients with poor ventricular function appear to be at higher risk of compromise at the time of testing.[18] Prior to initiation of DFT testing, roles and responsibility must be discussed amongst the team members. A plan must be in place if the first, and possibly second, internal defibrillation attempts fail. External defibrillation pads should be applied to the patient, and the defibrillator set to an appropriate energy in case both first and second ascending internal shocks fail. In the highest risk patients, such as those with severe ventricular

Table 7.1 *Treatment options for high DFTs*

Treat reversible causes	Non-invasive strategies	Invasive strategies
1 Medications: - remove or change anti-arrhythmic, anesthetic agents 2 Prolonged procedure time - repeat testing on another day may be appropriate 3 Pneumothorax 4 Metabolic and electrolyte derangements	1 Change in shock vector polarity 2 Tilt modification 3 Electronic removal of SVC coil if shock impedance <40 Ω 4 Addition of Sotalol or Dofetilide under careful observation	1 Reposition RV lead to a more apical or RVOT location 2 Addition of lead (subcutaneous, coronary sinus, azygos vein) 3 Placement of a separate proximal coil 4 Use high output ICD generator

dysfunction, it may be prudent to have mechanical support such as extracorporeal membrane oxygenation available, if it is felt that a DFT must be performed. Alternatively, it may be prudent to skip, or at least defer, DFT testing until this type of patient becomes more clinically stable.

Factors that affect DFTs

There are multiple factors that have been shown to be associated with higher DFTs. Patient based factors include higher body mass, younger age, nonischemic cardiomyopathy, cardiac hypertrophy, and cardiac dilation. Amiodarone is well recognized to potentially elevate DFTs, and consideration should be given to performing repeat DFT testing on any patient who requires initiation of this medication. Other medications that may increase DFT include lidocaine, verapamil, cocaine, sildenafil, and some anesthetic agents.[19-23] Conversely, Sotalol and Dofetilide are both associated with lowering of DFTs.[24, 25] The type of defibrillation lead, and the impact of recent fibrillation can alter defibrillation thresholds, suggesting a need to allow adequate time between testing.[26]

Approach to the patient with high DFTs

When faced with a patient with high DFTs, one should first evaluate for any possible reversible causes, such as pneumothorax or anesthetic agent. If no reversible causes are found, programming

changes can sometime find an acceptable defibrillation strategy (Table 7.1). Changes in the shock vector may improve DFT, as may modification of waveform tilt, which is programmable on some ICDs. Vector can also be shifted by removal or addition of an SVC coil. In patients with dual coil ICD leads this may be possible simply through programming; however, if the patient has a single coil lead as is more likely in the pediatric and congenital population, an independent SVC coil or conversion to a dual coil lead may be required. Lead repositioning can also lead to a better DFT if a position can be found that recruits more myocardial mass into the defibrillation vector. Addition of a subcutaneous high voltage lead or array has also been shown to assist in achieving an acceptable margin for defibrillation. As Sotalol has been associated with a drop in DFTs in many patients, adding this medication may improve DFTs, although repeat DFT testing may be required to confirm if the drop in DFT is adequate. Even still, this pharmacologic method is not very reassuring for reducing the threshold needed for terminating a spontaneous life-threatening arrhythmia.

Retesting of the DFT in pediatric and congenital heart disease

There is little data focused specifically on DFTs in the pediatric and congenital population. One study found that the majority of routine defibrillation threshold testing did not uncover any clinically significant findings. However, in patients in whom there was evidence of a clinical change which lead to the obtaining of the DFT (such as change on radiographic screening, inappropriate shocks, or a change in pacing or sensing parameters), threshold testing revealed abnormalities that led to important programming or hardware modifications.[27] Thus in this population routine defibrillation threshold testing is likely unnecessary, but any significant clinical changes should lead to consideration of repeat testing. There were important limitations of this study – it was a retrospective, small series with potential for selection bias, so it may not be directly extrapolated to a larger group of pediatric patients.

Follow-up DFTs in non-transvenous ICD configurations

In pediatric patients and those with congenital heart disease, implantation of cardioverter-defibrillators may be limited due to cardiac anatomy or patient size. Epicardial patches have been used historically in some of these patients, but these require a thoracotomy and may put patients at risk of a restrictive pericardial process. In the last 10 years, alternative configurations have been used in patients who are too small for traditional transvenous implantation, or those with intracardiac shunting. In 2001 these novel configurations were first described as three centers published cases where epicardial ventricular sensing leads were combined with a subcutaneously implanted high voltage coil and an active can which was placed in an abdominal position.[28–30] Evolving at the same time was a configuration that used a transvenous high voltage lead in an epicardial position, again with an abdominally positioned active generator. These and other alternative configurations have now been used in children and young adults with congenital heart disease, with reasonable success rates. However, these patients require close monitoring and follow-up, including routine testing of the defibrillation threshold, as they are new technologies and thus are prone to unanticipated complications.[31] These novel configurations may also have higher rates of failure compared to standard transvenous ICD systems.[32] However, many of the patients in whom these novel systems were implanted were not candidates for standard transvenous ICDs.

Conclusions

In conclusion, implanting defibrillators in pediatric and congenital heart disease patients entails a wide-range of techniques and a heterogeneous approach to evaluation. Defibrillation threshold testing is still utilized in some of these patient cohorts, particularly when suspicion is aroused due to clinical or radiographic changes. The risks and benefits of DFT testing should be considered when evaluating the functionality of an implanted device.

References

1 Silka MJ, Kron J, Dunnigan A, Dick M, 2nd., Sudden cardiac death and the use of implantable cardioverter-defibrillators in pediatric patients. The Pediatric Electrophysiology Society. *Circulation*. 1993; 87(3): 800–807.

2 Alexander ME, Cecchin F, Walsh EP, Triedman JK, Bevilacqua LM, Berul CI. Implications of implantable cardioverter defibrillator therapy in congenital heart disease and pediatrics [see comment]. *Journal of Cardiovascular Electrophysiology*. 2004; 15(1): 72–76.

3 Korte T, Koditz H, Niehaus M, Paul T, Tebbenjohanns J. High incidence of appropriate and inappropriate ICD therapies in children and adolescents with implantable cardioverter defibrillator. *Pacing Clin Electrophysiol*. 2004; 27(7): 924–932.

4 Samie FH, Berenfeld O, Anumonwo J, Mironov SF, Udassi S, Beaumont J, et al. Rectification of the background potassium current: a determinant of rotor dynamics in ventricular fibrillation. *Circ Res*. 2001; 89(12): 1216–1223.

5 Huang J, Zhou X, Smith WM, Ideker RE. Restitution properties during ventricular fibrillation in the in situ swine heart. *Circulation*. 2004; 110(20): 3161–3167.

6 Chen PS, Swerdlow CD, Hwang C, Karagueuzian HS. Current concepts of ventricular defibrillation. *J Cardiovasc Electrophysiol*. 1998; 9(5): 553–562.

7 Blatt JA, Poole JE, Johnson GW, Callans DJ, Raitt MH, Reddy RK, et al., Investigators SC-H. No benefit from defibrillation threshold testing in the SCD-HeFT (Sudden Cardiac Death in Heart Failure Trial). *J Am Coll Cardiol*. 2008; 52(7): 551–556.

8 Gula LJ, Massel D, Krahn AD, Yee R, Skanes AC, Klein GJ. Is defibrillation testing still necessary? A decision analysis and Markov model. *J Cardiovasc Electrophysiol*. 2008; 19(4): 400–405.

9 Birnie D, Tung S, Simpson C, Crystal E, Exner D, Ayala Paredes FA, et al. Complications associated with defibrillation threshold testing: The Canadian experience. *Heart Rhythm*. 2008; 5(3): 387–390.

10 Mainigi SK, Cooper JM, Russo AM, Nayak HM, Lin D, Dixit S, et al. Elevated defibrillation thresholds in patients undergoing biventricular defibrillator implantation: incidence and predictors. *Heart Rhythm*. 2006; 3(9): 1010–1016.

11 Russo AM, Sauer W, Gerstenfeld EP, Hsia HH, Lin D, Cooper JM, et al. Defibrillation threshold testing: is it really necessary at the time of implantable cardioverter-defibrillator insertion? *Heart Rhythm*. 2005;2(5):456–461.

12 Gold MR, Breiter D, Leman R, Rashba EJ, Shorofsky SR, Hahn SJ. Safety of a single successful conversion of ventricular fibrillation before the implantation of cardioverter defibrillators. *Pacing & Clinical Electrophysiology*. 2003; 26(1 Pt 2): 483–486.

13 Codner P, Nevzorov R, Kusniec J, Haim M, Zabarski R, Strasberg B. Implantable cardioverter defibrillator with and without defibrillation threshold testing. *Isr Med Assoc J*. 14(6): 343–346.

14 Berul CI, Van Hare GF, Kertesz NJ, Dubin AM, Cecchin F, Collins KK, et al. Results of a multicenter retrospective implantable cardioverter-defibrillator registry of pediatric and congenital heart disease patients. *J Am Coll Cardiol*. 2008; 51(17): 1685–1691.

15 Day JD, Doshi RN, Belott P, Birgersdotter-Green U, Behboodikhah M, Ott P, et al. Inductionless or limited shock testing is possible in most patients with implantable cardioverter-defibrillators/cardiac resynchronization therapy defibrillators: results of the multicenter ASSURE Study (Arrhythmia Single Shock Defibrillation Threshold Testing Versus Upper Limit of Vulnerability: Risk Reduction Evaluation With Implantable Cardioverter-Defibrillator Implantations). *Circulation*. 2007; 115(18): 2382–2389.

16 Radbill AE, Triedman JK, Berul CI, et al. Prospective evaluation of defibrillation threshold and post-shock rhythm in young ICD recipients. *Pacing Clin Electrophysiol*. 2012; 35(12): 1487–1493.

17 Swerdlow CD, Shehata M, Chen PS. Using the upper limit of vulnerability to assess defibrillation efficacy at implantation of ICDs. *Pacing Clin Electrophysiol*. 2007; 30(2): 258–270.

18 Steinbeck G, Dorwarth U, Mattke S, Hoffmann E, Markewitz A, Kaulbach H, Tassani P. Hemodynamic deterioration during ICD implant: predictors of high-risk patients. *Am Heart J*. 1994; 127(4 Pt 2): 1064–1067.

19 Moerman A, Herregods L, Tavernier R, Jordaens L, Struys M, Rolly G. Influence of anaesthesia on defibrillation threshold. *Anaesthesia*. 1998; 53(12): 1156–1159.

20 Cohen TJ, Lowenkron DD. The effects of pneumothorax on defibrillation thresholds during pectoral implantation of an active can implantable cardioverter defibrillator. *Pacing Clin Electrophysiol*. 1998; 21(2): 468–470.

21 Cohen TJ, Chengot T, Quan C, Peller AP. Elevation of defibrillation thresholds with propofol during implantable cardioverter-defibrillator testing. *J Invasive Cardiol*. 2000; 12(2): 121–123.

22 Fain ES, Lee JT, Winkle RA. Effects of acute intravenous and chronic oral amiodarone on defibrillation energy requirements. *Am Heart J*. 1987; 114(1 Pt 1): 8–17.

23 Jung W, Manz M, Pizzulli L, Pfeiffer D, Luderitz B. Effects of chronic amiodarone therapy on defibrillation threshold. *Am J Cardiol*. 1992; 70(11): 1023–1027.

24 Hohnloser SH, Dorian P, Roberts R, Gent M, Israel CW, Fain E, et al. Effect of amiodarone and sotalol on ventricular defibrillation threshold: the optimal pharmacological therapy in cardioverter defibrillator patients (OPTIC) trial. *Circulation*. 2006; 114(2): 104–109.

25 Simon RD, Sturdivant JL, Leman RB, Wharton JM, Gold MR. The effect of dofetilide on ventricular defibrillation thresholds. *Pacing Clin Electrophysiol*. 2009; 32(1): 24–28.

26 Berul CI, Callans DJ, Schwartzman DS, Preminger MW, Gottlieb CD, Marchlinski FE. Comparison of initial detection and redetection of ventricular fibrillation in a transvenous defibrillator system with automatic gain control. *J Am Coll Cardiol*. 1995; 25(2): 431–436.

27 Stephenson EA, Cecchin F, Walsh EP, Berul CI. Utility of routine follow-up defibrillator threshold testing in congenital heart disease and pediatric populations. *Journal of Cardiovascular Electrophysiology*. 2005; 16(1): 69–73.

28 Berul CI, Triedman JK, Forbess J, Bevilacqua LM, Alexander ME, Dahlby D, et al. Minimally invasive cardioverter defibrillator implantation for children: an animal model and pediatric case report. *Pacing & Clinical Electrophysiology*. 2001; 24(12): 1789–1794.

29 Gradaus R, Hammel D, Kotthoff S, Bocker D. Nonthoracotomy implantable cardioverter defibrillator placement in children: use of subcutaneous array leads and abdominally placed implantable cardioverter defibrillators in children [see comment]. *Journal of Cardiovascular Electrophysiology*. 2001; 12(3): 356–360.

30 Thogersen AM, Helvind M, Jensen T, Andersen JH, Jacobsen JR, Chen X. Implantable cardioverter defibrillator in a 4-month-old infant with cardiac arrest associated with a vascular heart tumor. *Pacing & Clinical Electrophysiology*. 2001; 24(11): 1699–1700.

31 Stephenson EA, Batra AS, Knilans TK, Gow RM, Gradaus R, Balaji S, et al. A multicenter experience with novel implantable cardioverter defibrillator configurations in the pediatric and congenital heart disease population. *Journal of Cardiovascular Electrophysiology.* 2006; 17(1): 41–46.

32 Radbill AE, Triedman JK, Berul CI, Fynn-Thompson F, Atallah J, Alexander ME, et al. System survival of nontransvenous implantable cardioverter-defibrillators compared to transvenous implantable cardioverter-defibrillators in pediatric and congenital heart disease patients. *Heart Rhythm.* 2010; 7(2): 193–198.

PART 3
Implantation Techniques

CHAPTER 8

Permanent transvenous pacemaker, CRT, and ICD implantation in the structurally normal heart

Akash R. Patel[1] and Steven Fishberger[2]

[1]Electrophysiologist, Pediatric and Congenital Arrhythmia Center, University of California – San Francisco Benioff Children's Hospital, Assistant Professor of Pediatrics, University of California – San Francisco, San Francisco, CA, USA
[2]Pediatric Electrophysiologist, Nicklaus Children's Hospital, Miami, FL, USA

Introduction

In children requiring pacemakers and implantable cardioverter defibrillators (ICDs), transvenous leads offer several advantages compared with epicardial leads: a less invasive approach, lower capture thresholds, and better lead and battery longevity. The approach to pediatric device implantation with a focus on single and dual chamber pacemakers, cardiac resynchronization therapy devices, and implantable cardioverter-defibrillators will be presented in this chapter.

The approach to transvenous device implantation in the pediatric patient with a structurally normal heart possesses a unique set of challenges.[1-5] These include the well-recognized factors such as patient size and ongoing somatic growth, along with adequacy of blood vessel caliber, and the need for long term therapy. Additionally, psychosocial concerns include cosmetic and body image issues, and as well as lifestyle considerations such as sports participation.

Procedural requirements and patient selection

Device implantation in pediatric patients with a structurally normal heart has additional considerations compared with adult patients. Planning should include availability and expertise of personnel, identification of a pediatric-centric procedural venue, accessibility of appropriate pediatric procedural and device equipment, and appropriate candidacy of the patient for transvenous device therapy.[2, 4]

Assessment of appropriate personnel should be undertaken prior to transvenous device implantation. This includes a trained electrophysiologist with expertise and comfort in caring for pediatric patients requiring device therapy. In some hospitals, an adult-trained electrophysiologist may be responsible for implanting transvenous devices in children. Additional expertise from a pediatric cardiologist, pediatric interventional cardiologist, and/or pediatric cardiothoracic surgeon

Cardiac Pacing and Defibrillation in Pediatric and Congenital Heart Disease, First Edition.
Edited by Maully Shah, Larry Rhodes and Jonathan Kaltman.
© 2017 John Wiley & Sons Ltd. Published 2017 by John Wiley & Sons Ltd.
Companion Website: www.wiley.com/go/shah/cardiac_pacing

may be required. They can provide assistance in assessing the impact of growth potential, management of psychosocial issues, obtaining venous access, and/or creating a device pocket. Other key personnel include nurses comfortable with pre- and post-procedural care of pediatric patients, a scrub nurse, a cardiac catheterization lab technician comfortable with assisting with device implantation; and a circulating nurse available to provide non-sterile assistance during the case. This may include obtaining supplies, medication administration, and patient monitoring. In addition, personnel knowledgeable in pediatric device implantation, such as a device manufacture representative, should be available for device analysis, programming, and testing. An anesthesiologist or nurse anesthetist with expertise in sedating and anesthetizing children is recommended.

The venue for cardiac rhythm device implantation should be a sterile environment, which can either be a cardiac catheterization/electrophysiology laboratory or an operating room. An advantage of the cardiac catheterization laboratory is familiarity with the fluoroscopy system and staff. In addition, there is availability of equipment that may be required for patients with difficult access or anatomy. The operating room typically provides a more sterile environment and increased venue familiarity for surgeons in the setting of catastrophic events that may require an open chest. The disadvantages of the operating room may potentially include less sophisticated arrhythmia monitoring, limited access to catheterization or electrophysiologic equipment, lack of cardiovascular expertise of support staff, and a less sophisticated fluoroscopy system. A hybrid cardiac catheterization/operating room provides the most ideal environment for device implantation especially in complex or high risk procedures. In addition, an appropriate location for recovery and post-operative antibiotics is necessary. Our practice has been to observe patients for a less than 23-hour observation period to receive post-operative intravenous antibiotics. This can be done in a post-anesthesia care unit or inpatient unit with pediatric experience.

All device and procedure related equipment should be readily available including a pacing

Table 8.1 *Equipment for device pocket creation including surgical tray*

Adison forceps with teeth
mouth-tooth forceps
smooth forceps
medium blunt Weitlaner retractor
small Weitlaner retractor
Senn Retractors
Army-Navy retractor
baby towel clips
curved mosquito clamps
Peers clamp
curved Kelly clamps
Metzenbaum scissors
curved Mayo scissors
knife handle
needle holder
Goulet rectractor
Bozeman uterine dressing forceps
coker
suture material
scalpel blade
sterile towel
gauze

Adapted from Ellenbogen et al. (9)

system analyzer, pulse generators, leads, introducing sheaths, and associated tools. In addition, surgical equipment should be appropriate for children including a surgical tray, electrocautery, wall suction, and vascular access supplies (Table 8.1). The room should also be prepared for pediatric emergencies including a code cart with pediatric dosing readily available, defibrillator with pediatric pads, pericardiocentesis kit, thoracentesis kit, and chest tube insertion tray. During any procedure, cardiopulmonary monitoring should be utilized and age appropriate equipment (i.e., blood pressure cuffs) should be used. Finally, a protocol for sterile procedures should be in place. This includes the use of povidone-iodine, chlorhexidine, or hexachlorophene scrub to disinfect the skin followed by standard draping of the pediatric patient. In addition, perioperative antibiotics with pediatric dosing should be administered prior to the skin incision and appropriate antibiotic irrigation solution should be used.[6]

Indication for device therapy is important in determining candidacy for transvenous device therapy. Patients who require dual chamber pacing or defibrillation capability may be excluded due to inadequate vessel caliber, large lead diameters, or suboptimal shock vector orientation.[5, 7] Single chamber pacing as a short-term strategy until adequate growth would accommodate additional lead placement may be considered.[8] Growth resulting in an increased intravascular distance between the lead insertion site and attachment site may result in dislodgement, changes in sensing and pacing thresholds, and changes in shock vector orientation in the setting of an implantable defibrillator (Figure 8.1).[9–11] In general, greater than 10 kg is considered adequate size for single chamber transvenous pacing and greater than 20 kg for ICD placement.[3] Since there is limited vascular access and concern for the development of venous occlusion, others have recommended a more conservative approach, utilizing epicardial leads and delaying transvenous device placement

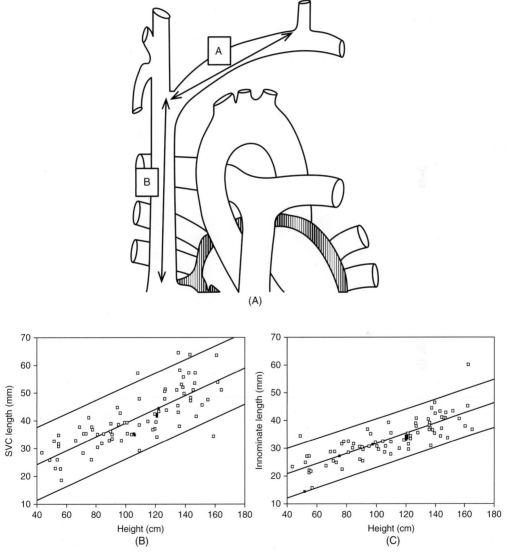

(A)

(B)

(C)

Figure 8.1 *Growth Potential of the Superior Vena Cava and Innominate Vein:Vessel Length. A. A = Length of Innominate Vein. B = Length of Superior Vena Cava B. Superior Vena Cava Length as a function of height C. Innominate Vein Length as a function of Height. (Adapted from Sanjeev and Karpawich (1).)*

until children are >3 or 4 years of age or at least 25 kg.[3, 5, 12–14] However, endocardial leads have consistently been shown to be more effective when compared with epicardial leads in children.[15–17]

Transvenous access and site selection

Several factors influence vascular access site location including venous anatomy, vessel caliber, lead size and quantity, and implanter preference.[2] The predominant vascular access sites in children are the subclavian and axillary vein. The cephalic vein may also be used in pediatric patients that approach adult size. In addition transfemoral and internal jugular approaches have been described.[18, 19]

The venous anatomy of children is similar to adults except for smaller caliber and shallower depth. Variants of venous anatomy can be seen with congenital heart disease and are discussed elsewhere. The vessel calibers of central venous structures such as the subclavian veins are adequate for single and possibly multiple lead placement and increase with age (Figure 8.2). The risk profile for children may be increased due to smaller anatomy, therefore it is essential to maintain emergency equipment.[20] Complications of vascular access include bleeding, hematoma, pneumothorax, hemothorax, laceration of blood vessel, inadvertent arterial access, AV fistula, brachial plexus injury, thoracic duct injury, chylothorax, and lymphatic fistulas.

Various techniques have been utilized to access the target vein including percutaneous puncture using surface landmarks, puncture using deep landmarks, direct visualization via surgical cut down, and image guided access using fluoroscopy, contrast venography, or ultrasound.[2] Contrast venography using a peripheral intravenous catheter in the upper extremity of interest allows for determination of vessel patency and caliber. A 10–20 cc bolus of radiopaque contrast is injected followed by a 10–20 cc saline flush. Under fluoroscopy or cineangiogrpahy the contrast bolus is followed to the point of interest, generally the axillary vein to the superior vena cava. The image can be stored and analyzed for vessel caliber to determine if the target vessel will accommodate the leads and introducer sheaths. The image can be used as a guide for percutaneous puncture (Figure 8.3).[21]

The Seldinger technique is used to obtain access to the blood vessel.[22] An 18 or 21 gauge needle attached to a non-leur lock 10 cc syringe is advanced towards the blood vessel with negative pressure on the syringe to assess for aspiration of blood. Once the vessel is entered, a wire is passed through the needle into the blood vessel and followed under fluoroscopy to confirm placement in the correct vessel. When an 18-gauge needle is used, an 0.035" J guidewire is placed, the needle removed, and a peel away sheath is advanced over the wire with a slight curve on the tip to provide optimal orientation toward the SVC- RA junction. If a 21-gauge needle is used for smaller children to minimize puncture size, than a 4Fr or 5Fr microintroducer set can be used to replace the 0.018" guidewire with the stiffer 0.035" J guidewire followed by sheath placement.

In the setting of dual chamber pacing or cardiac resynchronization therapy, additional wire and sheath placement is required.[2] This can be done by utilizing the method described above to obtain two or more separate puncture sites, wire insertion, and sheath placement. An alternative approach is a single puncture site with a retained guidewire. Following a single puncture, a sheath is placed over the guidewire. Through this sheath additional guidewires are placed and the sheath is removed leaving only the guidewires in place. Individual peel-away sheaths can be placed over each wire. This technique decreases complications related to vessel puncture. The disadvantage is that the leads course through the same opening resulting in a possible binding site, which may impair future lead extraction.

The subclavian vein can be accessed via a medial approach between the first rib and clavicle or an approach lateral to the intersection of the first rib and clavicle, generally at the intersection of the middle and outer third of the clavicle where it turns superiorly. The needle is inserted with the bevel side up and directed towards the sternal notch. If the needle abuts the clavicle, it should be angled under the clavicle to avoid tracking through the periosteum. The needle should be slowly advanced while aspirating the syringe until a flash of free flowing venous blood enters the syringe. Once

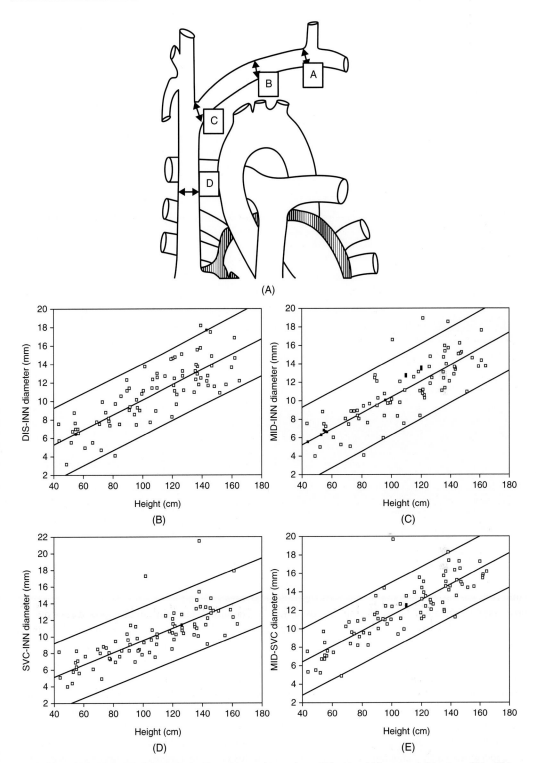

(A)

(B)

(C)

(D)

(E)

Figure 8.2 *Growth Potential of the Superior Vena Cava and Innominate Vein: Vessel Diameter. A. Diagram of identifying locations of venous diameter measurement. B-E. Venous Diameter as a function of Height. B. Distal Innominate Vein. C. Mid Innominate Vein. D. Proximal Innominate Vein at Insertion to Superior Vena Cava. E. Superior Vena Cava. (Adapted from Sanjeev and Karpawich (1).)*

(A)

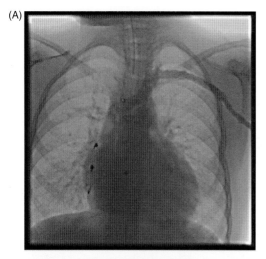

(B)

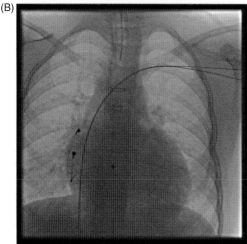

Figure 8.3 *Contrast Venography Road Map for Vascular Access. A. Contrast Venogram. B. Access with Guide wire placement. (Adapted from Silvetti et al. (2).)*

this occurs, the syringe should be removed and the guidewire placed using the Seldinger technique. The lateral approach minimizes the risk of pneumothorax and subclavian crush.

The axillary vein, which is extrathoracic and lateral to the first rib, can also be accessed (Figure 8.4). The axillary vein is a continuation of the basilica vein and terminates immediately beneath the clavicle at the outer border of the first rib. The venipuncture site is usually around 2.5 cm (~1 inch) medial to the deltopectoral groove and ~2.5 cm/1 inch inferior to the lateral third of the clavicle.[21] The needle should be almost parallel to

the tissue and angled approximately 60° from the cranial-caudal axis. Radiographically, the lateral axillary vein is located where the anterior portion of the second rib superimposes on the posterior portion of the third rib. The medial aspect of the axillary vein is usually just inferior to the intersection of the first rib and clavicle. Its location and anatomy are desirable for venous access because of easy accessibility and abundant capacity for multiple leads. Pneumothorax and subclavian crush syndrome rarely occur with axillary venous access.

Cephalic vein cut down has been recognized as a safe method for gaining venous access for lead implantation.[23] Direct visualization of the vein eliminates the risks associated with needle puncture including vascular and lung injury. The cephalic vein is located in the deltopectoral groove. Once it has been isolated, the distal end is tied and a venotomy is performed. The leads are introduced through the venotomy, though if this is not achievable, introduction of a guidewire is recommended. In adults, unsuccessful lead insertion may be observed in up to 40% due to inadequate size of the cephalic vein, the presence of venous stenosis, or extensive vessel tortuosity. The size limitation is even more pronounced in children.

Lead placement in the structurally normal heart

Lead placement in pediatric patients with structurally normal hearts is similar to adults, though increased consideration towards lead size and lead slack to accommodate patient growth is essential. Active fixation leads have become the preferred lead choice due to the ability to position the lead and for ease of future extraction.[24–26]

The right ventricular lead, pacing or defibrillation, tends to pose the easiest lead position and therefore is typically placed first. For active fixation leads with an inner lumen, a flexible straight stylet is placed through the lumen of the lead. The lead is advanced into the mid-right atrium via the peel away sheath. The straight stylet is removed and replaced with a hand-curved stylet. This can be formed using the thumb and index figure or thumb and handle of forceps to gently form a curve on the distal portion of the stylet which will assist in orienting the lead towards the tricuspid valve.

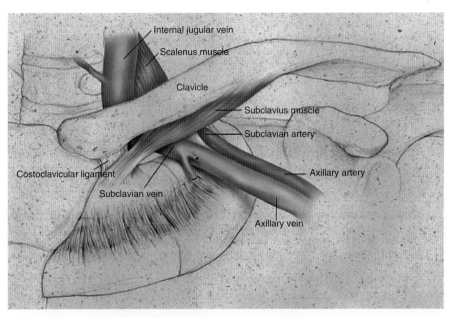

Internal jugular vein

Scalenus muscle

Clavicle

Subclavius muscle

Subclavian artery

Costoclavicular ligament

Axillary artery

Subclavian vein

Axillary vein

Figure 8.4 *Vascular Access Anatomy for Device Implantation. (Adapted From Ramza et al. (3).)*

The stylet is advanced and the lead is directed towards the tricuspid valve. The anterior-posterior fluoroscopy camera can be adjusted to a slight right anterior oblique projection to enhance visualization of the lead passing through the tricuspid valve. Once in the right ventricle or pulmonary outflow tract, the curved stylet is removed and a flexible straight stylet is placed not quite extending to the tip of the lead. The lead is withdrawn along with the stylet to facilitate dropping of the lead tip towards the right ventricular apex. When this occurs, the stylet is advanced fully and the lead is carefully advanced into the apex. This may require a back and forth motion of withdrawing the lead and then the stylet to reorient the tip to fall into the apex. Alternative sites of pacing include the mid and high septum which may require a hand curved stylet, preformed stylet, or steerable stylet, and positioning the fluoroscopy camera in a left anterior oblique projection. When the lead is in position, passive testing analysis of the lead may be performed using a pacing system analyzer connected via alligator clips to the lead. The active fixation lead is secured with a wrench tool that deploys the retractable helix. The tool is attached to the tip of the lead and rotated clockwise until the helix is fully extended.

The lumenless active fixation lead, the Medtronic SelectSecure 3830 lead, is advantageous in pediatric patients since the external diameter is 4 French, while standard pacing leads are 7 French.[27–29] Lumenless active fixation leads are delivered through a preformed delivery sheath directed to the area of interest. The entire lead is rotated clockwise to drive the helix into the myocardium. The tines of passive fixation leads are imbedded in the trabeculations of the right ventricle. The fixated lead should undergo testing through the pacing system analyzer to assess for adequate sensing, capture, impedance and lack of extracardiac stimulus at high outputs. Once the lead is secured with acceptable testing, the lead body should be adjusted to accommodate future growth by placing a "heel" on the lead in the right atrium. Gheissari et al. report that 190 mm of additional lead in an infant and 100 mm of additional lead in a 10 year old is required to have adequate lead slack at adult size.[30] For very small children, loops in the atrium have been advocated (Figure 8.5) but this may result in higher rate of dislodgement or prolapse across the tricuspid or pulmonary valve resulting in symptomatic valvar insufficiency.[30–32] Others propose prolapsing the lead into the inferior vena cava with limited success (Figure 8.6).[33, 34] For

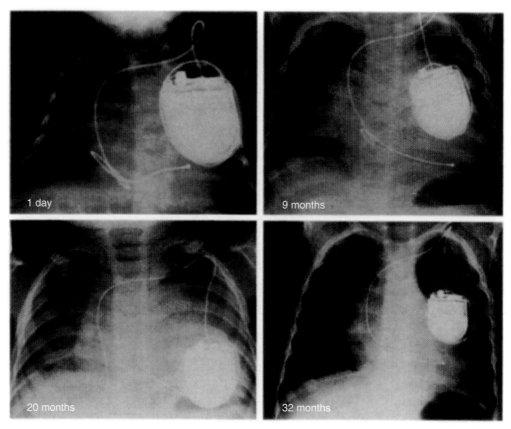

Figure 8.5 *Atrial Loop for Right Ventricular Lead Placement in Small Children. (Adapted from Rosenthal et al. (4).)*

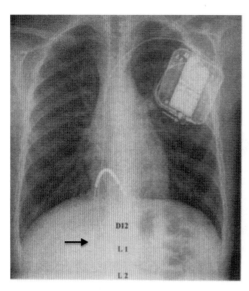

Figure 8.6 *Inferior Vena Cava Loop for Implantable Defibrillator Lead. (Adapted from Gasparini et al. (5).)*

implantable cardioverter-defibrillators, orientation of the shock coil to the device should be considered to optimize ideal shock vector. It is important to consider that future changes in body size may result in reorientation of the system and potentially provide diminished defibrillation efficacy.

The atrial lead can then be positioned if a left ventricular lead is not required. For an active fixation lead with an inner lumen, a flexible straight stylet is placed through the lumen of the lead. The lead is introduced into the mid right atrium. The stylet is removed and replaced with a preformed J curved stylet. The lead is gently pulled upwards with the curve facing slightly anterior and medial until in attaches into the right atrial appendage. The lead tip should be "wagging" side-to-side suggesting appropriate location in the appendage. Lead fixation is similar to that described for right ventricular leads. The lead should undergo testing before and after fixation and adjustment of lead slack. High output pacing should be performed to assess for phrenic stimulation. The slack should allow for the loop to extend towards the low right atrium in smaller children and mid atrium in older children taking care to avoid stenting open the tricuspid valve. An alternative site for atrial pacing that can be considered is Bachmann's bundle. This is located in the posterior high right atrial septum near the superior vena cava and is an option if there is significant far-field sensing in the atrial appendage.[5]

The left ventricular lead for cardiac resynchronization therapy can be placed via a variety of delivery systems that allow for coronary sinus and cardiac vein engagement. The first step in coronary sinus engagement is to utilize a special sheath and guidewire to gain access. A balloon occlusion injection can be performed to assess coronary sinus and cardiac vein anatomy (Figure 8.7). Using a guidewire or telescoping vein selector sheath, the vein of interest is engaged with the guidewire. The

left ventricular lead is placed over the guidewire and deployed into the cardiac vein. Since the lead is passive fixation, care should be taken to ensure the lead is lodged into the vessel and does not freely move, which increases the risk of dislodgement. The lead is tested to ensure adequate function. Though various locations for left ventricular lead placement have been reported in adults, the apex should be avoided and in general a reasonable target is the posterior lateral cardiac vein with a mid-basal location.[35, 36] The role of cardiac resynchronization therapy in pediatric patients without structural disease is limited and therefore expertise availability with left ventricular placement should be considered.

After each lead is placed, the peel away sheath is removed and the lead is secured to the fascia at the vessel entry site using the anchoring sleeve and non-absorbable suture. It has been suggested that using absorbable sutures will allow

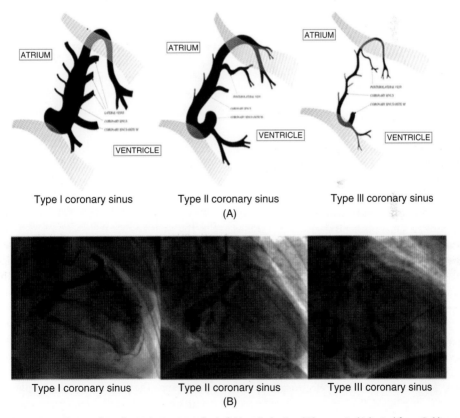

Type I coronary sinus   Type II coronary sinus   Type III coronary sinus
(A)

Type I coronary sinus   Type II coronary sinus   Type III coronary sinus
(B)

Figure 8.7 *Coronary Sinus and Cardiac Vein Anatomy for Left Ventricular Lead Placement. (Adapted from Gokhroo et al. (6).)*

for lead migration into the intravascular space with growth.[37] However, this assumes that the lead within the vessel and in the generator pocket is freely movable, which may not be the case after healing and fibrosis occurs.

Device location and pocket creation

Placement of the device pocket is dependent on device size, location of patent vascular access, patient preference, and cosmetics. The creation of the pocket can be done prior to or after venous access. The benefit of creating the pocket prior to lead implantation is to provide a longer period for hemostasis to avoid pocket hematoma, to allow for more direct access and possible visualization via cut down for vascular access, and to allow for the lead entrance to more likely be in the same plane as the device pocket. The disadvantage is that an unnecessary pocket may be created if venous access is not obtained. Either approach is reasonable and is based on implanting physician preference.

The location of the pocket is typically dependent upon the site of venous access to avoid tunneling of leads. The most common site is the infraclavicular region. Other sites include the retromammary, axillary, or in rare instances abdominal location.[38, 39] In addition, the pocket can be created in the subcutaneous or submuscular plane. The subcutaneous pocket has a decreased risk of bleeding/hematoma, procedural time, and need for additional expertise. A submuscular pocket has better cosmetics and increased protection from infection and trauma in children who lack adequate subcutaneous tissue.[40]

An infraclavicular pocket is started with a scalpel blade incision parallel to the clavicle at the level of the coracoid process and carried the width of the device. The incision is 1–2 fingerbreadths below the clavicle. In general, the subclavian vein is accessed lateral to the crossing of the first rib and clavicle, therefore the incision is located caudal to the middle third of the clavicle. For axillary access, this location can be used or one similar to a cephalic cut down approach depending on the site of insertion. Utilizing electrocautery, the incision is developed through the subcutaneous tissue and fat to the prepectoral facial layer. Use of a retractor or forceps to lift the subcutaneous tissue

away from the incision plane can assist in improved visualization and control. The electrocautery controls superficial bleeders maintaining hemostasis. A prepectoral subcutaneous pocket is fashioned using blunt and/or sharp dissection to create a cavity that will accommodate the size of the device and extra lead, which is common in pediatric patients. This can be done using electrocautery, blunt dissection with the implanter's fingers, or spreading of tissue using a pair of Metzenbaum scissors. It is important for the plane to remain just above the prepectoral fascia and ensure the depth of subcutaneous tissue remains constant to avoid any areas at increased risk for device erosion. Once the pocket has been created and hemostasis is achieved, antibiotic soaked gauze can be placed into the cavity until the pocket is needed.

An alternative is the creation of a subpectoral pocket for improved cosmetics, reduced tension of pocket margins for closure, decreased pressure points to avoid pocket erosion, and added protection for the more active lifestyles of children.[40] The same approach is taken as described previously though the dissection is extended through the preprectoral fascia plane. Care should be taken to ensure a clear linear incision and slight removal of the edge of the fascia off the pectoralis muscle to allow for clean margins, which will ease pocket closure. Once the pectoralis major is exposed, the muscle is examined to find a plane between muscle fibers. Use of Metzenbaum scissors, blunt dissection, or electrocautery can be used to disrupt the fibrous connections between the muscle bundles. The opening should be extended to accommodate the device. The dissection is advanced to the anterior chest wall and the pocket fashioned by using either blind blunt dissection with an index finger or direct visualization with retraction and electrocautery. The disadvantage of blunt dissection is the risk of disrupting blood vessels resulting in bleeding. This can be managed with electrocautery, vascular clips, suture ligation, or direct pressure. If direct visualization is used, it is important that adequate lighting is available, which may include a headlamp. The pocket should accommodate the device and excess lead, hemostasis achieved, and antibiotic soaked gauze placed in the cavity until the pocket is needed. Prior to placement of the new device, the gauze is removed and the pocket irrigated with antibiotic saline solution.

The leads are connected to the device by inserting the pins into the header of the pulse generator and tightening the set screws with a ratcheted screwdriver. An attempt is made to avoid acute lead angles which may pose a risk for fracture. The pin openings of the header may be oriented either medially or laterally depending on lead location. Extending the pocket more superiorly to allow for the leads to be placed behind the device may be necessary. Fluoroscopy should be undertaken to assess satisfactory lead and device position. The device can be secured with a non-absorbable suture if there is concern for movement. The pocket is typically closed in three layers using absorbable sutures, with polyfilament for the fascia and dermal layers, and a thinner monofilament for the subcuticular layer. The skin closure is reinforced with tincture of benzoin and sterile flexible skin closure strips. A dry dressing and light pressure dressing is applied. For new implants, the patient may be given an arm sling to prevent and remind against sudden arm movement to avoid acute lead dislodgement, and provide comfort.

The approach to the axillary implant is to make a vertical incision along the anterior axillary line and dissect to the retropectoral space, creating a pacemaker pocket (Figure 8.8).[38] The retromammary approach requires an incision in the inframammary fold with dissection taken to the prepectoral fascia posterior to the breast. Finally, the abdominal site can be either subcutaneous or submuscular under the abdominal rectus muscle. The assistance of a surgeon is useful if the operator lacks clinical expertise with alternative site implantation.

Approach to the generator change

Indications for pulse generator change include battery depletion, the need for device upgrade, pulse generator malfunction, pocket issues, device recall, and Twiddler's syndrome (Figure 8.9). The device should be interrogated prior to surgery to evaluate lead function. In the event the device has reached end of service prohibiting this evaluation, careful review of the device and lead history should be undertaken. In addition, leads should be reviewed to determine if they are the subject of recalls or warnings. Finally, chest radiography may provide additional assistance in determining if there is concern for device migration, reduction in lead slack, identification of abandoned transvenous leads, or suboptimal lead to device orientation with regards to implantable cardioverter-defibrillators that may raise concerns. The identification of additional unused leads in the vascular space may prevent vascular access for additional lead placement or require special procedures including extraction or tunneling.

All patients require similar pre- and postprocedural considerations as a new device implantation. A generator change requires peri-operative antibiotics and in our practice, the use of post procedural antibiotics. The previous incision is identified and the scar is excised, thus removing nonviable tissue and serving to enhance wound healing. Careful electrocautery, avoiding the cut

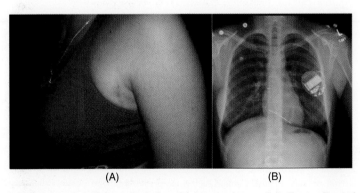

Figure 8.8 *Axillary Device Pocket. A. Axillary Implantation with improved cosmesis B. Chest radiography of axillary implant. (Adapted from Rausch et al. (7).)*

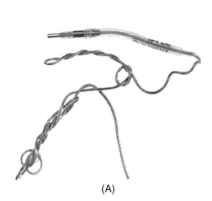
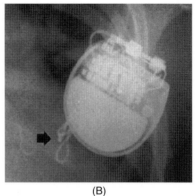

(A)   (B)

Figure 8.9 *Twiddler Syndrome. A. Coiled endocardial lead due to patient manipulation after explantation. B. Chest radiography demonstrating coiling of endocardial lead. (Adapted from Abrams et al. (8).)*

mode, and blunt dissection is performed to expose the device with special attention to avoid lead damage and bleeding. The device is explanted with care taken to remove adhesions with electrocautery or blunt dissection. A pair of cokers or a large curved hemostat can help facilitate this process by grabbing the generator body. The leads are disconnected by loosening the set screws in the header. Prior to disconnection, it is important to have an understanding of the underlying rhythm. In patients with inadequate escape rates, pacing cables and the pacing system analyzer should be readily available. Assessment of existing leads should be done through the pacing system analyzer prior to attachment to the new device.

Conclusion

Optimal transvenous device implantation in pediatric patients requires careful planning, patient assessment, and technical expertise. In addition, familiarity with special needs of growing children should always be taken in to consideration.

References

1 Antretter, H, Covin J, Schweigmann U, Hangler H, Hofer D, Dunst K, et al. Special problems of pacing in children. *Indian Pacing Electrophysiol* 2003; 3: 23–33.

2 Belott, PH. Permanent Pacemaker and implantable cardioverter-defibrillator implantation. In Ellenbogen GN, Lau C, Wilkoff BL, eds. *Clinical Cardiac Pacing, Defibrillation, and Resynchronication Therapy*. Saunders Elsevier. 2007: 561–652.

3 Berul CI. Unique aspects of pacemaker implantation. In Walsh EP; Triedman JK, eds. *Pediatric Patients, in Cardiac Arrhythmias in Children and Young Adults with Congenital Heart Disease*. Lippincott Williams & Wilkins. 2001: 303–320.

4 Berul CI, Walsh EP. Implantable cardioverter-defibrillators in pediatric patients, in cardiac arrhythmias. In Walsh EP, Triedman JK, eds. *Children and Young Adults with Congenital Heart Disease*. Lippincott Williams & Wilkins. 2001: 321–334.

5 Singh HR, Batra AS, Balaji S. Cardiac pacing and defibrillation in children and young adults. *Indian Pacing Electrophysiol* 2013; 13: 4–13.

6 Baddour LM, Epstein AE, Erickson CC, Knight BP, Levison ME, Lockhart PB, et al. Update on cardiovascular implantable electronic device infections and their management: a scientific statement from the American Heart Association. *Circulation* 2010; 121: 458–477.

7 Friedman RA, Collins E, Fenrich AL. Pacing in children: Indications and techniques. *Progress in Pediatric Cardiology*, 1995; 4: 21–29.

8 Silvetti MS, Drago F. Upgrade of single chamber pacemakers with transvenous leads to dual chamber pacemakers in pediatric and young adult patients. *Pacing Clin Electrophysiol* 2004; 27: 1094–1098.

9 Sanjeev S, Karpawich PP. Superior vena cava and innominate vein dimensions in growing children: an aid for interventional devices and transvenous leads. *Pediatr Cardio* 2006; 27: 414–419.

10 O'Sullivan JJ, Jameson S, Gold RG, Wren C. Endocardial pacemakers in children: lead length and allowance for growth. *Pacing Clin Electrophysiol* 1993; 16: 267–271.

11 Spotnitz HM. Endocardial pacemakers in children: lead length and allowance for growth. *Pacing Clin Electrophysiol* 1993; 16: 2074.

12 Gillette PC. Zeigler V, Bradham GB, Kinsella P. Pediatric transvenous pacing: a concern for venous thrombosis? *Pacing Clin Electrophysiol* 1988; 11: 1935–1939.

13 Figa FH, McCrindle BW, Bigras JL, Hamilton RM, Gow RM. Risk factors for venous obstruction in children with transvenous pacing leads. *Pacing Clin Electrophysiol* 1997; 20: 1902–1909.

14 Bar-Cohen Y, Berul CI, Alexander ME, Fortescue EB, Walsh EP, Triedman JK, Cecchin F. Age, size, and lead factors alone do not predict venous obstruction in children and young adults with transvenous lead systems. *J Cardiovasc Electrophysiol* 2006; 17: 754–759.

15 Sachweh JS, Vazquez-Jimenez JF, Schondube FA, Daebritz SH, Dorge H, Muhler EG, Messmer BJ. Twenty years experience with pediatric pacing: epicardial and transvenous stimulation. *Eur J Cardiothorac Surg*, 2000; 17: 455–461.

16 Udink ten Cate F, Breur J, Boramanand N, Crosson J, Friedman A, Brenner J, et al. Endocardial and epicardial steroid lead pacing in the neonatal and paediatric age group. *Heart* 2002; 88: 392–396.

17 Silvetti MS, Drago F, De Santis A, Grutter G, Rava L, Monti L, Fruhwirth R. Single-centre experience on endocardial and epicardial pacemaker system function in neonates and infants. *Europace* 2007; 9: 426–431.

18 Bevilacqua L, Hordof A. Cardiac pacing in children. *Current Opinion in Cardiology* 1998; 13: 48–55.

19 Costa R, Filho MM, Tamaki WT, Crevelari ES, Nishioka SD, Moreira LF, Oliveira SA. Transfemoral pediatric permanent pacing: long-term results. *Pacing Clin Electrophysiol* 2003; 26: 487–491.

20 Czosek RJ, Meganathan K, Anderson JB, Knilans TK, Marino BS, Heaton PC. Cardiac rhythm devices in the pediatric population: utilization and complications. *Heart Rhythm* 2012; 9: 199–208.

21 Silvetti MS, Placidi S, Palmieri R, Righi D, Rava L, Drago F. Percutaneous axillary vein approach in pediatric pacing: comparison with subclavian vein approach. *Pacing Clin Electrophysiol* 2013; 36: 1550–1557.

22 Seldinger SI. Catheter replacement of the needle in percutaneous arteriography; a new technique. *Acta Radiol* 1953; 39: 368–376.

23 Neri R, Cesario AS, Baragli D, Monti F, Danisi N, Glaciale G, Gambelli G. Permanent pacing lead insertion through the cephalic vein using an hydrophilic guidewire. *Pacing Clin Eletrophysiol* 2003; 26: 2313–2314.

24 Friedman RA, Moak JP, Garson Jr, A. Active fixation of endocardial pacing leads: the preferred method of pediatric pacing. *Pacing Clin Electrophysiol* 1991; 14: 1213–1216.

25 Kenny D, Walsh KP. Noncatheter-based delivery of a single-chamber lumenless pacing lead in small children. *Pacing Clin Electrophysiol* 2007; 30: 834–838.

26 Cecchin F, Atallah J, Walsh EP, Triedman JK, Alexander ME, Berul CI. Lead extraction in pediatric and congenital heart disease patients. *Circ Arrhythm Electrophysiol* 2010; 3: 437–444.

27 Campbell RM, Raviele AA, Hulse EJ, Auld DO, McRae GJ, Tam VK, Kanter KR. Experience with a low profile bipolar, active fixation pacing lead in pediatric patients. *Pacing Clin Electrophysiol* 1999; 22: 1152–1157.

28 Lapage MJ, Rhee EK. Alternative delivery of a 4Fr lumenless pacing lead in children. *Pacing Clin Electrophysiol* 2008; 31: 543–547.

29 Tuzcu V. Implantation of SelectSecure leads in children. *Pacing Clin Electrophysiol* 2007; 30: 831–833.

30 Gheissari A, Hordof AJ, Spotnitz HM. Transvenous pacemakers in children: relation of lead length to anticipated growth. *Annals of Thoracic Surgery* 1991; 52: 118–121.

31 Rosenthal E, Bostock J. Use of an atrial loop to extend the duration of endocardial pacing in a neonate. *Pacing Clin Electrophysiol* 1997; 20: 2489–2491.

32 Berul CI, Villafane J, Atkins DL, Cecchin F, Kirsh JA, Johns JA, Kanter RJ. Pacemaker lead prolapse through the pulmonary valve in children. *Pacing Clin Electrophysiol* 2007; 30: 1183–1189.

33 Gasparini M, Mantica M, Galimberti P, Coltorti F, Ceriotti C, Priori SG. Inferior vena cava loop of the implantable cardioverter defibrillator endocardial lead: a possible solution of the growth problem in pediatric implantation. *Pacing Clin Electrophysiol* 2000; 23: 2108–2112.

34 Antretter H, Hangler H, Colvin J, Laufer G. Inferior vena caval loop of an endocardial pacing lead did not solve the growth problem in a child. *Pacing Clin Electrophysiol* 2001; 24: 1706–1708.

35 Worley S. Left Ventricular lead implantation. In Ellenbogen GN, Lau C, Wilkoff BL, eds. *Clinical Cardiac Pacing, Defibrillation, and Resynchronization Therapy*. Saunders Elsevier. 2007; 653–826.

36 Dubin AM, Janousek J, Rhee E, Strieper MJ Cecchin F, Law IH, et al. Resynchronization therapy in pediatric and congenital heart disease patients: an international multicenter study. *J Am Coll Cardiol* 2005; 46: 2277–2283.

37 Stojanov P, Velimirovic D, Hrnjak V, Pavlovic SU, Zivkovic M, Djordjevic Z. Absorbable suture technique: solution to the growth problem in pediatric pacing with endocardial leads. *Pacing Clin Electrophysiol* 1998; 21: 65–68.

38 Rausch CM, Hughes BH, Runciman M, Law IH, Bradley DJ, Sujeev M, et al. Axillary versus infraclavicular placement for endocardial heart rhythm devices in patients with pediatric and congenital heart disease. *Am J Cardiol* 2010; 106: 1646–1651.

39 Rosenthal E. A cosmetic approach for pectoral pacemaker implantation in young girls. *Pacing Clin Electrophysiol* 2000; 23: 1397–1400.

40 Gillette PC, Edgerton J, Kratz J, Zeigler V. The subpectoral pocket: the preferred implant site for pediatric pacemakers. *Pacing Clin Electrophysiol* 1991; 14: 1089–1092.

CHAPTER 9

Permanent pacemaker, CRT, and ICD implantation in congenital heart disease

Ian Law[1] and Nicholas H. Von Bergen[2]

[1]Director, Division of Pediatric Cardiology, University of Iowa Children's Hospital, Clinical Professor of Pediatrics, University of Iowa College of Medicine, Iowa City, IA, USA
[2]Pediatric Electrophysiologist, The University of Wisconsin – Madison, Pediatric Cardiology, Associate Professor of Pediatrics, The University of Wisconsin – Madison, Madison, Wisconsin, USA

Pacemakers and ICDs in the pediatric and young adult population make up less than 1% of all device implants. An even smaller percentage is implanted in patients with congenital heart disease. However, with technology advancements including smaller devices, more durable epicardial leads, and more appropriate sensing and tracking capabilities, device implantation has become more feasible in this population. In these patients their size, their potential for growth, and variations in congenital and surgical anatomy challenges the implanting physician when device therapy is required in the unrepaired and post-operative congenital heart disease patient. The inevitable need for device and lead replacements in a patient population that has often undergone numerous previous cardiac surgeries further complicates initial device system selection, device follow-up, and subsequent generator and lead replacements. This chapter will focus on indications for pacemaker and ICD placement in patients with congenital heart disease, lead and device selection when implanting a device in patients with congenital heart disease, and unique issues for pacemaker, ICD, and cardiac resynchronization therapy device implantation in patients with congenital heart disease.

Indications for pacemaker placement in patients with congenital heart disease

Pacemakers

The indications for placement of the pacemaker are often similar to the indications in adult populations, though the etiology of the disease is often quite different. In general, pacemakers are implanted for sinus node dysfunction, congenital atrioventricular block, post-surgical complete AV block or advanced secondary block, and occasionally neurocardiogenic syncope secondary to prolonged episodes of extreme bradycardia or asystole. Additionally, patients with arrhythmias, often associated with congenital heart disease, are now having pacemakers placed for the suppression, treatment, and detection of arrhythmias.

Cardiac Pacing and Defibrillation in Pediatric and Congenital Heart Disease, First Edition.
Edited by Maully Shah, Larry Rhodes and Jonathan Kaltman.
© 2017 John Wiley & Sons Ltd. Published 2017 by John Wiley & Sons Ltd.
Companion Website: www.wiley.com/go/shah/cardiac_pacing

The current Cass I, Class IIA, IIB, and III indications for pacemaker placement as recommended by the 2008 guidelines from the ACC/AHA/HRS are discussed next as it relates to the congenital heart patient population. For further details, please refer to the Guidelines.[1] A Class I indication means that the benefit significantly outweighs the risk, and that device implantation is considered beneficial and effective. A Class IIa indication is given when there is conflicting data, but it is felt that the benefit outweighs the risk, and that it is reasonable to implant a device. A Class IIb indication implies that efficacy is less well-established and that further data may be needed. In this case the procedure may be considered. A class III indication indicates that implantation of a device is not useful and may be harmful.

Recommendations for pacemaker placement in pediatric and CHD

Sinus node dysfunction

Implantation of a pacemaker is a Class I indication in sinus node dysfunction with documented *symptomatic* bradycardia. This may be as a result of decreased sinus node function due to prior cardiac surgery, but may also be due to side effects from long-term medication therapy when there are no other acceptable alternatives. The definition of bradycardia in adults generally denotes heart rates less than 40 bpm while awake and systolic pauses greater than 3–4 seconds. In pediatrics, the definition of bradycardia is age dependent (Table 9.1). Furthermore, the patient's ability to tolerate bradycardia is greatly dependent on their hemodynamic status. For example, a newborn with a structurally normal heart should tolerate a heart rate of 70 bpm, however, if the newborn has complex congenital heart disease or a significant intracardiac shunt resulting in volume overload or profound cyanosis, a heart rate of 70 may be poorly tolerated. Thus, although sinus node dysfunction *without* symptoms generally warrants observation in adults (even with heart rates less than 30 or 40 bpm while awake), a pacemaker may be required in a patient in whom improved hemodynamics (i.e., single ventricle physiology) may be determined to prevent symptoms or worsening of hemodynamic status depending on the underlying heart disease.

Table 9.1 *Normal heart rate ranges for age. Generalized from the article "New normal limits for the paediatric electrocardiogram".[2] (Source: Rijnbeek 2001. Reproduced with permission of OUP)*

Age	Heart rate in bpm range (mean)
0–1 month	130–190 (155)
1–3 months	120–190 (155)
3–6 months	110–180 (135)
6–12 months	100–190 (130)
1–3 years	95–160 (120)
3–5 years	75–125 (100)
5–8 years	65–115 (90)
8–12 years	55–105 (80)
12–16 years	50–100 (75)

In addition to baseline bradycardia, post-operative patients or patients with atrial isomerism may require pacemaker implantation for chronotropic incompetence due to an inability to increase their heart rate during exertion; another Class I indication for pacemaker placement.

Given the higher risk of sinus node dysfunction in patients with congenital heart disease (both unrepaired and repaired), a baseline 24-hour ambulatory ECG can provide valuable information on subclinical rhythm disturbances and heart rate variability. If symptoms do not occur daily, a longer term event monitor (up to 1 month) may be necessary, and in some cases an implantable loop recorder is required for events that occur only a few times per year or less. If chronotropic incompetence is suspected, an exercise test may provide immediate feedback and is also an excellent method to evaluate the heart rate response to exertion. An electrophysiology study may aid in the evaluation of sinus node dysfunction but is a surrogate for the clinical studies mentioned previously.

Syncope as indication for pacemaker implantation

Patients with recurrent syncope with periods of asystole longer than 3 s and symptoms that have been correlated to the asystolic event fall into a Class I indication for pacemaker implant (Figure 9.1). A Class IIA indication is present if there is recurrent syncope with either sinus node dysfunction or significant vagal response

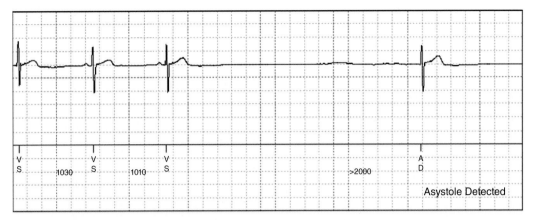

Figure 9.1 *Recording from of an episode of asystole and associated syncope documented on an implantable loop recorder.*

without a clear association between the two events. Distinguishing syncopal events secondary to asystole from other cardiac and non-cardiac causes is especially important in patients with congenital heart disease; their increased risk for abnormal, and occasionally life threatening arrhythmias warrants a thorough work-up. At times an electrophysiology study may be considered if the etiology of the syncope is uncertain, especially if an arrhythmia is suspected.

Atrioventricular block

AV block is a relatively common cause of pacemaker placement in the pediatric and congenital heart disease patient population. Infants with complete atrioventricular block (often due to maternal autoantibodies) are recommended for pacemaker placement with ventricular rates less than 50–55 bpm after birth. This recommendation is adjusted in patients with congenital heart disease and complete heart block to rates less than 70 bpm. Similar to the guidelines discussed for sinus node dysfunction, these recommendations should not be a strict cut-off as compromised ventricular function or significant shunts may require AV synchrony and higher heat rates to maintain an appropriate cardiac output. Therefore, the patient's clinical status should be considered with implantation of a pacemaker in this population.

In the older population, those with third degree heart block or with high grade secondary heart block associated with symptoms is a Class I indication for pacemaker placement. This is true both with and without congenital heart disease. It should be noted that it is common for patients to have second degree AV block with single dropped beats, typically at night and not associated with symptoms. In these patients, a pacemaker would not be indicated. Once again, it is important to correlate the electrocardiographic findings with symptoms.

It is estimated that the risk of heart block after cardiac surgery is around 1% for VSD closure;[3] therefore it remains a frequent cause of pacemaker implantation. If high grade second or third degree heart block is present post operatively then a pacemaker should be considered after 7–10 days if there has been no return of AV node function.

Pause dependent ventricular arrhythmias

A unique set of patients are those with Long QT syndrome and other diseases who may be at risk for pause dependent ventricular arrhythmias and who require medications that may cause sinus bradycardia. In patients with confirmed sustained pause-dependent VT (without QT prolongation) pacing is a class I indication (typically with an ICD). In other congenital long-QT syndrome patients who are considered high risk, permanent pacing is a Class IIA indication.

Hypertrophic cardiomyopathy

The current guidelines suggest giving consideration to pacing in hypertrophic cardiomyopathy with medically refractory, symptomatic LV outflow obstruction (class IIb). In this case the ventricular pacing is implemented to create ventricular dyssynchrony, thereby potentially decreasing the dynamic outflow obstruction.

Post cardiac transplant

In addition to the causes listed above, pacing is indicated (Class I) for persistent inappropriate or symptomatic bradycardia not expected to resolve in the heart transplant population. This may also be a sign of acute transplant rejection and should be evaluated accordingly.

Pacing to terminate atrial arrhythmias

Congenital heart disease and cardiac surgery place patients at increased risk of re-entry atrial arrhythmias. Intra-atrial reentrant tachycardia is the most common reentrant arrhythmia seen in patients who have undergone surgery, affecting as many as 40–50%.[4] Proposed mechanisms include underlying and surgically created anatomic barriers, the progression of myocardial fibrosis, myocardial changes associated with atrial stretch from volume or pressure overload, and sinus node dysfunction that may trigger the reentrant arrhythmia. In these cases, permanent pacing is a class IIa recommendation for symptomatic recurrent SVT that is reproducibly terminated by overdrive pacing when catheter ablation and/or medications fail to control the arrhythmia. This is seen most commonly in the older post-operative congenital heart disease patient. Caution should be exercised in patients that have an accessory pathway that has a short refractory period (Class III), or an AV node capable of conducting rapidly to the ventricle, as the rapid atrial pacing may result in an accelerated ventricular rate and cardiovascular compromise. For this reason, current atrial pace-termination protocols are automatically disabled when there is 1:1 AV conduction. In general, due to the risk of inadvertent ventricular arrhythmia induction should the atrial lead dislodge to the ventricle, atrial arrhythmia pacing protocols are not enabled until 6 weeks post implant when lead placement is confirmed.

Pacing to prevent atrial arrhythmias

Arrhythmias, such as intra-atrial reentrant tachycardia or atrial fibrillation can be suppressed with

atrial pacing maneuvers; such as preferential pacing above the sinus rate to establish a uniform atrial activation site, or increasing the atrial pacing rate after a premature atrial complex, to prevent atrial pauses that may trigger pause dependent arrhythmias. There are currently no recommendations for implantation of a pacemaker in attempt to suppress atrial arrhythmias, though if a device is needed or in place for other indications, it should be optimized in attempt to decrease atrial arrhythmia burden.

Recommendations for implantable cardioverter defibrillator placement in patients with CHD

Cardiac indications for ICD placement in pediatric and young adults include electrical disease (i.e., long QT syndrome, CPVT), cardiomyopathies (i.e., hypertrophic cardiomyopathy, ARVC) and congenital heart disease. It is estimated that between 27%[5] and 46%[6] of young patients who undergo ICD placement have congenital heart disease. Over half of these are implanted for secondary prevention (patient already experienced a significant ventricular arrhythmia, concerning syncopal event, or sudden cardiac arrest)[5] At 5 years, the estimated appropriate shock rate for ICDs in patients with CHD was ~42%.[5] It has also been suggested that patients with CHD may be at increased risk for inappropriate shocks[5,7] (Figure 9.2).

The indication for ICD implantation is relatively clear in patients who are survivors of a cardiac arrest and in patients with symptomatic VT due to a non-reversible cause (Class I). In patients who are considered at high risk for a cardiac event, and who have unexplained syncope an ICD may also be indicated, and an EP study may be indicated to assist with ventricular arrhythmia risk (Class I if VT is induced during an EP study). Though less common in the congenital heart disease population, patients with a LVEF <35% due to a prior MI, or due to non-ischemic dilated cardiomyopathy with NYHA functional class II or III fall into the Class I indication.

The indications are less clear when implanting an ICD for primary prevention in patients with congenital heart disease. Decisions must be made on an individual basis with consideration of patient

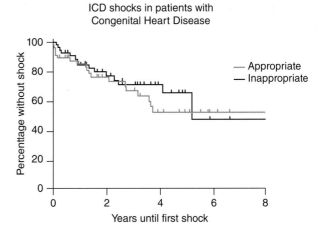

Figure 9.2 *Freedom from an ICD shock after implantation of an ICD in patients with congenital heart disease. (Source: Von Bergen 2011. Reproduced with permission of Springer[5].)*

disease, family history and patient and family input. Congenital heart disease substrate may play a key role in risk stratification for ICD implant, with certain forms of congenital heart disease having a higher risk of ventricular arrhythmia (i.e., tetralogy of Fallot, palliated systemic right ventricles). For further details concerning the indication for ICD implantation see the ACC/AHA/HRS 2008 guidelines[1] and Chapter 8 in this book.

Implanting the device

Selecting the device, leads, and device location

In this section we will discuss placement of a transvenous and epicardial devices in patients with congenital heart disease, and the decisions that surround choosing the correct device, leads and approach for each patient.

Transvenous versus epicardial leads

In patients with congenital heart disease the size of the patient (and consequently their vessels and cardiac chambers), and the anatomy of cardiovascular system are two of the major determinants to guide lead placement.

Patient size

The variable age and size in patients with congenital heart disease who require a device mandates the consideration of patient and vessel size. Though there is limited data evaluating vessel size in younger patients, the literature supports using smaller or fewer leads in smaller patients.[8-10] While controversy exists about how large a patient must be to accommodate transvenous leads, patients above 15–20 kg will usually have a subclavian, and/or axillary vein of large enough caliber to accommodate at least one lead. Above 20–30 kg, then consideration may be given to dual chamber transvenous systems. If the patient is less than ~15–20 kg, epicardial lead placement is often the best choice, though institutions vary on this recommendation. Factors that may sway one toward epicardial lead placement include; smaller subclavian vein and superior vena cava size due to the presence of a persistent left superior vena cava, stenotic systemic venous drainage secondary to past surgeries (e.g., partial anomalous vein repair requiring venous/cardiac baffle placement near the SVC-right atrial junction), or a history of recurrent venous thrombosis. Factors that may favor transvenous lead placement include numerous past cardiac surgeries or a history of pericarditis that increase the risk of epicardial fibrosis. However, in general, if there are concerns regarding small patient or vessel size, the epicardial approach is recommended.

Patient size and anatomy has further implications when implanting an ICD due to the inherently larger transvenous lead size and the shock vector created by the varied anatomy. Surprisingly, placing the ICD generator on the contralateral side of the chest in comparison to the heart (e.g., left pectoral implant in patient with dextrocardia) does not appear to be detrimental.[11] Nevertheless, the shock vector should ideally course through as much ventricular myocardium as possible.

At the time of this publication the smallest pacing lead on the market is an active fixation 4 Fr system making it seemingly ideal for smaller patients, although the 8 Fr introducing catheter limits its applicability. Attempts at reducing ICD leads have been met with mixed results, as evidenced by the higher lead failure rate seen in the Medtronic Sprint Fidelis Lead.[12]

Patient anatomy

Intracardiac anatomy and vascular anomalies may limit transvenous access to the heart. The wide variability of anatomy in the congenital heart disease population necessitates detailed knowledge of the current anatomy, prior surgical procedures, intracardiac shunting, and history of vascular access difficulties. Prior surgical notes and prior catheterization data can provide vital information to allow appropriate lead selection and placement and should be reviewed and available for each procedure. A cardiac CT or MRI, or heart catheterization with venograms prior to device implant may prove extremely valuable when evaluating for venous anomalies and stenosis. At times intervention may be required such as balloon dilation and/or stent placement prior to transvenous lead placement. In some cases, such as long segment SVC occlusion, epicardial lead placement should be considered.

In the single ventricle population, such as those who may have undergone an extracardiac Fontan procedure (IVC and SVC drain directly to the pulmonary arteries bypassing the heart) there may be no viable transvenous route to obtain access to the atrial (or ventricular) myocardium. However, in other Fontan variations, such as patients with a lateral tunnel Fontan (the IVC baffles via the RA to drain into the pulmonary arteries), there may be access to the atrial wall, allowing placement of a single atrial lead. Implanting centers have varying philosophies regarding the advisability of placing a transvenous lead in this population, however, with appropriate anticoagulation this can be a consideration[13, 14] (Figure 9.3).

Another important consideration is presence of an intracardiac lesion which may result in a right to left shunt. In these cases, even with

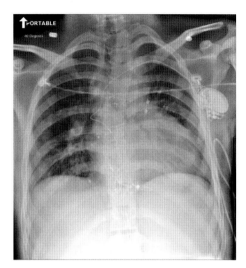

Figure 9.3 *Single chamber pacemaker with a transvenous atrial lead placed in a patient with a lateral tunnel Fontan.*

anticoagulation, epicardial lead(s) should be considered, or if possible closure of the shunt.

Extrathoracic ICDs have been developed and can be considered in patients who do not require pacing. This device generator is placed in the axilla with subcutaneous leads placed extrathoracic parallel to the sternum. Though avoiding the need for intravascular or epicardial lead placement, these devices are currently large, and are not feasible in smaller patients.

Location of device

The most common location for placement of a transvenous device generator is the pectoral area, placing an incision below the clavicle, or just medial to the delta-pectoral groove. A pocket can then be created either above or below the pectoralis major muscle. This approach allows ease of lead placement and securing the sewing sleeves and a more straight-forward approach for generator replacements. Generator placement below the pectoralis muscle may be more cosmetically appealing for children and young adults (especially those who are relatively thin) but requires more extensive dissection at the time of implant and replacement.

Interestingly, even in patient with scars due to prior cardiac surgery, we have found that many of our young adult patients are less satisfied with an anterior pectoral approach due to cosmetic reasons.[15] It is for this reason that we may

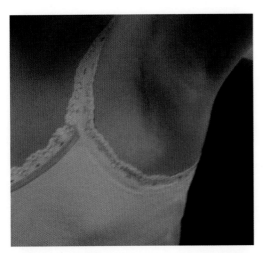

Figure 9.4 *Fully healed anterior axillary line incision for placement of a subpectoral ICD in a 10-year-old female.*

Table 9.2 *Considerations when selecting a pacemaker or ICD in a patient with congenital heart disease*

Arrhythmia history
Risk for life-threatening arrhythmias
Congenital heart disease
Battery longevity
AV node conduction
Device size
Upper tracking rate
Rate responsive mode
Need for resynchronization
MRI compatibility

consider an approach on the anterior axillary line (Figure 9.4).[15] This approach may require additional time, in part due to slightly more challenging vascular access (usually the proximal axillary vein). The generator may be placed either above or below the pectoral muscle, or in the axilla. Additionally, care must be taken when securing the sewing sleeve and tunneling the lead to the pocket (if subpectoral or axillary). Securing the lead as close to the vein entrance site will reduce the possibility of lead dislodgement. This approach typically also requires slightly more lead slack when compared to a more medial subclavian approach, due to potential greater caudal movement of the device when the patient is upright. Despite the more axillary position, no difference has been found in pocket infection or lead dislodgement.[15]

When an axillary pocket is used for placement of the device generator a smaller incision may be placed near the delta pectoral groove and the lead is tunneled to a larger incision near the anterior axillary line. The larger incision allows a pocket to be created in the axilla.[15] This axillary placement is also used with the leadless extrathoracic device (Cameron Health), which is placed in the axilla with subcutaneous sensing and defibrillation lead parallel to the sternum.[16]

Pacemaker/ICD generator selection

To select the appropriate device for patients with congenital heart disease the implanting physician must consider the patient's current arrhythmias and risk of disease progression. Some considerations are included in Table 9.2. For example, you may wish to consider a dual chamber device in a patient with sinus node dysfunction who may be at risk for AV block in the future. Additionally, variable features on the devices must be considered – such as over drive pacing, rate stabilization as well as maximum upper tracking rate.

Standard approach to placement of a pacemaker or an ICD

In many cases the approach to lead and generator placement for patients with congenital heart disease is identical to those with a structurally normal heart, discussed in Chapter 8.

Unique scenarios for pacemaker or ICD implantation in patients with congenital heart disease

High thresholds with epicardial device placement

Due to diseased myocardium it is not uncommon to have elevated pacing thresholds in patients with prior cardiac surgery. When placing epicardial leads, significant effort and patience is required on the part of the cardiac surgeon to remove adhesions and avoid scar tissue. If the epicardial sensing or pacing thresholds are inappropriately high, a unipolar surface lead or a screw-in lead may be considered. While unipolar leads may allow for improved sensing, they may have a lower impedance (resulting in higher pacing current drain), and some devices require a bipolar lead for sensing (e.g., atrial anti-tachycardia pacemakers, ICDs). The current penetrating unipolar lead also lack steroid elution technology, potentially reducing lead longevity. In some instances, consideration may be given to placing a transmyocardial endocardial lead by making a purse string suture within the atrium, advancing a transvenous lead through that purse string, and affixing it to the endocardium within the atrium or ventricle.[17]

Bioprosthetic tricuspid valves and a transvenous pacemaker

Lead placement through a mechanical valve is contraindicated. However, the appropriateness of placing leads across a bio-prosthetic valve is uncertain. There is limited information to guide therapy, though it is known that the presence of a permanent pacemaker is a risk factor for tricuspid regurgitation after annuloplasty.[18] As this would also place the patient at increased risk for clot and valve stenosis we typically choose to place epicardial leads if possible. In appropriate patients the ventricular lead may be placed within the coronary sinus, instead of through the tricuspid valve.[19]

Left sided superior vena cava and lead placement

The presence of a persistent left superior vena cava draining to the coronary sinus is more common in patients with complex congenital heart disease.[20, 21] In patients where a transvenous approach from the right subclavian vein is not feasible, placement through the coronary sinus is possible but is more challenging, especially for the ventricular lead due to the relatively acute angle needed to cross the tricuspid valve (Figure 9.5). Using a steerable sheath with smaller leads may allow improved ability to navigate the leads into appropriate atrial and ventricular sites.

Though implantation in patients with a LSVC is generally reasonably straightforward special attention needs to be taken with removal of the leads as the vessel wall is likely more pliable than the superior vena cava and the number of direction changes of the lead may place increased pressure onto those walls during removal. Therefore, removal of these leads should be performed by

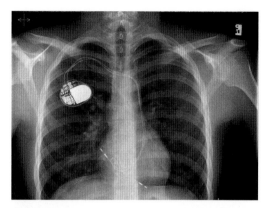

Figure 9.5 *A dual chamber pacemaker placed through a LSVC to coronary sinus.*

a physician experienced in lead extraction, with appropriate surgical back-up.

Placement of leads in a patient with D-transposition of the great arteries post Mustard or Senning procedure

Patients with dextro-transposition of the great arteries after a Mustard or Senning procedure frequently require pacemakers due to sinus node dysfunction and atrial arrhythmias. Additionally, due to the systemic right ventricle they are also at increased risk for ventricular arrhythmias or cardiac dysfunction prompting an ICD or cardiac resynchronization (Figure 9.6).

At the time of device implantation in patients post Mustard or Senning procedure a hemodynamic catheterization with an interventional pediatric cardiologist is prudent to evaluate for baffle leaks, stenosis, or occlusion that may not be seen on echocardiogram. Cardiac imaging by CT or MRI may also be appropriate to evaluate the anatomy. In the case of venous or baffle stenosis or other underlying anatomical concerns the decision for device placement may be altered. In the case of a baffle leak or stenosis, device occlusion, or stent placement has been successfully performed in the same setting though care must be taken to avoid entrapment or dislodgement during lead placement (Figure 9.7A–C). There is also the theoretic concern of lead insulation damage by device-lead interaction, although this appears to be a rare occurrence.

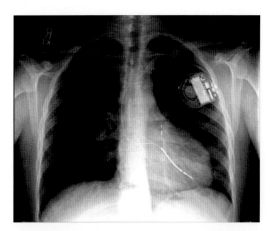

Figure 9.6 *Placement of a dual chamber ICD through a stent in the superior baffle in a patient with D-TGA post Mustard procedure. The atrial lead is at the base of the left atrial appendage, and the ventricular lead near the left ventricular apex.*

When placing transvenous leads in patients in this population, the left atrial portion of the systemic venous atrium is often the best site for stable lead attachment. A steerable sheath, such as that used in the smaller diameter non-stylet driven lead systems, may allow for improved site selection through the atrial baffle. Placing the lead tip near the dome of the left atrium greatly reduces the risk of phrenic nerve capture; though high output pacing should be performed to evaluate for phrenic nerve stimulation. The ventricular lead usually is directed toward the left ventricular apex after passing through the baffle system. In patients who require chronic ventricular pacing, directing the lead toward the septum may reduce ventricular dyssynchrony.

Placement of an implantable cardioverter defibrillator in patients with challenging vascular access

Congenital heart disease patients often have vascular access or intracardiac anatomy anomalies that may make the transvenous route infeasible. This has resulted in the development of novel implant techniques. Optimal ICD function requires a thorough understanding of the patient's anatomy, past surgical history, arrhythmia history, and pacing requirements. Often "hybrid systems" are required to allow appropriate sensing, pacing, and defibrillation. In place of standard transvenous defibrillation

leads, physicians have used epicardial patches, subcutaneous array(s), or transvenous leads placed into the pericardial or pleural space.[11, 22] While effective, these novel ICD systems tend to have higher defibrillation thresholds. In addition, more intensified device follow-up should be considered due to reported higher failure rate secondary to lead movement, elevated DFT, or early failure.[11]

Resynchronization therapy

Recommendations for cardiac resynchronization

Class I indication: Patients with a LVEF <35% and QRS duration >120 ms and sinus rhythm. NYHA functional class III or IV despite optimized pharmacological therapy.[1]

Cardiac resynchronization is now an established technique to improve overall heart function and ejection fraction in patients with evidence of electrical and mechanical dyssynchrony. In adult patients with left ventricular failure and a wide QRS complex (typically due to a left bundle branch block) both acute and chronic hemodynamic improvement in left ventricular ejection fraction has been reported.[23–25] Though usually reserved for patients with severely diminished function and significant heart failure, resynchronization has also been shown to improve LVEF even in those with mild heart failure.[26]

The use of CRT in pediatric patients was first described in 2001 as an alternative therapy for dilated cardiomyopathy in patients with congenital heart disease.[27] However, there is currently limited data in the congenital heart disease population to provide guidance for patient selection, effectiveness or risks associated with cardiac resynchronization. The guidelines from the European Society of Cardiology, published in *Europace* in 2007, report "pacing for heart failure in this complex heterogenous sub-population is supported by limited evidence and requires further investigation to identify who may benefit the most from which pacing modality."[28] Acknowledging that we have not developed adequate guidelines to assist with patient selection, we can follow some basic guidance based on interpretation of adult data, as well as pediatric case reports and retrospective studies.

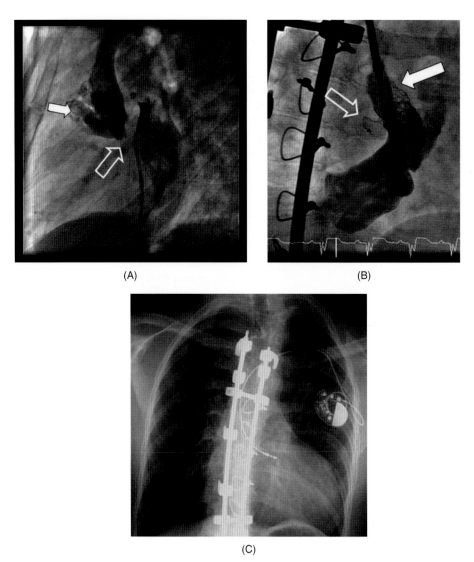

Figure 9.7 *(A) Angiography (Lateral view) with simultaneous contrast injection in the superior and inferior limb of the systemic venous baffle in a patient with D-TGA, s/p Mustard procedure and sinus node dysfunction prior to transvenous atrial pacemaker placement. A complete discontinuation between the superior and inferior limb is noted (open arrow) and a baffle leak is present (closed arrow). (B) Angiography (PA) view in the same patient after re-establishing baffle patency with a stent and baffle leak closure with an Amplatzer™ occlude. Note the patient also has Harrington rods implanted after a spinal fusion procedure, which are visualized. (C) Chest X-ray (PA view) of the same patient after transvenous atrial lead placement through the baffle stent.*

Effectiveness of cardiac resynchronization therapy (CRT)

The efficacy of cardiac resynchronization is less predictable as the heterogeneity of the population increases. Currently, the two largest studies in patients with congenital heart disease each retrospectively evaluated over 100 pediatric and congenital heart patients who underwent CRT.[29, 30] Though both studies evaluated a broad age range, the median age was in the second decade for both studies, suggesting that the data would be relevant to both pediatric and adult patients with CHD. These and other smaller studies describe a widely variable population including systemic left ventricles, systemic right ventricles, and univentric-ular hearts. In general, the patient population that has a more favorable response to CRT were those with systemic left ventricles, showing between a 10–13% increase in ejection fraction. The sub-set of patients who had a history of heart block and chronic ventricular pacing responded most favorably,[30] results echoed in other studies.[31–34] Though not described by Janousek, improvement after CRT was noted in patients with a systemic right ventricle by Dubin, with increases in ejec-tion fraction from 7–13% on echocardiogram. In patients with univentricular hearts, Cecchin et al. reported a benefit of 11% in ejection fraction, along with continued long term benefit, though Dubin et al. showed no significant increase in ejection fraction for these patients.[34]

Unlike some adult studies, pediatric and congenital heart patients may have significant dyssynchrony without signs of heart failure[29] sug-gesting that NHYA heart failure classification is an inadequate marker for screening patients in the congenital heart population. The benefit of CRT appears to be inversely related to the ejection fraction at time of implantation, and in general, those with lower EF derive greater benefit.[29, 34] Interestingly, though meta-analysis of adult data has suggested diminished benefit with CRT in patients with a shorter QRS duration,[35] there may be a role for CRT in patients with CHD and a normal QRS. Patients with CHD may have sig-nificant dyssynchrony in spite of a QRS complex <120 m.[36] The potential for an improvement in ventricular function with CRT and a narrower QRS complex has been supported by studies evaluating temporary biventricular pacing in post-operative patients with a narrow QRS complex.[37, 38]

Unfortunately, there is occasional worsen-ing of heart function after placement of a CRT device, and 20% or more patients may be non-responders.[29, 30, 34, 39] Janousek noted that the only independent multivariable predictor of a non-responder was primary dilated cardiomyopa-thy with an initially poor NYHA class. Additionally, the placement of a CRT device has been reported to be associated with frequent complications (18–22%), including post-operative arrhythmias, lead dislodgements, bleeding, and even death.[29, 34] Therefore, though there does appear to be benefit

from cardiac resynchronization in patients with CHD, these patients must be carefully selected.

Assessment of dyssynchrony in congenital heart disease

Patients with congenital heart disease are at risk for an abnormal ventricular filling in addition to inter-and intraventricular dyssynchrony. Cardiac resynchronization attempts to address each of these abnormalities.

Evaluation of AV synchrony

Heart block, prolonged PR interval, variable AV conduction and a widened QRS complex can result in suboptimal AV synchrony. Echocardiogram imaging allows evaluation of trans-mitral (or systemic AV valve) flow to confirm appropriate ventricular filling as measured by the E and A wave. Though there is sparse data in the pediatric population to guide appropriate settings in this population,[40] data from adult studies suggests that LV filling time should be greater than 40% of the R to R interval.[41] In optimal resynchronization the A wave should follow the E wave without truncation of the A wave (too short AV time with mitral valve closure prior to completing the A wave), or fusion of the E and A wave (too long of an AV time with mitral valve closure late after spontaneous closure) (Figure 9.8). Failure to appropriately time the atrial and ventricular contractions can cause lack of the full atrial filling, diastolic valve regurgitation and occasionally loss of bi-ventricular pacing. Cur-rently these settings are optimized while the patient is stationary, and there is currently a paucity of data evaluating optimal A-V timing during activity.

Evaluation of Intra-ventricular synchrony

There are many techniques used for evaluation of intra-ventricular synchrony. The echocardiogram is the most commonly used, though the optimal technique has yet to be determined. Recently, 3D echocardiography has gained acceptance to evaluate cardiac dyssynchrony by merging LV wall segment time-volume loops. These loops when compared against one another determine the systolic dyssynchrony index (SDI), a measure

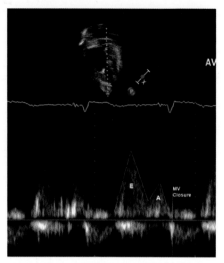

Figure 9.8 *E and A waves for evaluation of atrio-ventricular synchrony by evaluation of mitral inflow in a patient with congenital heart disease.*

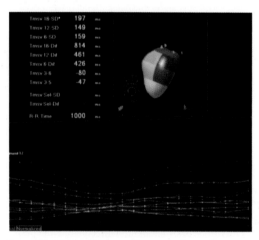

Figure 9.9 *Left ventricular wall segment time volume loops by 3D echocardiogram.*

suggestive of dyssynchrony when segments have greater variability[39, 42, 43] (Figure 9.9).

More traditionally, pulse wave Doppler is used to assess the velocity time integral (VTI) of the outflow jet, typically measured in the ascending aorta. A higher VTI is taken as a surrogate of improved ventricular ejection and thus improved synchrony. Additionally, tissue Doppler imaging (TDI) may be used to evaluate segmental wall movement and wall velocity abnormalities as well as myocardial strain and velocity[44] (Figure 9.10). M mode may be

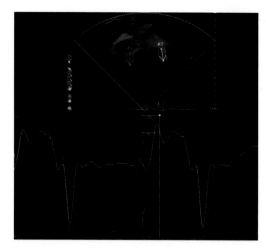

Figure 9.10 *Tissue Doppler imaging to evaluate segmental wall movement.*

used to evaluate the symmetry of movement of the septum and the posterior wall[45], and newer techniques continue to be developed, such as speckle tracking to evaluate wall movement and regional strain,[46, 47] and evaluating LV twisting.[48, 49]

The variability in cardiac anatomy in patients with congenital heart disease makes the use of any one technique for determination of heart function more difficult, especially in those with a systemic right ventricle or a single ventricle. In these patients an MRI or CT scan can be considered to assist with cardiac function, as well as resynchronization planning. Information regarding coronary sinus location, size, and branching can be obtained with high resolution CT or MRI scans, and may assist determining the feasibility of a transvenous system. It should be noted, that with current technology most pacing devices are not currently compatible with MRI scans, and CT imaging can produce significant artifact around epicardial and transvenous leads that may limit initial or follow-up evaluation.

Evaluation of inter-ventricular dyssynchrony

Though less commonly used, pulsed wave Doppler measurements in the aorta and pulmonary artery may be used to evaluate differences in timing of ventricular contractions in patients with two ventricles. Though this has been used in adult studies there is limited data in pediatric patients to confirm its predictive value to assess responsiveness to CRT.[32, 47, 50, 51]

Single ventricular lead for CRT

There is currently limited information regarding the effectiveness and appropriateness of single lead pacing in patients with CHD. The European Heart Journal consensus statement indicates that biventricular pacing is preferable, but isolated LV pacing may be acceptable in selected patients.[28] Currently, indications for single lead pacing are not clearly defined in the adult population and there is significantly less information in the pediatric and congenital heart disease population. Nevertheless, a number of case reports and adult studies suggest that the response to single lead pacing (traditionally left ventricular lead placement) may not be inferior to bi-ventricular pacing.[52, 53] As one might predict, there have been limited studies showing feasibility in the pediatric and CHD population and no significant data comparing effectiveness to bi-ventricular pacing.[47, 54]

Implantation of a CRT device

Transvenous versus epicardial approach

Cardiac resynchronization in the congenital heart population can be approached by the transvenous, epicardial or a hybrid route. The transvenous route may be considered for patients who have a systemic left ventricle and normal coronary sinus anatomy that drains into the right atrium. As discussed previously, each patient must be considered individually due to potential intrinsic or post-operative variations such as vascular or baffle stenosis, intracardiac shunting, variable intracardiac anatomy, and degree and location of dyssynchrony.

As is most common in the adult population, the standard approach for a transvenous system consists of a single atrial lead, a right-sided ventricular lead placed in a "traditional" position, and a left-sided ventricular lead placed within a branching coronary vein. The coronary sinus lead position is typically chosen in the lateral LV mid-distant between the coronary sinus and apex of the ventricle. This is chosen in an attempt to be near the expected point of greatest dyssynchrony. However, it remains important to carefully evaluate the coronary sinus anatomy and compare it to regional wall motion. Ideally, the location of the LV lead should be placed in an area near maximal dyssynchrony and care should be taken to keep the LV lead away from the apex of the ventricle, as this will typically place the lead in close proximity to the RV lead limiting the ability to improve synchrony. High output pacing should also be performed to assess for phrenic nerve stimulation. Unfortunately, the absence of phrenic nerve capture in the supine position does not ensure that phrenic nerve pacing will not occur when the patient is prone or in another position.

Traditionally, wedge venography using balloon occlusion angiography has been used for CS evaluation, and is commonly used during implantation.[55] Some operators incorporate pre-procedural coronary sinus imaging with CT or MRI evaluation.[56, 57] Given the marked variability of venous anatomy in congenital heart disease, especially in those patients with systemic right ventricles or abnormal ventricular looping, pre-procedural anatomic evaluation has played a greater role in pre-procedural planning. Unfortunately, often the diameter and branching of the CS can be difficult to assess with these modalities, especially in smaller patients. Interestingly, some centers have attempted to use 3D mapping systems for evaluation of coronary sinus anatomy, and facilitate lead placement in the appropriate CS branch.[58] This 3D mapping may also be used to measure the greatest electrical delay to assist with lead placement.

In patients who have anatomy that is unfavorable for placement of a transvenous left ventricular lead, a hybrid approach can be considered. The hybrid approach may be necessary in anatomy such as seen after the atrial switch procedure as the coronary sinus lies on the pulmonary venous side of the atrial baffle. For a typical hybrid approach, a transvenous atrial and pulmonary ventricular lead is placed, with epicardial lead placement on the systemic ventricle. Depending on the patients' anatomy, a left lateral thoracotomy approach may allow adequate access to a lateral ventricular location and may allow the surgeons the ability to reach the heart unencumbered by scar from previous surgeries. In the case of patients who have undergone and Mustard or Senning atrial switch, the transvenous lead will be in the posterior left ventricle and a sternotomy will be required to place the right ventricular lead. When possible, the best location for epicardial lead placement can be guided by pre-procedural imaging as mentioned previously. The area of latest electrical activation can be determined while pacing from the endocardial ventricular lead and "mapping" for the area of latest ventricular activation. While in theory this technique has merit, there is no prospective data to indicate improved synchrony and in practice the ideal location must take into consideration anatomic variability including adhesions, scar tissue, coronary arteries, and adequate surgical exposure to the site of interest. Ideally a bipolar steroid eluding epicardial lead is chosen to allow maximum flexibility in pacing vectors, however, at times a bipolar lead is impractical or impossible in which case a unipolar lead or screw in lead can be used.

In patients with single ventricle anatomy, which typically does not allow a transvenous system, epicardial lead placement is preferable. In these instances, an anterior sternotomy approach will allow lead placement on the right atrium and right ventricular free wall. Depending on adhesions, the anterolateral or lateral LV wall may be reached for the second ventricular lead, although a left lateral thoracotomy may be required. Again, the selection of lead location should be adjusted in an attempt to provide optimal mechanical (and electrical) synchrony; therefore, intra-procedural evaluation of lead location may be necessary. As there are no standards for lead placement in a univentricular heart, evaluation by TEE may guide lead placement, evaluating for the latest area of ventricular contraction while pacing through the first ventricular lead. Pacing in a "biventricular" fashion following temporary lead placement may also allow intraoperative assessment of improvements in mechanical (improved function and coordinated ejection) and electrical dyssynchrony (shorter QRS duration).

References

1 Epstein AE, DiMarco JP, Ellenbogen KA, et al. ACC/AHA/HRS 2008 guidelines for device-based therapy of cardiac rhythm abnormalities: A report of the American College of Cardiology/American Heart Association Task Force on Practice Guidelines (writing committee to revise the ACC/AHA/NASPE 2002 guideline update for implantation of cardiac pacemakers and antiarrhythmia devices) developed in collaboration with the American Association for Thoracic Surgery and Society of Thoracic Surgeons. *J Am Coll Cardiol.* 2008; 51(21): e1–62.

2 Rijnbeek PR, Witsenburg M, Schrama E, Hess J, Kors JA. New normal limits for the paediatric electrocardiogram. *European Heart Journal.* 2001; 22(8): 702–711.

3 Tucker EM, Pyles LA, Bass JL, Moller JH. Permanent pacemaker for atrioventricular conduction block after operative repair of perimembranous ventricular septal defect. *J Am Coll Cardiol.* 2007; 50(12): 1196–1200.

4 Fishberger SB, Wernovsky G, Gentles TL, et al. Factors that influence the development of atrial flutter after the Fontan operation. *J Thorac Cardiovasc Surg.* 1997; 113(1): 80–86.

5 Von Bergen NH, Atkins DL, Dick M, 2nd, et al. Multicenter study of the effectiveness of implantable cardioverter defibrillators in children and young adults with heart disease. *Pediatr Cardiol.* 2011; 32(4): 399–405.

6 Berul CI, Van Hare GF, Kertesz NJ, et al. Results of a multicenter retrospective implantable cardioverter-defibrillator registry of pediatric and congenital heart disease patients. *J Am Coll Cardiol.* 2008; 51(17): 1685–1691.

7 Yap SC, Roos-Hesselink JW, Hoendermis ES, et al. Outcome of implantable cardioverter defibrillators in adults with congenital heart disease: A multi-centre study. *Eur Heart J.* 2007; 28(15): 1854–1861.

8 Bar-Cohen Y, Berul CI, Alexander ME, et al. Age, size, and lead factors alone do not predict venous obstruction in children and young adults with transvenous lead systems. *J Cardiovasc Electrophysiol.* 2006; 17(7): 754–759.

9 Figa FH, McCrindle BW, Bigras JL, Hamilton RM, Gow RM. Risk factors for venous obstruction in children with transvenous pacing leads. *Pacing Clin Electrophysiol.* 1997; 20(8 Pt 1): 1902–1909.

10 Sanjeev S, Karpawich PP. Superior vena cava and innominate vein dimensions in growing children: An aid for interventional devices and transvenous leads. *Pediatr Cardiol.* 2006; 27(4): 414–419.

11 Stephenson EA, Batra AS, Knilans TK, et al. A multicenter experience with novel implantable cardioverter defibrillator configurations in the pediatric and congenital heart disease population. *J Cardiovasc Electrophysiol.* 2006; 17(1): 41–46.

12 Hauser RG, Kallinen LM, Almquist AK, Gornick CC, Katsiyiannis WT. Early failure of a small-diameter high-voltage implantable cardioverter-defibrillator lead. *Heart Rhythm.* 2007; 4(7): 892–896.

13 Johnsrude CL, Mullins CE, Vincent J, Fagan TE, Friedman RA. Novel approach to transvenous

pacemaker implantation in a post-Fontan adolescent. *Pediatr Cardiol.* 1997; 18(4): 309–311.

14 Lopez JA. Transvenous right atrial and left ventricular pacing after the Fontan operation: Long-term hemodynamic and electrophysiologic benefit of early atrioventricular resynchronization. *Tex Heart Inst J.* 2007; 34(1): 98–101.

15 Collins KK, Runciman M, Rausch CM, Schaffer MS. Toward improved cosmetic results: A novel technique for the placement of a pacemaker or internal cardioverter/defibrillator generators in the axilla of young patients. *Pediatr Cardiol.* 2009; 30(8): 1157–1160.

16 Bardy GH, Smith WM, Hood MA, et al. An entirely subcutaneous implantable Cardioverter–Defibrillator. *N Engl J Med.* 2010; 363(1): 36–44.

17 Hoyer MH, Beerman LB, Ettedgui JA, Park SC, del Nido PJ, Siewers RD. Transatrial lead placement for endocardial pacing in children. *Ann Thorac Surg.* 1994; 58(1): 97–101; discussion 101–102.

18 McCarthy PM, Bhudia SK, Rajeswaran J, et al. Tricuspid valve repair: Durability and risk factors for failure. *J Thorac Cardiovasc Surg.* 2004; 127(3): 674–685.

19 Grimard C, Clementy N, Fauchier L, Babuty D. Ventricular pacing through coronary sinus in patients with tricuspid prosthesis. *Ann Thorac Surg.* 2010; 89(6): e51–52.

20 Porcellini S, Rimini A, Biasi S. Pacemaker implantation in a patient with persistent left superior vena cava using a steerable catheter-delivered lead. *J Cardiovasc Med (Hagerstown).* 2012 Oct; 13(10): 653–655.

21 Frangini P, Vergara I, Gonzalez R, Fajuri A, Casanegra P. Permanent pacemaker implantation in patients with persistent left superior vena cava and absent right superior vena cava. report of three cases. *Rev Med Chil.* 2006; 134(6): 767–771.

22 Gradaus R, Hammel D, Kotthoff S, Böcker D. Nonthoracotomy implantable cardioverter defibrillator placement in children: Use of subcutaneous array leads and abdominally placed implantable cardioverter defibrillators in children. *J Cardiovasc Electrophysiol.* 2001; 12(3): 356–360.

23 Blanc JJ, Etienne Y, Gilard M, et al. Evaluation of different ventricular pacing sites in patients with severe heart failure: Results of an acute hemodynamic study. *Circulation.* 1997; 96(10): 3273–3277.

24 Cazeau S, Leclercq C, Lavergne T, et al. Effects of multisite biventricular pacing in patients with heart failure and intraventricular conduction delay. *N Engl J Med.* 2001; 344(12): 873–880.

25 Young JB, Abraham WT, Smith AL, et al. Combined cardiac resynchronization and implantable cardioversion defibrillation in advanced chronic heart failure: The MIRACLE ICD trial. *JAMA.* 2003; 289(20): 2685–2694.

26 Linde C, Abraham WT, Gold MR, Daubert C, REVERSE Study Group. Cardiac resynchronization therapy in asymptomatic or mildly symptomatic heart failure patients in relation to etiology: Results from the REVERSE (REsynchronization reVErses remodeling in systolic left vEntricular dysfunction) study. *J Am Coll Cardiol.* 2010; 56(22): 1826–1831.

27 Rodriguez-Cruz E, Karpawich PP, Lieberman RA, Tantengco MV. Biventricular pacing as alternative therapy for dilated cardiomyopathy associated with congenital heart disease. *Pacing Clin Electrophysiol.* 2001; 24(2): 235–237.

28 Vardas PE, Auricchio A, Blanc J, et al. Guidelines for cardiac pacing and cardiac resynchronization therapy. *Europace.* 2007; 9(10): 959–998.

29 Dubin AM, Janousek J, Rhee E, et al. Resynchronization therapy in pediatric and congenital heart disease patients: An international multicenter study. *J Am Coll Cardiol.* 2005; 46(12): 2277–2283.

30 Janousek J, Gebauer RA, Abdul-Khaliq H, et al. Cardiac resynchronisation therapy in paediatric and congenital heart disease: Differential effects in various anatomical and functional substrates. *Heart.* 2009; 95(14): 1165–1171.

31 Moak JP, Hasbani K, Ramwell C, et al. Dilated cardiomyopathy following right ventricular pacing for AV block in young patients: Resolution after upgrading to biventricular pacing systems. *J Cardiovasc Electrophysiol.* 2006; 17(10): 1068–1071.

32 Janousek J, Tomek V, Chaloupecky V, Gebauer RA. Dilated cardiomyopathy associated with dual-chamber pacing in infants: Improvement through either left ventricular cardiac resynchronization or programming the pacemaker off allowing intrinsic normal conduction. *J Cardiovasc Electrophysiol.* 2004; 15(4): 470–474.

33 Adelstein E, Schwartzman D, Gorcsan J, 3rd, Saba S. Predicting hyperresponse among pacemaker-dependent nonischemic cardiomyopathy patients upgraded to cardiac resynchronization. *J Cardiovasc Electrophysiol.* 2011; 22(8): 905–911.

34 Cecchin F, Frangini PA, Brown DW, et al. Cardiac resynchronization therapy (and multisite pacing) in pediatrics and congenital heart disease: Five years experience in a single institution. *J Cardiovasc Electrophysiol.* 2009; 20(1): 58–65.

35 Sipahi I, Carrigan TP, Rowland DY, Stambler BS, Fang JC. Impact of QRS duration on clinical event reduction with cardiac resynchronization therapy: Meta-analysis of randomized controlled trials. *Arch Intern Med.* 2011; 171(16): 1454–1462.

36 Ghosh S, Silva JN, Canham RM, et al. Electrophysiologic substrate and intraventricular left ventricular dyssynchrony in nonischemic heart failure patients undergoing cardiac resynchronization therapy. *Heart Rhythm.* 2011; 8(5): 692–699.

37 Pham PP, Balaji S, Shen I, Ungerleider R, Li X, Sahn DJ. Impact of conventional versus biventricular pacing on hemodynamics and tissue Doppler imaging indexes of resynchronization postoperatively in children with congenital heart disease. *J Am Coll Cardiol*. 2005; 46(12): 2284–2289.

38 Zimmerman FJ, Starr JP, Koenig PR, Smith P, Hijazi ZM, Bacha EA. Acute hemodynamic benefit of multisite ventricular pacing after congenital heart surgery. *Ann Thorac Surg*. 2003; 75(6): 1775–1780.

39 Kleijn SA, van Dijk J, de Cock CC, Allaart CP, van Rossum AC, Kamp O. Assessment of intraventricular mechanical dyssynchrony and prediction of response to cardiac resynchronization therapy: Comparison between tissue Doppler imaging and real-time three-dimensional echocardiography. *J Am Soc Echocardiogr*. 2009; 22(9): 1047–1054.

40 Janousek J, Tomek V, Chaloupecky V, et al. Cardiac resynchronization therapy: A novel adjunct to the treatment and prevention of systemic right ventricular failure. *J Am Coll Cardiol*. 2004; 44(9): 1927–1931.

41 Cazeau S, Bordachar P, Jauvert G, et al. Echocardiographic modeling of cardiac dyssynchrony before and during multisite stimulation: A prospective study. *Pacing Clin Electrophysiol*. 2003; 26(1 Pt 2): 137–143.

42 Baker GH, Hlavacek AM, Chessa KS, Fleming DM, Shirali GS. Left ventricular dysfunction is associated with intraventricular dyssynchrony by 3-dimensional echocardiography in children. *J Am Soc Echocardiogr*. 2008; 21(3): 230–233.

43 Raedle-Hurst TM, Mueller M, Rentzsch A, Schaefers HJ, Herrmann E, Abdul-Khaliq H. Assessment of left ventricular dyssynchrony and function using real-time 3-dimensional echocardiography in patients with congenital right heart disease. *Am Heart J*. 2009; 157(4): 791–798.

44 Ypenburg C, Westenberg JJ, Bleeker GB, et al. Noninvasive imaging in cardiac resynchronization therapy: part 1: Selection of patients. *Pacing and Clinical Electrophysiology*. 2008; 31(11): 1475–1499.

45 Pitzalis MV, Iacoviello M, Romito R, et al. Cardiac resynchronization therapy tailored by echocardiographic evaluation of ventricular asynchrony. *J Am Coll Cardiol*. 2002; 40(9): 1615–1622.

46 Suffoletto MS, Dohi K, Cannesson M, Saba S, Gorcsan J. Novel speckle-tracking radial strain from routine black-and-white echocardiographic images to quantify dyssynchrony and predict response to cardiac resynchronization therapy. *Circulation*. 2006; 113(7): 960–968.

47 Tomaske M, Breithardt OA, Balmer C, Bauersfeld U. Successful cardiac resynchronization with single-site left ventricular pacing in children. *Int J Cardiol*. 2009; 136(2): 136–143.

48 Sade LE, Demir Ö, Atar I, Müderrisoglu H, Özin B. Effect of mechanical dyssynchrony and cardiac resynchronization therapy on left ventricular rotational mechanics. *Am J Cardiol*. 2008; 101(8): 1163–1169.

49 Bertini M, Delgado V, Nucifora G, et al. Effect of cardiac resynchronization therapy on subendo- and subepicardial left ventricular twist mechanics and relation to favorable outcome. *Am J Cardiol*. 2010; 106(5): 682–687.

50 Jauvert G, Rousseau-Paziaud J, Villain E, et al. Effects of cardiac resynchronization therapy on echocardiographic indices, functional capacity, and clinical outcomes of patients with a systemic right ventricle. *Europace*. 2009; 11(2): 184–190.

51 Dreger H, Antonow G, Spethmann S, Bondke H, Baumann G, Melzer C. Dyssynchrony parameter-guided interventricular delay programming. *Europace*. 2012 May; 14(5): 696–702.

52 Gasparini M, Bocchiardo M, Lunati M, et al. Comparison of 1-year effects of left ventricular and biventricular pacing in patients with heart failure who have ventricular arrhythmias and left bundle-branch block: The bi vs left ventricular pacing: An international pilot evaluation on heart failure patients with ventricular arrhythmias (BELIEVE) multicenter prospective randomized pilot study. *Am Heart J*. 2006; 152(1): 155.e1–155.e7.

53 Boriani G, Kranig W, Donal E, et al. A randomized double-blind comparison of biventricular versus left ventricular stimulation for cardiac resynchronization therapy: The biventricular versus left univentricular pacing with ICD back-up in heart failure patients (B-LEFT HF) trial. *Am Heart J*. 2010; 159(6): 1052–1058.e1.

54 Dodge-Khatami A, Kadner A, Dave H, Rahn M, Prêtre R, Bauersfeld U. Left heart atrial and ventricular epicardial pacing through a left lateral thoracotomy in children: A safe approach with excellent functional and cosmetic results. *European Journal of Cardio-Thoracic Surgery*. 2005; 28(4): 541–545.

55 Gilard M, Mansourati J, Etienne Y, et al. Angiographic anatomy of the coronary sinus and its tributaries. *Pacing Clin Electrophysiol*. 1998; 21(11 Pt 2): 2280–2284.

56 Gerber TC, Sheedy PF, Bell MR, et al. Evaluation of the coronary venous system using electron beam computed tomography. *Int J Cardiovasc Imaging*. 2001; 17(1): 65–75.

57 Mao S, Shinbane JS, Girsky MJ, et al. Coronary venous imaging with electron beam computed tomographic angiography: Three-dimensional mapping and relationship with coronary arteries. *Am Heart J*. 2005; 150(2): 315–322.

58 Del Greco M, Marini M, Bonmassari R. Implantation of a biventricular implantable cardioverter-defibrillator guided by an electroanatomic mapping system. *Europace*. 2012 Jan; 14(1): 107–111.

CHAPTER 10

Permanent epicardial pacing: When, how, and why?

Larry Rhodes[1] and Maully Shah[2]

[1] Professor of Pediatrics, West Virginia University School of Medicine and Chair, Department of Pediatrics, West Virginia University Children's Hospital, Morgantown, WV, USA

[2] Professor of Pediatrics, Perelman School of Medicine, University of Pennsylvania and Director, Cardiac Electrophysiology, The Children's Hospital of Philadelphia, Philadelphia, PA, USA

Introduction

For the past 40 years, the standard approach for placement of pacing systems in adults has been transvenous, utilizing veins that drain into the SVC. Although this approach has also been used in pediatric patients for more than 30 years,[1] there are issues that preclude this approach in smaller children and patients with congenital heart disease. This, in addition to the fact that these young patients will require pacing systems for decades, has led to an increased interest in the placement of epicardial pacing systems to maintain vascular access. The indications for consideration of placement of epicardial pacing systems are listed in Table 10.1.

Patient size

It is not difficult to understand that a newborn baby weighing 3 kg with congenital heart block and hydrops is not large enough for the placement of a transvenous lead. Not only are the vessels too small for even a 4 French lead, there is not enough room to place a pacemaker in the infraclavicular area. Implanting physicians have placed transvenous leads in the subclavian vein, tunneled the lead outside the thorax and placed the pacer in the abdomen. This procedure requires two surgical fields and frequently sacrifices the blood vessel. Leads tunneled over ribs to reach the abdomen can be dislodged or fractured as the infant grows and becomes mobile.

The slightly more debatable patient population is children at 5–15 kg requiring single chamber pacing. A child of this size has a subclavian vein that would likely receive a 4 or 5 French pacing lead and possibly have space enough for placement of a pacemaker in the infraclavicular area. The issue in this size patient is the potential for the subacute loss of the vessel secondary to venous obstruction. This is thought to be related to the size of the lead relative to the internal diameter of the vessel. The risk of vessel loss has been evaluated by comparing the cross sectional area of lead or leads(s) and indexed them to the patient's body surface area at time of implant. Patients with a higher mean index had a higher incidence of obstructions. An index value of >6.6 mm^2/m^2 was used to predict obstruction, with a sensitivity of 90% and specificity of 84%.[2]

A follow up study by Bar-Cohen et al.[3] demonstrated there were factors independent of patient

Cardiac Pacing and Defibrillation in Pediatric and Congenital Heart Disease, First Edition.
Edited by Maully Shah, Larry Rhodes and Jonathan Kaltman.
© 2017 John Wiley & Sons Ltd. Published 2017 by John Wiley & Sons Ltd.
Companion Website: www.wiley.com/go/shah/cardiac_pacing

Table 10.1 *Primary indications for epicardial pacing*

1.	Small patient size
2.	Venous abnormalities that prevent transvenous lead implantation
3.	Congenital malformations or surgical barriers that prevent endocardial lead implantation
4.	Right-to-left shunt
5.	High endocardial pacing and sensing thresholds due to endocardial scarring
6.	Concurrent cardiac surgery
7.	Prosthetic tricuspid valve that precludes lead placement in right ventricle

size that led to venous obstruction. They evaluated 85 patients undergoing repeat pacemaker or ICD procedures with venograms looking for complete or partial obstruction. Obstruction was seen in 21 of the 85 patients with 11 being complete and 10 partial. When these patients were divided into age related groups 3–12 years, (n = 35) and 13 years and older (n = 50) there was no significant difference noted in the incidence of obstruction. The younger patients had a larger lead indexed to BSA ratio (6.82 vs 5.05, P = 0.005) but they found no significant differences between obstruction and nonobstruction relative to age or size.

Growth is another important size related factor in infants and toddlers. A newborn child will normally double its height and weight in the first 6 months of life and frequently triple it by 1 year of age. There is continued growth throughout the preschool and primary grade years with another growth spurt during puberty. Longitudinal growth occurs primarily in the limbs and thorax with very little from the epigastric region to the xiphoid. With this growth there is potential for dislodgement or fracture of the lead. There is also a significant increase in a child's activities including many not frequently employed by adults and not pacemaker friendly, that is, swinging on monkey bars, wrestling, wrecking bicycles, and so on.

In the past 10 years, there has been a growing effort to remove existing nonfunctional leads when upgrading pacing systems in an attempt to preserve vascular access in this population. This has had a reasonable success rate but is not without an incidence of morbidity. There have been a number of failures to extract the lead and on occasion loss of the vessel after successful extraction.

Patient anatomy and physiology

Many patients with congenital heart disease require the placement of a pacing system or implantable defibrillator prior to or following palliation. Indications include sinus node dysfunction, AV block, ventricular dysfunction, and ventricular arrhythmias. In addition to patient size there are frequently anatomical or physiological issues prohibiting the placement of transvenous systems. A primary anatomical and physiologic contraindication is right to left shunting prior to or following palliation. Pacing leads have the potential to be thrombogenic and can lead to embolization. It is an established contraindication to place a transvenous lead in a patient with an intracardiac right to left shunt. This is also an issue with the placement of transvenous atrial leads in patients that have undergone Fontan operations in that a pulmonary embolus could be life threatening in their physiology. This concern is compounded by the sluggish blood flow seen in patients with Fontan physiology and other anomalies such as cardiomyopathies wherein decreased ventricular function can also lead to an increased risk of thrombus formation.

Another relative contraindication is the placement of a transvenous lead across the tricuspid valve in a patient with significant pulmonary insufficiency. A pacing lead or a defibrillator lead can stent a tricuspid valve partially open leading to no competent valve on the right side of the heart.

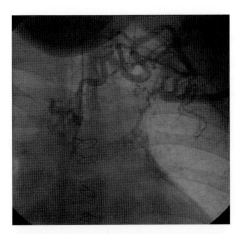

Figure 10.1 *Contrast injection through a left peripheral i.v. shows complete occlusion of left subclavian vein with venous collaterals in a patient with a long standing left internal jugular venous catheter.*

In some patients with a normal or abnormal cardiac anatomy, epicardial pacing is mandatory because there is complete loss of venous access into the heart (Figure 10.1).

A number of purely anatomical issues preclude the use of transvenous leads due to a lack of access to the chamber that requires pacing. Some of these are present prior to palliation, that is, tricuspid atresia, but the majority is seen in the post-op patient. Patients with single ventricle physiology who have undergone staged palliation including a Fontan have no direct systemic venous access to their ventricle. In the extracardiac conduit Fontan it is impossible to pace the atrium via a transvenous approach. Although the lateral tunnel Fontan does not prohibit transvenous atrial pacing it is difficult secondary to the decreased surface area of "living" tissue available for pacing. Patients with a Glenn shunt (SVC to pulmonary artery anastomosis) have no direct access from head and neck vessels to the heart. Patients with prosthetic valves, whether metal or bio prosthetic should not have leads placed across them.

Lead placement and cardiomyopathy

There has been concern over the past decade about the use of chronic pacing and the development of cardiomyopathies. Tantengco et al.[4] looked at the effect of apical right ventricular pacing on left ventricular function. In their study they evaluated 24 patients with normal anatomy paced from the RV apex with a mean follow up of 9.5 years with noninvasive assessment of LV function. They had 33 age and BSA-matched controls. This study identified a significant difference in both systolic and diastolic function between the groups. Based on these findings they suggested that alternate sites of ventricular pacing to simulate normal biventricular electrical activation should be sought. A similar publication from the Netherlands in 2004[5] reported that the left ventricular apex was a superior pacing site. This study involving 11 healthy dogs and 8 children undergoing cardiac surgery evaluated dual chamber pacing performed at the RV apex, LV apex, and LV lateral free wall. The results showed hemodynamic measurements as good as during sinus rhythm during LV apex pacing, but pulse pressure was reduced during RV apex and LV free wall pacing. They noted LV apical pacing enabled synchronous activation of the LV and was associated with superior hemodynamic performance. Another publication in 2004 showed that upgrading pacing systems in patients with advanced heart failure and RV pacing to a biventricular system led to significant improvement in systolic function as well as electrical and LV mechanical synchrony.[6]

Epicardial pacing affords one the opportunity to use "pace mapping" to evaluate ventricular activation and function prior to permanent placement of the lead. This technique also has a utility when placing an LV lead in biventricular pacing.

Lead longevity and implantation

There is significant concern in pediatric pacing about the longevity of pacing systems. Growing, active children have a greater propensity for lead fracture and the development of exit block than seen in the adult population. The group at Boston Children's Hospital reported on factors related to pacing lead failure wherein they evaluated over 1000 leads placed in 497 patients. They noted lead failure in 155. In this study they noted epicardial leads were more likely to fail due to fracture or exit block and felt they were a significant contributor to lead failure. Based on their data they suggested an "expanded utilization of transvenous systems in smaller patients seems justified when anatomy permits."[7] This is somewhat different from what Cohen et al. reported in 2001[8] where they evaluated 1239 outpatient visits in patients with epicardial pacing systems from 1983 and 2000. Lead failure was defined similar to the Boston study with the addition of phrenic nerve or muscle stimulation. There were 207 leads implanted in 123 patients (60 atrial and 147 ventricular). In this group 40 % had steroid eluting leads. With a mean follow up of 29 months they reported a 1, 2, and 5 year lead survival at 96, 90, and 74%, respectively. They concluded that steroid eluting epicardial leads demonstrated stable acute and chronic pacing and sensing thresholds with results similar to those found with historical conventional endocardial leads.

The group from The Children's Hospital of Michigan presented data in 2003 regarding the use of steroid-eluting epicardial leads in children. They presented data relative to 10-year performance of steroid eluting leads in growing children compared with standard epicardial leads implanted from 1990 to 2000. There were 51 steroid eluting leads (27 ventricular and 24 atrial) in 35 patients compared to 28 standard epicardial leads (27 ventricular and 1 atrial). Standard measurements of pacing threshold, impedance, and energy were measured at implant and during follow-up. In this study the steroid eluting leads out performed standard epicardial leads in each of the parameters measured. They reported that fracture or dislodgement occurred in 4% of steroid eluting and 14% in standard epicardial leads. They concluded that steroid eluting epicardial leads show stable, chronic low thresholds over time in growing children.[9]

Finally, Lau et al. evaluated the long-term permanent epicardial pacing lead survival in 155 patients with congenital heart disease who had permanent epicardial pacing systems implanted in association with surgical repair and found that over 946 lead-years of follow up, the overall atrial lead survival at 1, 2, 5, and 10 years was 99, 93, 83, and 72%, respectively, and the ventricular lead survival was 97, 90, 74, and 60%, respectively, despite the potential for myocardial scarring from multiple cardiac operations.[10]

Epicardial pacing in specific patient substrates

High risk patient with complete congenital atrio-ventricular (AV) block

Patients born with congenital complete AV block and associated prematurity, low birth weight, hydrops, low ventricular rates, low cardiac output, and congenital heart disease are a high risk group in whom medical therapy is often ineffective, pacing is technically challenging, and mortality exceeds 80%. Single and dual chamber permanent pacemakers can be implanted in small neonates (Figure 10.2) and there are case reports of implanting epicardial pacemakers in extremely low birth weight infants.[11, 12] However, these strategies are not always without complications such as pericardial effusion, infection and wound dehiscence. An alternative approach is to utilize temporary pacing leads as the initial mode of pacing.[13] This approach obviates the immediate need to perform a larger-scale operation on a tenuous neonate. Glatz et al. described their institutional practice of placing three or four temporary epicardial wires plus at least one skin wire in high risk neonates

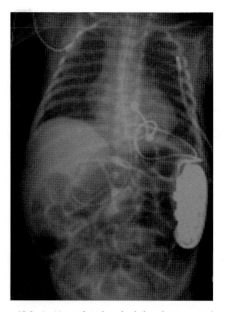

Figure 10.2 *An X-ray showing dual chamber pacemaker placement utilizing unipolar atrial and ventricular pacing leads in a 2.2 kg infant born with complete congenital heart block. Note the significant relative surface area of the pacemaker generator on the patient's abdomen.*

requiring pacing in the first 24 hours of life and showed effective electrical pacing for up to 67 (33.8 ± 18.3) days in a small subset of patients.[13] Once hemodynamic stability has been achieved and tissue integrity has improved, a permanent epicardial pacing system can be implanted.

Permanent pacing after multiple cardiac surgeries

Surgically induced myocardial inflammation, scarring and adhesions that occur after multiple sternotomies and thoracotomies, along with the cardiac surgical repair itself make epicardial lead implantation challenging, and lead survival is often thought to be suboptimal in this patient substrate. There are centers that have developed a practice

of placing epicardial pacing leads prophylactically in patients with a propensity to require them in the future (Figure 10.3). This population would include patients with single ventricle physiology or intra-atrial baffling procedures that are likely to develop sinus node dysfunction in the future or patients with L-TGA that have with the propensity for AV block. In 2004 Cohen et al.[14] reported on the Children's Hospital of Philadelphia (CHOP) experience of this practice. In this study they compared pacing thresholds and sensing in 13 patients with placement of epicardial pacing lead(s) at the time of congenital heart surgery to epicardial leads placed as a primary pacemaker surgery. They report that 86% prophylactic epicardial leads had acceptable pacing and sensing thresholds at

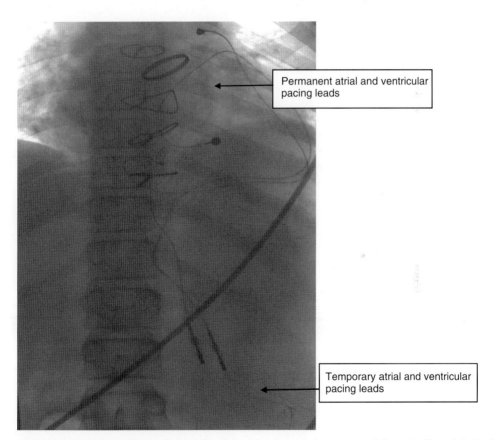

Permanent atrial and ventricular pacing leads

Temporary atrial and ventricular pacing leads

Figure 10.3 *X-ray showing unipolar permanent epicardial atrial and ventricular pacing leads implanted "prophylactically" without concomitant pacemaker generator placement at the time of Fontan surgery in a patient with single ventricle physiology. The permanent leads are tunneled to the abdomen where they can be connected to a pacemaker generator in the future without the need for a repeat sternotomy or thoracotomy if permanent pacing is required. In this case the permanent leads were also connected to temporary extension wires to allow for peri-operative pacing if required. The temporary wires can easily be pulled out in the routine manner prior to discharge from the hospital.*

retrieval at a median of 252 days after implant. Therefore, epicardial pacing leads can be successfully placed at the time of cardiac surgery and retrieved when needed with reasonable pacing and sensing threshold and therefore prevent the patient from a second sternotomy or a thoracotomy.

There are occasionally situations in which an epicardial approach may be superior to transvenous/endocardial approach when there is significant right atrial scarring such as after the Fontan palliation. Ramesh et al.[15, 16] described the use of epicardial pacing of the left atrium in patients where there may be with possible significant scarring in the right atrium from previous surgical interventions. In each of these procedures there are frequently significant suture lines and scarring secondary to the atrial baffles. This makes it difficult to locate tissue that allows acceptable pacing thresholds and sensing. When compared to right atrial epicardial leads they found energy thresholds (ET) were lower in the LA than RA at 6 months, 1 and 2 years (p < 0.05). There was no direct comparison in this study to transvenous pacing in that such patients had a lower incidence of structural abnormalities. The transvenous leads had a higher impedance than either atrial epicardial lead but the LA energy threshold approached the transvenous value at 2.5 years' follow-up.

Recent data from Lau et al.[10] described follow-up of epicardial leads in single ventricle patients showing the overall incidence of epicardial lead malfunction was 27% at 5 years and 44% at 10 years after lead implantation. There was no significant difference between patients with a bi-ventricular versus single ventricle physiology. Improvement of epicardial lead performance is attributed to steroid eluting mechanisms.[9, 10, 17]

An approach that has been adopted by some is the use of a transvenous steroid lead placed in an epi-intramyocardial fashion in the atrium or ventricle in patients with excessive surface myocardial scarring in whom transvenous pacing is not possible.[18] This technique utilizes creation of a small intra myocardial puncture to place the electrode via an epicardial approach into the intra-myocardial or endocardial region. The electrode is then secured with pledgetted sutures.

Types of epicardial pacing leads and implantation approaches

Epicardial pacing leads are either passive fixation, where the electrode lies along the surface of the heart and stay sutures hold the lead in place or active fixation that may use a "fish hook" or "cork screw or helix" mechanism to anchor the lead to the myocardium (Figure 10.4A–C). The active fixation leads have a myocardial penetration of 2–3.5 mm. The passive fixation and the cork screw active fixation leads are available in unipolar and bipolar models with steroid elution from different manufacturers (e.g., Myodex™ is a bipolar, steroid-eluting epicardial pacing lead

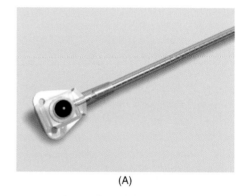

(A)

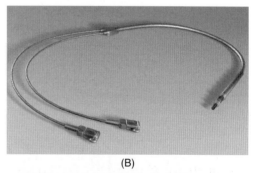

(B)

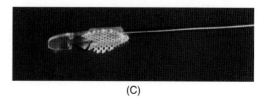

(C)

Figure 10.4 *(A) Image of a steroid eluting unipolar epicardial pacing lead. (B) Image of a steroid eluting bipolar epicardial pacing lead. (C) Image of a unipolar fish-hook epicardial lead.*

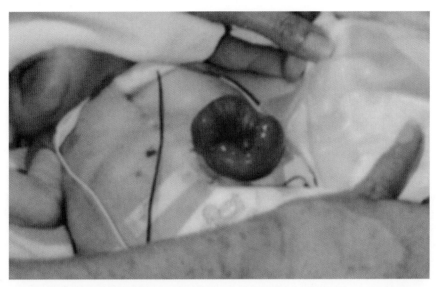

Figure 10.5 *Image showing a rare complication of skin necrosis and complete pacemaker pocket dehiscence after sepsis in a neonate with complete congenital AV block who received an epicardial permanent pacemaker on the second day of life. At the time of sub-rectus muscle pocket creation, an inadvertent tear in the peritoneum had ostensibly occurred allowing bowel loops to extrude through the pocket dehiscence.*

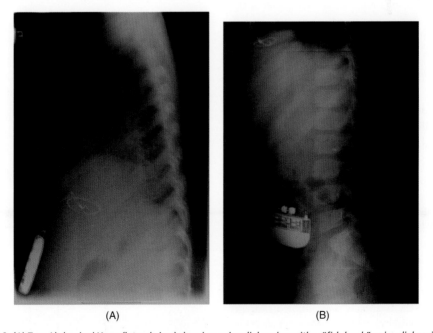

(A)   (B)

Figure 10.6 *(A) Top: Abdominal X-ray (lateral view) showing epicardial pacing with a "fish hook" epicardial pacing lead connected to a sub-rectus abdominal pacemaker generator. (B) Bottom: 1 year later, a repeat abdominal X-ray (lateral view) revealed that the generator had migrated into the abdominal intra-peritoneal cavity without any disturbance in ventricular pacing. The generator was removed via laparotomy because of risk of bowel obstruction from the pacing lead and the pacing system was revised.*

with an active fixation mechanism from St. Jude Medical, Capsure® 4698 is a bipolar steroid eluting epicardial passive fixation lead from Medtronic).

Typically, the atrial lead is implanted via a thoracotomy or a sternotomy and the ventricular lead can be implanted by a sub-xyphoid approach, limited thoracotomy, or sternotomy.

The pacemaker generator may be implanted in a pocket created in the subrectus, subcutaneous or retrocostal region. The subrectus pocket is the most common site for generator placement and is fashioned in the abdominal wall within the rectus abdominus muscle sheath. The epicardial leads are tunneled to the site of the pocket containing the pacemaker generator.

Bipolar leads are preferable to unipolar leads due to decreased potential for oversensing, but implantation of bipolar leads is not always feasible due to the limited "real estate" of healthy myocardial tissue. Another advantage of bipolar leads is that if one of the lead conductors fractures, there is potential to use the other conductor and reprogram the pacemaker in a unipolar mode.

In certain situations, where epicardial surface scarring is excessive, an active fixation lead has an advantage over the passive fixation lead by achieving greater myocardial penetration and "bypassing" the layer of fibrosis in the epicardium.

Complications after epicardial pacemaker implantation

There is little doubt that there is a significant difference in operative pain and potential morbidity with the placement of an epicardial pacing system versus transvenous leads. A thoracotomy and/or sternotomy cannot be performed without at least heavy sedation and, particularly in children, general anesthesia. Apart from the potentially longer recovery, significant complications may occur from lead or generator placement.

Epicardial lead placement can cause myocardial trauma which is usually self- limited. Rarely, a hemo-pericardium or pericardial effusion may develop. In addition, a pacing lead has a chance to migrate and encircle the heart before adhering to it. Thus progressive entrapment of the myocardium by a pacing lead may occur causing myocardial ischemia, progressive dilated cardiomyopathy or

death.[19, 20] In patients with multiple sternotomies, the myocardium may be stuck to the chest wall and there is a rare risk of cardiac laceration while performing a sternotomy for epicardial lead placement, which may have fatal consequences. Inadvertent diaphragmatic pacing may occur if leads are placed close to the phrenic nerve that might not be apparent at the time of implantation, especially if the patient is paralyzed under anesthesia.

Pacemaker pocket complications include infection, erosion and wound dehiscence (Figure 10.5). Rarely, instances of generator migration have been noted especially when a peritoneal tear has occurred at the time of creating the pacemaker pocket under the abdominal rectus sheath (Figure 10.6A, B). This allows the pacemaker generator to migrate into the peritoneal cavity over time and there is a risk of intestinal strangulation if there is concurrent migration of excess lead loops.

Conclusion

Epicardial leads have acceptable mid-term longevity in a heterogeneous population of patients including those with complex congenital heart disease who have undergone multiple surgeries suggesting the reliability of this pacing method. Steroid eluting leads are key to maintaining low pacing thresholds and reducing incidence of exit block.

References

1 Gillette PC, Shannon C, Blair H, Garson A Jr, Porter CJ, McNamara DG. Transvenous pacing in pediatric patients. *Am Heart J.* 1983 May; 105(5): 843–847.

2 Figa FH, McCrindle BW, Bigras JL, Hamilton RM, Gow RM. Risk factors for venous obstruction in children with transvenous pacing leads. *Pacing Clin Electrophysiol.* 1997 Aug; 20(8 Pt 1): 1902–1909.

3 Bar-Cohen Y, Berul CI, Alexander ME, Fortescue EB, Walsh EP, Triedman JK, Cecchin F. Age, size, and lead factors alone do not predict venous obstruction in children and young adults with transvenous lead systems. *J Cardiovasc Electrophysiol.* 2006 Jul; 17(7): 754–759.

4 Tantengco MV, Thomas RL, Karpawich PP. Left ventricular dysfunction after long-term right ventricular apical pacing in the young. *J Am Coll Cardiol.* 2001 Jun 15; 37(8): 2093–2100.

5 Vanagt WY, Verbeek XA, Delhaas T, Mertens L, Daenen WJ, Prinzen FW. The left ventricular apex is the optimal site for pediatric pacing: correlation with animal experience. *Pacing Clin Electrophysiol.* 2004 Jun; 27(6 Pt 2): 837–843.

6 Horwich T, Foster E, De Marco T, Tseng Z, Saxon L. Effects of resynchronization therapy on cardiac function in pacemaker patients "upgraded" to biventricular devices. *J Cardiovasc Electrophysiol.* 2004 Nov; 15(11): 1284–1289.

7 Fortescue EB, Berul CI, Cecchin F, Walsh EP, Triedman JK, Alexander ME. Patient, procedural, and hardware factors associated with pacemaker lead failures in pediatrics and congenital heart disease. *Heart Rhythm.* 2004 Jul; 1(2): 150–159.

8 Cohen MI, Bush DM, Vetter VL, Tanel RE, Wieand TS, Gaynor JW, Rhodes LA. Permanent epicardial pacing in pediatric patients: seventeen years of experience and 1200 outpatient visits. *Circulation.* 2001 May 29; 103(21): 2585–2590.

9 Horenstein MS, Hakimi M, Walters H 3rd, Karpawich PP. Chronic performance of steroid-eluting epicardial leads in a growing pediatric population: a 10-year comparison. *Pacing Clin Electrophysiol.* 2003 Jul; 26(7 Pt 1): 1467–1471.

10 Lau KC, William Gaynor J, Fuller SM, Karen A Smoots, Shah MJ. Long-term atrial and ventricular epicardial pacemaker lead survival after cardiac operations in pediatric patients with congenital heart disease. *Heart Rhythm.* 2015 Mar; 12(3): 566–573.

11 Roubertie F, Le Bret E, Thambo JB, et al. Intradiaphragmatic pacemaker implantation in very low weight premature neonate. *Interact Cardiovasc Thorac Surg* 2009; 9: 743–745.

12 McCrossan B, d'Udekem Y, Davis AM, Pflaumer A. Successful implantation of a dual-chamber pacemaker in an ELBW infant for long QT syndrome. *Cardiol Young.* 2015 Mar; 25(3): 600–602.

13 Glatz AC, Gaynor JW, Rhodes LA, Rychik J, Tanel RE, Vetter VL, et al. Outcome of high-risk neonates with congenital complete heart block paced in the first 24 hours after birth. *J Thorac Cardiovasc Surg.* 2008 Sep; 136(3): 767–773.

14 Cohen MI, Rhodes LA, Spray TL, Gaynor JW. Efficacy of prophylactic epicardial pacing leads in children and young adults. *Ann Thorac Surg.* 2004 Jul; 78(1): 197–202; discussion 202–203.

15 Ramesh V, Gaynor JW, Shah MJ, Wieand TS, Spray TL, Vetter VL, Rhodes LA. Comparison of left and right atrial epicardial pacing in patients with congenital heart disease. *Ann Thorac Surg.* 1999 Dec; 68(6): 2314–2319.

16 Kucharczuk JC, Cohen MI, Rhodes LA, Karl TR, Spray TL, Gaynor JW. Epicardial atrial pacemaker lead placement after multiple cardiac operations. *Ann Thorac Surg.* 2001 Jun; 71(6): 2057–2058.

17 Tomaske M1, Gerritse B, Kretzers L, Pretre R, Dodge-Khatami A, Rahn M, Bauersfeld U. A 12-year experience of bipolar steroid-eluting epicardial pacing leads in children. *Ann Thorac Surg.* 2008 May; 85(5): 1704–1711.

18 Karpawich PP1, Walters H, Hakimi M. Chronic performance of a transvenous steroid pacing lead used as an epi-intramyocardial electrode. *Pacing Clin Electrophysiol.* 1998 Jul; 21(7): 1486–1488.

19 Takeuchi D1, Tomizawa Y. Cardiac strangulation from epicardial pacemaker leads: diagnosis, treatment, and prevention. *Gen Thorac Cardiovasc Surg.* 2015 Jan; 63(1): 22–29.

20 Watanabe H1, Hayashi J, Sugawara M, Hashimoto T, Sato S, Takeuchi K. Cardiac strangulation in a neonatal case: a rare complication of permanent epicardial pacemaker leads. *Thorac Cardiovasc Surg.* 2000 Apr; 48(2): 103–105.

CHAPTER 11

Managing device related complications and lead extraction

Avi Fischer[1] and Barry Love[2]

[1] Vice President, Global Education and Medical Director, St. Jude Medical, Austin, Texas, USA
[2] Assistant Professor of Pediatrics and Medicine, Icahn School of Medicine Director, Pediatric Electrophysiology and Adult Congenital Heart Disease, Mount Sinai School of Medicine/Mount Sinai Medical Center, New York, NY, USA

Introduction

The superiority of endocardial pacing systems compared to epicardial systems along with the increasing availability of smaller leads and generators has led to a marked increase in the number of transvenous pacemaker and implantable defibrillator systems in the pediatric patient population. For patients with congenital heart disease, cardiac rhythm device therapy has been a lifesaving therapy, however, complications associated with device-placement in this patient population are common. There are a unique set of challenges faced in this population and complications are encountered in the setting of acquired heart disease due to a variety of factors (Table 11.1). These include the current size of the patient, the expected growth of the patient, if and what type of congenital anomalies are present and the need for long-term pacing. Many device related considerations in pediatric patients (such as lead type, lead length, location of the pulse generator, etc.) persist long after the initial implant, but must be considered at the time of initial device placement as well as during any upgrade of system revision (Figure 11.1). As a result of improvements in the medical care given to

the pediatric population with complex congenital heart disease, patients are living longer and more normal lives.

Complications associated with cardiac rhythm devices may occur at implant and during follow-up. Operator experience and surgical technique are important in reducing the risk of acute complications and while complications are rare and unwanted, the reality is that every implanting physician has had complications. Some are not device-specific and may occur with any of the devices implanted and others are specific to select devices such as implantable cardioverter defibrillators (ICDs) and cardiac resynchronization (CRT) devices. Recognizing the potential for complications can help minimize their occurrence and help mitigate untoward effects if and when they occur. Complications may arise at the time of implantation, early in the post-implant period, or late after implantation. The three main categories of complications are implant-related, device-related, and lead-related.

In addition to the complications associated with the implant procedure, the importance of proper programming of the device, the functionality and integrity of the leads and the presence of

Cardiac Pacing and Defibrillation in Pediatric and Congenital Heart Disease, First Edition.
Edited by Maully Shah, Larry Rhodes and Jonathan Kaltman.
© 2017 John Wiley & Sons Ltd. Published 2017 by John Wiley & Sons Ltd.
Companion Website: www.wiley.com/go/shah/cardiac_pacing

Table 11.1 *Considerations for cardiac rhythm device implantation in pediatric and congenital heart disease patients*

- Age and size of the patient
  - pectoral versus abdominal implant
  - epicardial versus transvenous leads
- Expected growth of the patient
  - appropriate lead selection
  - sufficient redundant lead to allow for growth related stress
- Unique cardiovascular anatomy
  - access to cardiac chambers
  - non-standard placement and configuration of leads
- Need for long-term atrial and/or ventricular pacing
- Expected patient longevity
  - multiple revisions, upgrades and generator replacements
- Activity level of the patient
  - appropriate pacing modes and rates
  - tailored tachyarrhythmia therapy

Table 11.2 *Recommendations for monitoring device performance*

- Greater transparency in post-market surveillance, analysis and reporting
- Establishment of systems to identify malfunctioning devices more quickly
- Standard notification and communication to physicians and patients when device malfunction is identified Manufacturers, the FDA and physicians are encouraged to work together to prevent adverse events due to device malfunctions
- The global scope of device performance issues Cooperation among industry, physicians, government authorities and national health care systems to reduce the risk of injuries and deaths due to device malfunctions.

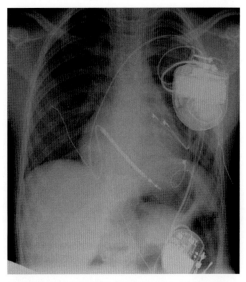

Figure 11.1 *PA chest radiograph of a 7-year-old with long QT syndrome (LQTS) who had an abdominal epicardial pacemaker system placed. After an episode of torsades de pointes, thoracic ganglionectomy was performed and a single chamber, single coil transvenous ICD implanted. Atrial pacing was provided via the epicardial system minimizing intravasacular hardware. Note the redundant slack present in the RV lead to allow for growth.*

a central component of managing this complex patient population. Understanding and appreciating the potential complications associated with each of these aspects of patient care is important so that appropriate discussions can take place with the patient and family prior to any planned procedure.

Implant-related complications

For pediatric patients and those with congenital heart disease, leads may be placed from an epicardial approach or a transvenous approach. While some complications encountered are specific to the implant approach used, other complications are common to both approaches.

Epicardial leads

Epicardial pacing via permanently implanted leads fixed to the epicardial surface of the atrial and ventricular myocardium can be performed. Currently these systems account for a small percentage of device implantation procedures but remain important for the neonate and infant. Additionally, this

permanently implanted hardware in the vascular system are becoming increasingly recognized and appreciated. It is widely accepted that the leads represent the "weak link" in all pacemaker and defibrillator systems and that lead failure is an anticipated problem over time. Managing cardiac rhythm device patients now includes managing lead-related issues and lead extraction has been method of pacing is often considered in patients with a prosthetic tricuspid valve or tricuspid valve atresia as well as in other conditions that preclude entering the right ventricle through the tricuspid valve. Traditionally, pacing and sensing thresholds of epicardial leads tended to deteriorate over time and older literature demonstrated a decreased lead survival compared to endocardial leads. Improvements in lead design have improved the longevity of these leads to the extent that the survival of epicardial and endocardial leads is now quite similar. The use of bipolar epicardial leads may be partially responsible for reduction in the incidence of sensing and pacing failures, particularly with atrial leads.[1] Complications associated with epicardial lead placement include all of the potential complications associated with surgical exposure of the heart (sternotomy or thoracotomy). For patients who have not had prior cardiac surgery, or in whom cardiac surgery was performed very recently, identifying anatomic landmarks on the epicardial surface of the heart used when placing leads is rarely difficult. For patients who have had multiple reoperations, fibrous adhesions, and scar tissue may obscure normal anatomic landmarks and relationships. Dissection to the epicardial surface of the heart carries a significant risk of inadvertent entry into an unwanted location such as into a cardiac chamber or coronary artery, both of which may potentially be catastrophic. We are aware of at least one instance where an experienced pediatric cardiac surgeon inadvertently placed an epicardial ventricular screw-in pacing lead into a coronary artery in a patient with hypoplastic left heart syndrome following the Fontan procedure. This led to severe myocardial dysfunction that ultimately required cardiac transplantation.

Transvenous leads

Venous access related complications

Inherent in any approach to venous access is the potential for damage to adjacent structures such as neural or arterial structures, excessive bleeding, thrombosis, and air embolism. Complications may occur at any stage of the procedure and may become evident immediately or hours or even days after implant. Typically, transvenous access for placement of endocardial pacing and defibrillator leads includes the subclavian, cephalic, jugular, and ileofemoral veins.[2, 3]

Pneumothorax

Pneumothorax may manifest acutely during the implant procedure or late after implantation. Aspiration of air into the syringe used for access during the attempted venous puncture may increase the suspicion of pneumothorax, but this is neither sensitive nor specific. During the procedure, the occurrence of agitation, chest pain, respiratory distress, hypoxia, hypotension, and tachycardia often suggest the presence of pneumothorax. Any symptom that arises during the procedure should prompt assessment of blood pressure, pulse, oximetry and even blood gas analysis. Fluoroscopy can quickly identify the presence of pneumothorax during the implant and chest radiography after the procedure can assist in identifying pneumothorax (Figure 11.2). Depending on the size of pneumothorax, placement of a chest tube may be required.

Knowledge of venous anatomy is important to reduce the risk of pneumothorax associated with venous access. The route of the axillary vein and subclavian vein and the relationship of these veins to the clavicle, first rib and apex of the lung is crucial to minimize the risk of pneumothorax associated with venous puncture. The axillary vein is an extra-thoracic structure that terminates at the lateral margin of the first rib. Contrast venography may aid in identifying the desired vein and for identifying branches such as the cephalic vein, axillary vein and subclavian vein (Figure 11.3). Direct cephalic vein cutdown has virtually no risk of pneumothorax.

Hemothorax

Although rare, this complication is known to occur if the subclavian vein is lacerated or if a larger-bore dilator or sheath is inadvertently introduced into the subclavian artery and then removed. As a result, bleeding occurs into the surrounding tissues and even into the thorax itself. Compression over the site of the laceration to stop the bleeding must be performed; rarely vascular surgical assistance is required to identify the location of the laceration and repair the damaged vascular structure. If a

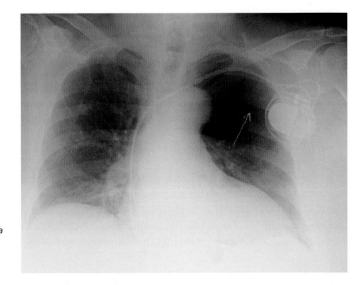

Figure 11.2 *PA chest radiograph immediately after insertion of a dual chamber pacemaker. The patient complained of chest discomfort, nausea and vomiting along with oxygen desaturation. Green arrow indicates a clearly visible pneumothorax.*

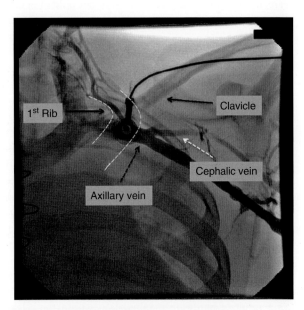

Figure 11.3 *Contrast venography through a left brachial intravenous line. Venous structures lateral to the first rib are extra-thoracic.*

large sheath is inserted into the artery, strong consideration for surgical repair should be considered and the sheath left in place.[2] The possibility of endovascular repair with balloon tamponade or stent graft repair has been reported.[4, 5] When hemothorax is identified, chest tube placement is required.

Air embolism

When introducing leads through a sheath placed in a central vein, air may enter the venous system.[6]

Air enters the venous system as it is sucked into the sheath during inspiration when intrathoracic pressure is negative. Air embolism may lead to chest pain, hypoxia, hypotension, and even respiratory distress. Air bubbles can often be seen traveling through the right heart ultimately dissipating. The use of sheaths with a one-way hemostatic valve, leg elevation, and having the patient Valsalva when the sheath is open to air minimize this risk. Although the sequela of air embolism in the venous system are transient, supportive measures such as supplemental oxygen and inotropic support are often utilized.

Miscellaneous access related complications

As all of the veins utilized for access are adjacent to other critical structures, a variety of other potential complications should not be forgotten. Rarely as a result of the proximity of the veins to their corresponding arteries, inadvertent puncture of both the vein and adjacent artery may result in formation of an arteriovenous fistula.[7] Other adjacent structures that have the potential for being damaged during venous access include the thoracic duct, regional nerves including the brachial plexus, and even, rarely, a left internal mammary artery graft.[8] All of these complications are quite rare, but the implanter must be aware not only of these structures, but of potential injury to these structures.

Arrhythmias during implantation

Tachyarrhythmias

During manipulation and placement of leads and/or guidewires used for implantation tachyarrhythmias may be induced. These are usually transient and self-limited, terminating either spontaneously or with change in the guidewire or lead position. Occasionally, tachyarrhythmias may sustain and require defibrillation. It is therefore advocated that all patients be attached via transcutaneous pads to an external defibrillator and life-support equipment be present in the room during device implantation.

The most common tachyarrhythmias to occur as a result of hardware manipulation within the atrium are atrial tachycardia, atrial flutter, and atrial fibrillation. Both atrial flutter and tachycardia can often be pace-terminated by overdrive pacing through the pacing system analyzer (PSA) or occasionally with further manipulation of the lead against the wall of the right atrium. Atrial fibrillation when sustained may require cardioversion. Ventricular tachycardia may also occur during lead manipulation. As is the case with supraventricular tachyarrhythmias, further lead manipulation in the ventricle, overdrive pacing, and defibrillation may be necessary to terminate a sustained arrhythmia.

Bradyarrhythmias

As is the case with implant-related tachyarrhythmias, bradyarrhythmias that occur during device implantation are frequently transient and self-limited. A common mechanism of bradycardia during lead placement is overdrive suppression of a ventricular escape focus during threshold testing. Reducing the pacing rate gradually via the PSA will allow the escape focus to reappear in the event that suppression occurs with threshold testing. Patients with intermittent AV block and those with a left bundle branch block (LBBB) are prone to mechanical trauma to the right bundle resulting in complete AV block. Care must be exercised when implanting CRT devices, where the presence of a LBBB is almost universal. Attaching the lead to the PSA with backup pacing readily available will aid in preventing asystole should AV block occur with lead manipulation. In the patient at high risk for development of AV block or asystole during the procedure, a temporary transvenous pacemaker can be placed prior to the procedure.

Lead perforation

Acute perforation

The incidence of lead perforation varies widely depending on the series and type of lead evaluated. Perforation may occur acutely during lead implantation (and the true incidence is probably greater than reported), but many perforations go unrecognized as clinical sequela often do not occur. Asymptomatic but radiographically apparent lead perforation has been reported to occur in up to 15% of patients.[9] Perforation may occur with placement of either the right ventricular lead or the right atrial lead; rarely coronary venous perforations occur with LV lead placement during a CRT implant. Findings that suggest the presence of a perforation include poor sensing and capture thresholds, an extremely distal lead tip location on fluoroscopy, chest pain, a right bundle branch block (RBBB) morphology during RV pacing and contrast outlining the cardiac borders after venography in the case of LV lead placement (Figure 11.4A–C). Anodal pacing compared with cathodal pacing may help determine whether the lead tip has perforated; cathodal pacing will not capture myocardium while anodal pacing will capture if the lead tip is

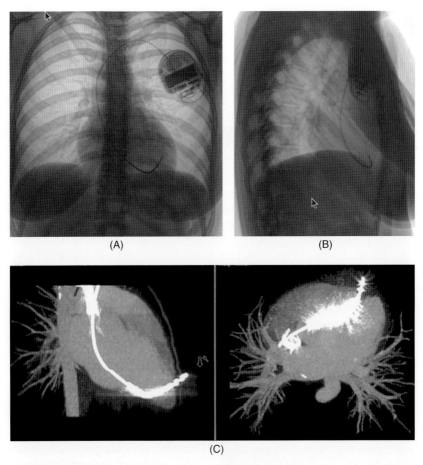

(A)   (B)

(C)

Figure 11.4 *PA (A) and lateral (B) chest X-rays of an 18-year-old girl with long QT syndrome who developed excruciating chest pain one week after transvenous ICD implantion. Chest X-ray in both views show the entire ICD lead contained in the cardiac silhouette. Transthoracic echocardiogram did not show a pericardial effusion and the tip of the lead did not appear to be out of the pericardium.* **(C)** *A chest computed tomography (CT) scan was performed, which confirmed RV perforation and showed the tip of the lead traversing the RV apical myocardium extending 7 mm past the epicardial surface with the tip terminating in the left anterolateral fifth-six intercostal muscles. (Source: Dr. Maully Shah, Division of Cardiology, The Children's Hospital of Philadelphia, U.S.A. Reproduced with permission of Dr. Maully Shah.)*

through the myocardium.[10] Progressive tachycardia and hypotension along with fluoroscopic clues suggest the possibility of cardiac tamponade as a result of perforation. In addition to tamponade, reports of right-sided pneumothorax have been reported with right atrial lead perforation.[11] Coronary sinus perforation rarely causes tamponade due to the fact that intravenous pressure (pressure within the coronary veins) is considerably lower than RV pressure. As a result, blood flows into the proximal portion of the vein rather than into the pericardial space.

Management of acute lead perforation depends on the clinical course. If perforation is thought to have occurred, echocardiography should be performed to identify the presence or absence of a pericardial effusion and assess for tamponade physiology. Pericardiocentesis and placement of a pigtail catheter into the pericardial space will prevent recurrent hemodynamic compromise and allow for monitoring of drainage. Timing of removal of the pigtail catheter depends on the presence or absence of reaccumulating fluid. A slow pericardial leak may occur as a result of perforation with symptoms occurring only days after the implant. As a result of the perforation, signs and symptoms of pericarditis may occur within 5–7 days and non-steroidal anti-inflammatory agents may be required for analgesia.

Chronic perforation

Occasionally, patients seen during routine follow-up are found to have lead perforation (Figure 11.5). The presence of recurrent pericardial effusions, pericarditis, poor sensing and pacing thresholds as well as lead position on chest X-ray may raise the suspicion of a lead perforation. Pericardial effusions should be drained when present and symptoms of pericarditis treated. Lead repositioning should be performed under hemodynamic monitoring in a facility and location capable of treating tamponade and cardiac surgery back up should be considered. Often a chronic lead can be repositioned, but depending on the age of the lead, the entire lead may need to be removed if manipulation and repositioning is difficult. When this occurs, it is recommended that venous access be obtained prior to removal of the old lead.

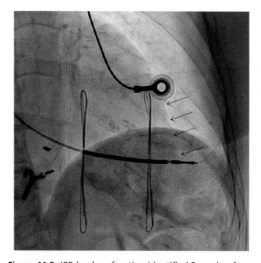

Figure 11.5 *ICD lead perforation identified 3 weeks after implantation during routine follow-up. The patient offered no complaints but device interrogation demonstrated poor sensing and elevated pacing threshold. Red arrows indicate the location of the left heart border with the lead tip clearly visible beyond this location. The lead was repositioned without incident.*

Lead placement into the systemic circulation

Early recognition of systemically placed leads along with lead repositioning are critical as the thromboembolic risk associated with systemic leads is high even for patients treated with anti-platelet agents.[12] Rarely, unintended placement of leads in the systemic circulation may occur through a patent foramen ovale or a VSD, or if inadvertent cannulation of the subclavian artery is performed with retrograde lead placement (Figure 11.6A–C). Knowledge of the typical course of anatomic structures in the thorax may is critical to early identification of such errors. Advancement of the guidewire used for venous access into the IVC confirms the vascular structure as being venous and that the right heart will be used for lead placement. Lead placement into the LV may not be readily apparent on the antero-posterior radiographic image, however, lateral or oblique views will clearly identify the ventricular lead in a posterior characteristic of the LV. Additionally, the morphology of the paced QRS complex should indicate which ventricle is being paced. For this reason, transvenous leads are not typically chosen for patients with anatomy where right-to-left shunting is present such as unrepaired common atrium and VSD with Eisenmeinger's. Long-term anticoagulation may be necessary in a chronically implanted lead found to be located in the systemic circulation.[12, 13] Cardiac surgery intervention should be considered for chronic LV leads, as percutaneous lead extraction is more complex and the thromboembolic consequences of removal of leads present in the systemic circulation are more serious.[14]

Lead dislodgement

A common complication of transvenous lead placement is lead dislodgement. The rate of dislodgement of atrial leads tends to be slightly higher than ventricular leads. Dislodgements are thought to correspond to implanter experience, with less experienced operators having higher dislodgement rates.[14] With current lead design, the dislodgement rate is <2–3%; however, some experienced operators believe that the rate should be even lower.[14] Generally, dislodgement is the result of migration prior to stabilization of the lead via fibrosis and thrombus formation. Dislodgement may be readily

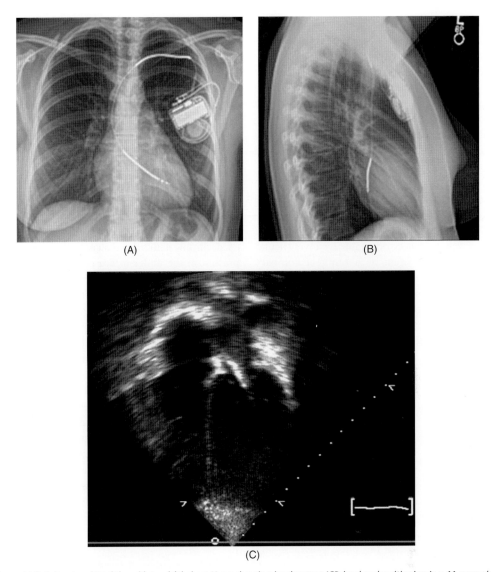

(A)

(B)

(C)

Figure 11.6 *Lateral and PA (A) and lateral (B) chest X-ray showing inadvertent ICD lead malpositioning in a 11-year-old girl with long QT syndrome at the time of evaluation for a lead fracture, 2 years after implantation. The lateral view had not been obtained at the time of implantation. On the PA view, the lead takes a leftward course high in the cardiac silhouette indicating suggesting passage through a patent foramen ovale into the left atrium and left ventricle. The lateral view shows a posterior location of the ICD lead. (C) Echocardiogram confirmed that the ICD lead traversed the mitral valve. These observations were confirmed by direct visualization at the time of ICD lead removal which was performed via a median sternotomy under cardio-pulmonary bypass. (Source: Dr. Maully Shah, Division of Cardiology, The Children's Hospital of Philadelphia, U.S.A. Reproduced with permission of Dr. Maully Shah.)*

visible on radiographic images or often with no clear radiographic evidence of lead migration, but pacing and sensing thresholds indicative of lead tip migration. Ensuring that the leads have adequate slack, anchoring the leads with the suture sleeves and limiting elevation and extreme flexion and extension of the ipsilateral upper extremity for several weeks after implant help reduce the incidence of dislodgement. Most important, however, is ensuring that a stable position is obtained at implant. The presence of ectopy, changing or worsening sensing or pacing thresholds and even loss of capture or sensing should raise the suspicion that the lead has migrated. Chest radiography should be obtained and compared with previously obtained radiographs. Repositioning of acutely implanted leads is usually not difficult, as the leads have not had sufficient time to fibrose to the endothelium and endocardium. Worsening function of a chronically implanted lead may ultimately require placement of a new lead as mobilizing and repositioning chronic leads can be challenging.

Coronary sinus lead dislodgement is one of the difficulties faced when treating patients with CRT devices. Occasionally, LV lead dislodgement manifests as diaphragmatic or extra-cardiac stimulation. Rarely, ventricular ectopy and even ventricular arrhythmias may occur as a result of coronary venous lead dislodgement. Although rates of dislodgement have been significantly reduced through improved lead technology and design, coronary venous leads continue to have a higher dislodgement rate than RA and RV leads. Unfortunately, LV leads are not easily repositioned without support from the sheaths and coronary sinus guides employed during implantation. Invariably the dislodged lead must be removed and another LV lead implanted.

The pulse generator pocket

The importance of creating an appropriately sized pocket cannot be over-stated as the location and size of the pocket must ensure comfort and mobility. The pulse generator pocket should be made to easily accommodate the pulse generator and leads. Too small a pocket may result in erosion and too large a pocket in device migration. With most transvenous pacemaker and defibrillator systems, a pectoral pocket is used, while an abdominal pocket is more often used for epicardial systems with leads that are placed surgically. The abdominal pocket is formed superficial to the deep fascia of the abdomen and lateral to the umbilicus. With pectoral implants in larger children and adults, the pulse generator pocket should be made in the prepectoralis fascia beneath the adipose layer. The pulse generator should be placed in a location inferior to the clavicle and medial to keep it from moving into the anterior axillary fold and causing discomfort with arm movements. For pectoral implants in smaller children and infants who lack adequate subcutaneous tissue, the pulse generator can be placed in a submuscular pocket created beneath the pectoralis major muscle.

Late complications such as pulse generator erosion and migration are often the result of suboptimal pocket placement during the initial implant. A variety of potential pulse generator pocket complications may occur including ecchymosis, hematoma formation, migration of the generator, generator or lead erosion, chronic pain, infection, and rarely dehiscence. With either a pectoral or abdominal pocket, when the wrong tissue plane (subcuticular above the adipose layer) is used, chronic pain may result as the pulse generator presses on the undersurface of the skin. Revision of the pocket and placement in the correct tissue plain will relieve this discomfort.

Ecchymosis

Local ecchymosis is common after device implantation even in patients not treated with anticoagulants or antithrombotic agents. Most often observation alone is sufficient even for large ecchymoses as long as the ecchymotic area is not rapidly expanding. Substantial bruising may be seen when devices are implanted in patients treated with agents such as aspirin, warfarin and clopidogrel, thus care must be taken to achieve adequate hemostasis. Low molecular weight heparin, in particular, will almost always lead to pocket hematoma formation and thus should not be used at all post-operatively.

Pocket hematoma formation

One should always remember that with every opening of a pocket, the rate of infection increases. Therefore, management of hematoma formation in the pulse generator pocket depends on the sequela associated with bleeding into the pocket. One of the most effective means of dealing with a pocket hematoma is the use of a pressure dressing applied over the pulse generator pocket. Hematoma evacuation should be considered only when continued bleeding (particularly arterial), vascular compromise to the overlying tissue (impaired capillary refill), extreme pain despite analgesics and threatened dehiscence of the incision occur. Aspiration is not advised, as sterility will be compromised by introduction of a needle and thus the incidence of infection increased.

Chronic pocket pain

When pain at the implant site is present chronically, there are several possibilities that should not be overlooked. Pocket infection may present with chronic pain even in the absence of other signs of infection and as is the case with pocket hematomas, needle aspiration is not advised. Antibiotics may be used and if the pocket is opened and explored, cultures should be taken and swabs of the local tissue should be sent for microbiology analysis. In addition to infection, chronic pain may indicate improper positioning of the pulse generator pocket, and rarely allergy to the pulse generator or components exposed in the pocket. There are a number of components present in the pocket (titanium, nickel, cadmium, chromate, polyurethane and silicone to name a few) to which allergies have been identified. In addition, suture material may cause an allergic reaction. As the diagnosis of "allergy" is difficult to make it should not be considered until infection is ruled out.

Device erosion

Erosion is caused by pressure necrosis or most commonly infection. Generally, discomfort, discoloration and thinning of tissue overlying the device will occur prior to overt erosion. Overlying tissue becomes tense and thin over the device and ultimately a portion of the generator or leads protrudes through the skin (Figure 11.7). Identification of impending erosion during the stages before the skin is broken allows for salvage of the pacing system by repositioning of the hardware. Once erosion has occurred, the entire system (generator and all intravascular components) must be removed in order to resolve completely eradicate the infection. When erosion is present for some time, the skin margins may appear clean and uninfected with little or no erythema or purulence, however, the device and pocket should be treated as if it is actively infected. While local debridement, irrigation and/or antibiotics are often attempted this approach is generally not accepted and more often than not, does not work. Current guidelines recommend removal of both the generator and any existing leads in the event of pocket infection.[15] Features that make erosion more likely to occur include lack of sufficient subcutaneous tissue, improper pocket location (too superficial), extra hardware such as adapters and abandoned leads, irritation by the patient or irritation/rubbing by clothing overlying the device.

Infection

There has been a significant increase in the incidence in the number of cardiac rhythm device infections worldwide.[16] The incidence of infection varies widely and depends on the type of device (ICDs have a higher incidence than PPMs), the

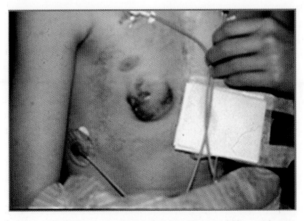

Figure 11.7 *Pacemaker migration and of the pacemaker pocket in a 12-year-old boy with post-operative complete heart block. Note that the generator has migrated from the infraclavicular region to a mid-thoracic location. Pressure necrosis ultimately led to erosion and system infection. The entire system – generator and leads – was removed. (Source: Dr. Maully Shah, Division of Cardiology, The Children's Hospital of Philadelphia, U.S.A. Reproduced with permission of Dr. Maully Shah.)*

experience of the implanting physician, the site of implantation and the underlying medical conditions of the patient.[16-18] One-third to one-half of infections affect new implants; the remainder during generator replacement or lead revision.[19] This is particularly important in the pediatric population where multiple pulse generator changes and revisions/upgrades can be expected over the course of the patient's life. Infections are generally classified as localized pocket infections, isolated lead infection, isolated valve infection or a combination.[19]

Acute bacterial infection usually presents within weeks and is usually secondary to *Staphylococcus aureus* that adhere to the insulation of pacing hardware. Pus formation in the generator pocket is not uncommon and dehiscence of the incision may occur. Antibiotics are rarely curative and removal of the infected hardware is required. More slowly growing bacteria such as *Staphylococcus epidermidis* often lead to device and/or pocket infection months to years after implantation.

Sepsis and endocarditis may result from pocket or lead infection and generally occur later than isolated pocket infection. The source of infection may be from introduction of organisms during the implant or from metastatic spread. The presence of vegetation mandates removal of the all hardware after initiation of antibiotics. The appropriate antibiotic regimen is dictated by the organisms cultured from either the blood or the hardware. Recurrent sepsis in a device patient after completion of an appropriate course of antibiotics without an etiology should prompt consideration of removal of the device and leads (Tables 11.3 and 11.4).[20] Encasing the pacemaker in an absorbable antibacterial envelope at the time of implantation may stabilize the generator and can help reduce the risk of surgical site infections in high risk patients.

Dehiscence

Wound dehiscence is rare and occurs within days or weeks after implant usually secondary to stress on the suture line from hematoma or fluid collection within the pocket. When dehiscence occurs in the absence of an underlying cause, surgical technique is responsible. To avoid contamination

Table 11.3 *Recommendations for antimicrobial management of CIED infection. Source: Baddour 2010. Reproduced with permission of Wolters Kluwer[20]*

Class I	
1.	Therapy should be based on the identification and *in vitro* susceptibility results of the infecting pathogen
2.	Duration of antimicrobial therapy should be 10–14 days after CIED removal for pocket-site infection
3.	Duration of antimicrobial therapy should be at least 14 days after CIED removal for bloodstream infection.
4.	Duration of antimicrobial therapy should be at least 4–6 weeks for complicated infection (i.e., endocarditis, septic thrombophlebitis, or osteomyelitis or if bloodstream infection persists despite device removal and appropriate initial antimicrobial therapy

Notes Class I – indicated, Class IIa – probably indicated, Class IIb – may be considered, Class III – should not be performed, CIED – cardiac implantable electronic device

and infection, immediate intervention needs to occur. Exploration and irrigation followed by closure is usually sufficient to prevent long-term complications. To reduce the risk of dehiscence of the entire incision and suture line, some operators advocate the use of interrupted sutures for the deep layers.

Venous thrombosis

Acute thrombosis

As a result of placement of leads through the subclavian vein, thrombus may form on or around the leads and cause venous occlusion[21] (Figure 11.8). Studies have demonstrated a high rate of asymptomatic thromboses that are related to the number of leads present.[22] The ratio of lead diameter to vein diameter is also likely to be important and one of the reasons transvenous systems may be less favorable in infants and small children. Symptomatic thrombosis usually presents within days to weeks after implant and is marked by pain and swelling of the upper extremity. Extension of the thrombus may occur and include the innominate vein, the superior vena cava (SVC), or even contra-lateral

Table 11.4 *Recommendations for removal of infected CIED. Source: Baddour 2010. Reproduced with permission of Wolters Kluwer[20]*

Class I	
1.	Complete device and lead removal is indicated for:
	– definite CIED infection, as evidenced by valvular and/or lead endocarditis or sepsis
	– abscess formation, device erosion, skin adherence, or chronic draining sinus without clinically evident involvement of the transvenous portion of the lead system
	– valvular endocarditis without definite involvement of the lead(s) and/or device
	– occult *staphylococcal* bacteremia
Class IIa	
1.	Complete device and lead removal is reasonable in patients with persistent occult Gram-negative bacteremia despite appropriate antibiotic therapy
Class III	
1.	CIED removal is not indicated for a superficial or incisional infection without involvement of the device and/or leads.
2.	CIED removal is not indicated for relapsing bloodstream infection due to a source other than a CIED and for which long-term suppressive antimicrobials are required.

Notes Class I – indicated, Class IIa – probably indicated, Class IIb – may be considered, Class III – should not be performed, CIED – cardiac implantable electronic device

veins. Clinically significant pulmonary embolism as a result of the thrombus has been reported but this phenomenon is rare.[23] Rarely SVC syndrome may manifest if thrombosis extends to the SVC and causes occlusion.

When thrombus leads to symptoms, there are several options. Use of heat and extremity elevation may reduce swelling and allow for collateralization to occur. Anti-coagulants such as Heparin and Warfarin as well as thrombolytic agents that allow for dissolution of the thrombus or recanalization or the vessel may cause rapid improvement in symptoms without an increased risk of bleeding complications. The role of long-term anticoagulation in these patients remains controversial.

Chronic venous occlusion

Asymptomatic thrombosis is not uncommon and the incidence of venous occlusion seems to be increasing.[21, 22] It is not necessary to treat an asymptomatic occlusion. There have been no significant risk factors found, but the rise in venous occlusions seen is in part attributed to more multi-chamber devices being implanted. In most patients, venous occlusion becomes apparent during the process of obtaining venous access for a device upgrade and/or when additional leads are placed as a result of lead failure. Alternative routes of venous access may be required to gain access to central veins. When partial venous occlusion is present, venoplasty has been used, with the lead placed immediately, as thrombosis of the vein often occurs as a result of the endothelial damage associated with the procedure. Obtaining contra-lateral access with tunneling across the chest has been used, but this method is not advised because of the potential for bilateral upper extremity occlusion. Extraction of functional leads has been employed to gain access to central veins in the presence of venous occlusion in order to upgrade devices.[24] A variety of techniques and tools exist to accomplish this.[25] Rarely, in patients with very limited venous access, implantation via femoral veins with abdominal generator placement may be required.[26]

"Asymptomatic" chronic SVC stenosis and atresia is encountered in patients with Mustard-type atrial repairs who also have one or more pacing leads traversing the SVC baffle limb. These patients rarely present with symptoms, although once treated and the SVC obstruction relieved, patients will often describe that in comparison, they previously had less exercise tolerance and symptoms of head and neck "fullness."

Device related failures and management

Of all the components of the cardiac rhythm device, the pulse generator has proven to be the most reliable. Nonetheless, device failures do occur

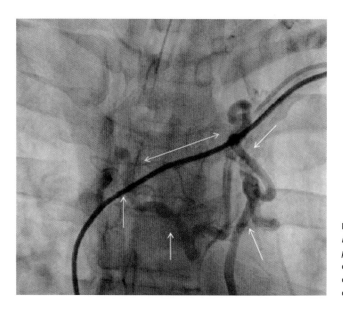

Figure 11.8 *Brachiocephalic vein occlusion in a patient with a single chamber pacemaker. White arrows point to venous collaterals present as a result of complete occlusion of the vein. The length of the occlusion is marked by the yellow arrow.*

and physicians should consider this when evaluating a patient with a suspected pacemaker/ICD problem. Most often, unanticipated device behavior can be explained by programming issues, lead malfunction or specific patient factors. Device malfunction should be considered only when other explanations have been excluded.

Battery depletion

All devices use a battery as a power source. Historically, some of the earliest pacemakers employed a nickel-cadmium rechargeable battery. However, longevity of device operation between charges (6 weeks at most) made this clinically problematic. Pacemaker batteries from the 1960s used zinc-mercury, but the hydrogen gas produced as a byproduct of the electrolysis reaction needed to be vented. As a result, the pacemaker generator could not be hermetically sealed (made impervious to water) and fluid could therefore enter the pacemaker generator leading to an electrical short-circuit and premature battery failure. In the 1970s, certain pacemaker designs incorporated nuclear batteries to maximize battery longevity. As opposed to the electrolytic chemical reaction of other batteries, nuclear batteries use a nuclear source (usually plutonium) to generate heat, which is converted to an electrical current. These nuclear-thermoelectric batteries are very long-lasting because the half-life of plutonium is 87

years. Unfortunately, these pacemakers were large, created problems when patients traveled due to the radioactive fuel and special disposal practices were required when the pacemaker is explanted or the patient expired. These pacemakers became obsolete with the introduction of lithium batteries in the mid-1970s.

All modern cardiac rhythm devices now use lithium as the anode and a cathode (typically iodine-polyvinylpyridine) as a power source. The advantages of the lithium-based cell include no gas generation, adaptable shape and size, corrosion resistance, light weight, and excellent current drain characteristics. The battery also has a long shelf-life with minimal current drain. In addition, the battery has relatively predictable voltage decay characteristics, which allow for relatively accurate prediction of battery depletion. The battery life of a cardiac rhythm device depends on a number of factors including the battery size, lead impedance, the programmed pacing output, the amount of pacing required, number of capacitor charges (for ICDs) and other battery uses for activities such as electrogram storage. The current battery longevity estimates for most pacemakers are 7–10 years and for ICDs 5–7 years although the actual battery longevity may vary considerably based on the aforementioned variables. This is particularly important to consider in pediatric and young adult patients, as the anticipated battery longevity means several anticipated generator replacements even without other complicating factors.

Device malfunctions

Although all device manufacturers have had a limited number of their products malfunction through the years, device malfunction became a well-known phenomenon. In 2005 ICD malfunction was highlighted on the front-page of the New York Times and a recall of several ICD models was announced. This device malfunction was brought to attention by the death of a then 21-year-old college student who collapsed and died despite having an ICD. The device had failed due to an internal short circuit while trying to deliver a high-voltage therapy for a malignant ventricular arrhythmia. Since then, numerous additional advisories have occurred in the cardiac rhythm device industry. The Heart Rhythm Society, working with device manufacturers, the FDA and the American College of Cardiology Foundation (ACCF), the American Heart Association (AHA), and the International Coalition of Pacing and Electrophysiology Organizations (COPE) issued a series of broad recommendations in 2006 related to device performance (Table 11.2). These industry-standard criteria are now in-place to alert physicians and patients to issues that affect the performance of pacemakers and defibrillators.

When device-related issues are identified, the options available for patient management include programming changes to mitigate against the potential issue, increased frequency of device follow-up and device removal and replacement. The risk-assessment calculus is roughly the incidence of the device-related problem multiplied by potential severity and outcome associated with the failure. Recommendations are formulated using this modeling, however, it is important to remember that these recommendations are just that, and that the final medical decision-making is a product of a full and informed discussion between the patient and his/her physician(s) regarding all of the options available taking into account the risks and benefits of any intervention along with individual patient characteristics and preferences.

Lead-related failures
Failure to capture

To provide its intended function, proper connection of the pacemaker or defibrillator system (leads to the generator) is critical. The terminal pin must be inserted properly into the connector block and the lead tip placed distally prior to tightening the set screw. In the event that the lead is not seated properly in the connector block, intermittent contact may be present causing loss of capture and/or inappropriate sensing of electrical signals causing inhibition of pacemaker output or in the case of an ICD, inappropriate therapies. Equally important is confirming that the terminal pin of each lead is correctly placed into the device header (Figure 11.9). A

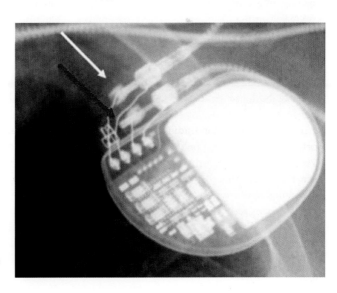

Figure 11.9 *Dual chamber pacemaker with atrial lead not inserted appropriately into the connector block in the device header. The white arrow points to terminal pin of the atrial lead that is not past the terminal portion of the connector block. The red arrow points to appropriate insertion of the ventricular lead terminal pin.*

full device interrogation, with evaluation of the lead connections as well as sensing and pacing thresholds after the system is placed into the pocket prior to closing the incision insures proper connections and function of the system and minimizes inadvertent errors.

Lead failure

Pacemaker and defibrillator leads are typically the "weakest-link" in the system and the source of many pacemaker and defibrillator problems especially in young patients. Implantable cardioverter-defibrillator lead design is more complex than that of a pacemaker lead, and thus the propensity for failure is increased. During follow-up at 10 years, the failure rate of an ICD lead may be as high as 20%.[27] Factors that affect lead performance include the implanting physician, the patient, and specific characteristics related to lead design. Chronic lead issues can usually be attributed to problems with wire integrity (fracture) or insulation. If a lead problem arises in a non-dependent portion of the system, the problem can often be managed with programming changes until an opportunity arises to replace the malfunctioning lead. If a lead problem arises in a critical portion of the system, it usually needs to be addressed immediately. All pacemaker and ICD leads if sufficiently stressed with malfunction over time. As with devices, all manufacturers have had leads that perform less-well than expected. Two of the most well recognized examples of major lead advisories are the Teletronics Accufix pacemaker lead and more recently the Medtronic Fidelis ICD lead.

In November 1994, after two deaths and two nonfatal injuries related to protrusion of an electrically inactive J retention wire had been reported the Accufix pacing lead was recalled. Due to design flaws, the J retention wire was prone to fracture and protrude from the polyurethane insulation. Compared with other pacing lead models that had been recalled for unacceptably high failure rates, the risk posed by this lead was different. In contrast to other pacing leads that exhibited insulation failure or conductor fracture, due to the potential risk of injury associated with this lead, many of leads were extracted. Through vigorous data collection and surveillance, it was ultimately concluded that

despite the high risk of J-retention wire fracture, the probability of injury from lead failure was considerably lower than the risks associated with lead extraction using the then available tools for lead extraction. In 2007, Medtronic recalled its Sprint Fidelis ICD lead over concerns about increased risk of pace-sense lead fracture that could lead to inappropriate sensing and ICD discharge, or failure to sense or pace leading to loss of pacing output or inability to detect and treat tachyarrhythmias. As a result of industry efforts and concerns related to lead failure, algorithms and alert systems have been implemented to reduce the risks associated with lead fracture. Many impeding lead failures can be detected in advance of overt failure and patient alerts can indicate the presence of a problem prior to any untoward events (such inappropriate ICD shocks) occurring to the patient. Unfortunately, this lead continues to have an increasing rate of failure over time. While each patient needs to be considered and evaluated on a case by case basis taking into account the underlying cardiac condition, risk of arrhythmia as well as the risk of lead fracture, many patients and physicians have opted for lead extraction especially at the time of generator change or device upgrade. A large multicenter study on the safety and efficacy of extraction of the Fidelis lead has shown that in experienced centers, the risk of complication associated with extraction of the Fidelis lead is quite low.[28]

Lead fracture

Fracture of the pace-sense portion of a pacemaker or ICD lead usually occurs adjacent to the pulse generator, near the site of venous access or at other points of stress. Fracture is usually manifest by the inability to pace or sense appropriately. For a transvenous lead, the cathode is most prone to fracture because in most leads, this is a single straight wire as opposed to the anode that is usually wound around a layer of insulation. Prior to an overt fracture, impending lead fracture may be heralded and present with increased pacing impedance. In the circumstance of anode fracture of a pacemaker lead, pacing may be maintained by changing the pacing polarity to unipolar. In ICD systems, leads cannot be programmed to a unipolar sensing polarity and the fractured lead ends "brushing" against each other may be detected as ventricular fibrillation by the ICD resulting in inappropriate shocks (often multiple). When ICD lead fracture occurs, electrograms typically demonstrate the presence of non-physiologic R-R intervals (Figure 11.10). This can be distinguished from the electrogram findings seen with electromechanical interference (EMI) which is typically seen on all leads (Figure 11.11).

With epicardial pacing systems, the anode and the cathode are equally prone to fracture. The anode and cathode, however, are not programmable and thus with fracture of the cathode, polarity reprogramming cannot resolve the problem. We prefer to place an extra ventricular lead at time of initial implant epicardial lead implant and leave the "spare" lead capped in the pacemaker pocket. In the event of lead failure, this "spare" lead can be mobilized from within the pocket and used. If this lead is functional, the significant risk of epicardial lead replacement is avoided.

Insulation break

Insulation defects often occur at stress points; at the site of the anchoring sleeves in the pulse generator pocket, near the costoclavicular ligament and near the tricuspid valve. As opposed to presenting with an increase in pacing impedance, insulation break is characterized by a decrease in pacing impedance. Insulating materials must ensure proper lead function taking into account the interaction of the leads with adjacent materials present in the vascular system (such as other leads) and in the pulse generator pocket (lead-lead and lead-pulse generator interactions). For more than 50 years, the most common materials used as insulators for pacemaker and defibrillator leads

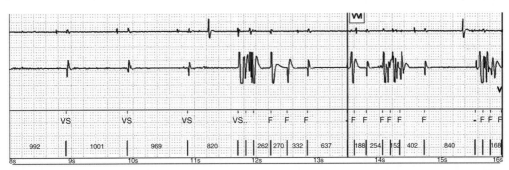

Figure 11.10 *Electrograms demonstrating high frequency, non-physiologic signals on the ventricular lead of an ICD system.*

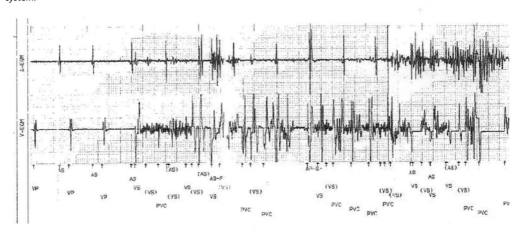

Figure 11.11 *Electomechanical interference (EMI) in a pacemaker patient. Top electrograms represent atrial signals and electrograms on the bottom represent ventricular signals. The presence of "noise" on both the atrial and ventricular channels suggest an external source of interference.*

have been silicone and polyurethane. Both silicone and polyurethane have excellent longevity, but each material has a unique set of characteristics that provide advantages and disadvantages to each compound. Silicone is flexible, has a long "track record" for performance, excellent biostability and can be repaired with medical adhesive and silicone film. However, silicone abrades easily (Figure 11.12), tears easily, cuts easily and is subject to cold flow failure. Polyurethane has the advantage of having a higher resistance for abrasion, higher tear strength, superior compressive properties, and is relatively stiff allowing for increased maneuverability during implant. However, polyurethane is subject to environmental stress cracking and metal ion oxidation and can be damaged by electrocautery. Optim® is a unique silicone polyurethane co-polymer created by St. Jude Medical, Inc. specifically for use with cardiac leads that combines the beneficial properties of both silicone and polyurethane and has been shown to be 50 times more abrasion resistant than silicone.[29]

Lead extraction

With the increase in implantable cardiac rhythm device implantation in the pediatric population, there has been an increasing need for lead extraction. As opposed to adults, where cardiac rhythm device infection represents the predominant indication for lead extraction, the most common indication for lead extraction in the pediatric patient population is lead malfunction.[30] This is often the result of patient growth, vigorous physical activity, and longer lifespan seen in this group of patients. Stretching and distortion of the lead and increased tension on the conducting elements occurs with longitudinal growth. Fibrous scar tissue begins to develop on the endothelial surface of the leads several weeks after implantation and progresses over time. This is particularly true with ICD leads and the presence of high voltage coils used for delivery of high voltage shocks (Figure 11.13). The presence of focal points of fibrous attachment, particularly with ICD leads (related to the high voltage coils) may prevent the unwinding of intentionally placed redundant loops of lead with growth. It is widely accepted that younger, more active patients have higher rates of lead failure and fracture.[31, 32] The challenges faced when managing leads in these younger patients incorporates the future requirement for multiple pulse generator changes, the need for repeated revisions and upgrades, the risks associated with abandoning leads and the expected longevity of these patients (Figure 11.14).

The complex vascular and cardiac anatomy seen in this patient population is unique and may even add additional indications for lead extraction. Increasingly patients are being identified with stenoses and occlusions at venous entry sites and along conduits and baffles created during corrective surgical intervention for complex congenital conditions and extraction to facilitate opening of the occluded or stenosed sites along with balloon and stent dilatation is being increasingly utilized (Figure 11.15). When considering the option

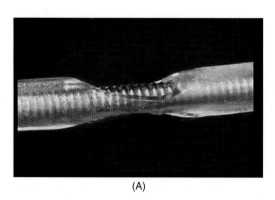
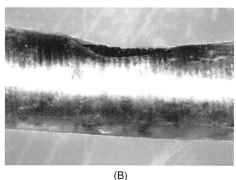

(A)   (B)

Figure 11.12 *Photographs of erosion of silicone insulation on pacemaker leads. Erosion is the result of lead-to-lead or can-to-lead mechanical contact. (A) Erosion present on a lead implanted for 4 years. (B) Erosion present on a lead implanted for 11 months.*

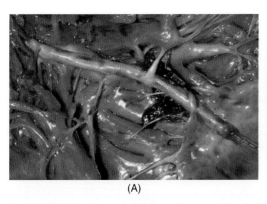

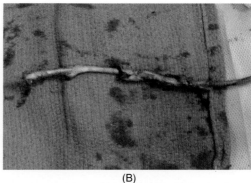

(A)   (B)

Figure 11.13 *Fibrosis seen on intravascular leads. (A) Pathologic specimen of an ICD lead in the trabeculations of the right ventricle. Fibrous encapsulation of the lead is seen with adhesions present along the lead and the high voltage coil is covered by fibrous tissue. (B) Photograph of an extracted pacemaker lead. Dense regions of fibrous adhesions are present where the lead was adherent to the vascular system and myocardium.*

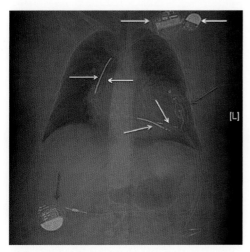

Figure 11.14 *PA radiograph of a patient with three pulse generators and multiple leads in-situ. Red arrows identify an abdominal pacemaker with epicardial leads both attached and abandoned. White arrows point to a left pectoral pacemaker system with a transvenous lead. Yellow arrows identify a left pectoral ICD system.*

of lead extraction, it is important to weigh the risks and benefits associated with the intended procedure. In addition to individual patient and physician preference, an understanding of the complex anatomy and physiology as well as proper equipment, experienced staff, and mandatory cardiac surgical backup are necessary to safely perform these procedures. Because of the nature of lead extraction and the potential risks associated with lead extraction in any patient, it is recommended that the procedure be performed under general anesthesia with the with the chest and abdomen prepared for emergency sternotomy and femoral arterial and venous access obtained for hemodynamic monitoring and access to the central circulation.

There are numerous approaches and tools employed to extract transvenous leads. Typically, leads are removed via the transvenous access site through which they were inserted (the implant vein). In cases where this approach is unsuccessful or impossible, alternative transvenous approaches via the femoral, jugular or subclavian veins can be used or occasionally surgical intervention via a trans-atrial or ventriculotomy approach is required. Regardless of the route, there are a standard set of techniques that are used to assist in lead removal. Traction, counterpressure and countertraction, progressive dissection, and mechanical dislodgement are all techniques used in lead extraction. Traction tools include specialized locking stylets, snares, or devices used to engage or entrap and remove a lead or lead fragments. Locking stylets are designed to hold onto the engage the inside of the conductor coil along its length or near the distal electrode, improve tensile properties, and prevent elongation of the lead body during traction (Figure 11.16). Any sheath or combination of sheaths may be used to apply counterpressure and countertraction on a lead. Mechanical sheaths composed of metal, Teflon, polypropylene, or other materials rely on mechanical force along with the

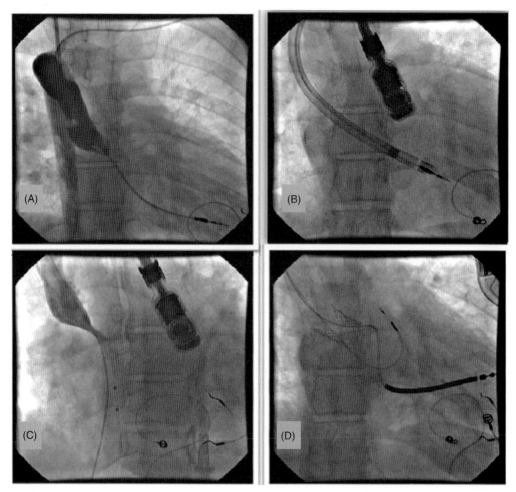

Figure 11.15 *Series of images in a patient s/p Mustard repair with baffle stenosis and a single chamber pacemaker. Patient had symptoms related to baffle obstruction and required upgrade to a dual chamber ICD system. (A) Baffle stenosis and functional single chamber pacemaker present. (B) Extraction sheaths used to pass the level of baffle stenosis and remove the pacing lead prior to baffle stenting. (C) Stenosis of the baffle seen after removal of the pacemaker lead in preparation for stent placement. (D) Stented baffle with dual chamber ICD system placed.*

properties of the sheath to disrupt fibrotic attachments (Figure 11.17). These sheaths are designed to disrupt and dilate tissue surrounding leads and to free the lead from fibrous adhesions via mechanical manipulation of the sheath over the lead either alone or via a telescoping system. With one sheath coaxially placed inside a second larger sheath, both flexibility and strength are provided, and the system can be passed over the lead breaking up fibrous scar tissue. Regardless of the type of sheath used, mechanical manipulation of the sheath is used to assist in disrupting fibrous adhesions.

There are a number of powered sheaths equipped with an energy source that in addition to the mechanical properties of the sheath, assist in lead extraction (Figure 11.18). Electrosurgical sheaths use bipolar radiofrequency energy emitted between two Tungsten electrodes located at the leading edge of the bevel of the sheath tip (Figure 11.18A). The application of radiofrequency energy produces a thermal effect allowing fibrous adhesions to be disrupted. Another powered sheath used in lead extraction is equipped with a rotationally powered mechanism that bores through and disrupts fibrotic

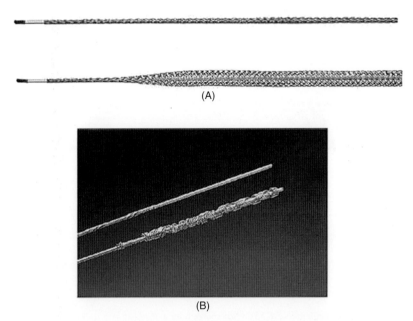

Figure 11.16 *A and B. Locking stylets used during lead extraction. By engaging the inner conductor coil of the lead, these stylets prevent elongation and unraveling of the lead when traction is placed and provide control of the lead as it is removed.*

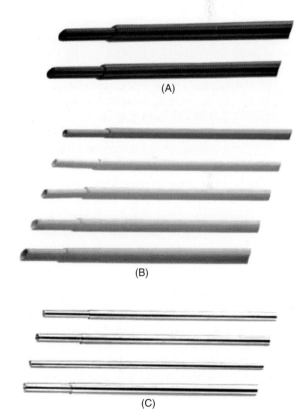

Figure 11.17 *Mechanical sheaths of different materials and sizes are available for use in lead removal and extraction. Sheaths made of (A) TFE, (B) polypropylene, or (C) stainless steel.*

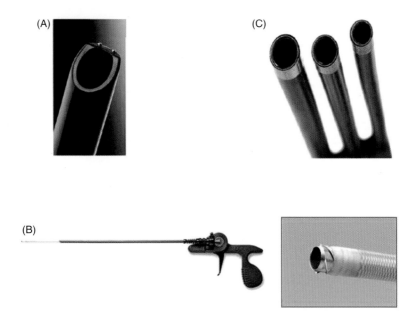

Figure 11.18 *Powered sheaths equipped with an energy source used in lead extraction. (A) Tungsten electrodes at the sheath tip emit radiofrequency energy producing a thermal effect. (B) A mechanical sheath with a rotating threaded stainless steel tip dissects through tissue. This sheath is particularly useful with calcified adhesions. (C) An excimer laser sheath utilizes ultraviolet light to ablate fibrous adhesions.*

attachments using a threaded screw mechanism at the sheath tip. This system is composed of an inner sheath with a threaded stainless steel tip and a telescoping outer sheath (Figure 11.18B). The device is shaped like a pistol with a trigger capable of rotating the sheath. This sheath is particularly useful for calcified adhesions and is capable of dissecting through all types of tissue. A short version called Evolution® Shortie (Cook Medical Inc., Bloomington, IN) is available for use under the clavicle at the venous entry site. A similar new addition is the TightRail™ and TightRail Mini™ (Spectranetics Inc, Colorado Springs, CO), which is a rotating dilator sheath that has a flexible shaft and a bidirectional mechanism to negotiate tortuous vessels. In contrast to the Evolution®, its dilating blade remains shielded until activated. These sheaths are recent additions to the list of tools available for extraction, reports on the efficacy and utility of this device in the literature are limited, but the efficacy and utility of this sheath is clear. The most commonly used powered sheath for lead extraction is the laser sheath. This sheath uses a fiberoptic system to transmit laser or ultraviolet light (wavelength 308 nm) in a circumferential

fashion at the sheath tip to ablate tissue to a depth of 50 μm (Figure 11.18C). As a result of solid photochemical destruction and liquid vaporization, photoablation occurs and scar tissue surrounding leads is disrupted. The sheath can be advanced over a lead and laser energy delivered at specific sites of tissue binding using mechanical manipulation of the sheath as it advances over the lead. The safety and efficacy of the laser system has been demonstrated and this is often the sheath of choice for many extractors.

Recently, a series of 144 patients was published demonstrating the safety and efficacy of lead extraction in young patients.[33] The majority of patients had structural heart disease with d-transposition of the great arteries and Tetralogy of Fallot being the most frequently encountered anomalies. As expected, lead failure was the indication for extraction in 65% of patients. Importantly, simple traction was sufficient for extraction in 29% of leads in this cohort. This report, along with others performed in the pediatric population, demonstrates that complete extraction of targeted leads can be successfully accomplished in a large number of patients. The overall complication rate (even in this highly experienced center) was 5.6% with an even distribution of major and minor complications occurring and no peri-procedural deaths.

Summary

While the technique of cardiac rhythm device implantation has evolved and become simpler and safer, it is still an invasive procedure fraught with complications even in for the most experienced implanter. Knowledge of the patient's cardiovascular history and anatomy as well as awareness of the potential complications possible at every step of the procedure is critical. The potential for problems exists beyond the immediate peri-operative period, throughout the longevity of the device.

References

1 Scherhag A, Gulbins H, Lange R, Saggaw W. Improved reliability of postoperative cardiac pacing by use of bipolar temporary pacing leads. *Eur JCPE* 1995; 5: 101–108.

2 Brinker J, Midei M. Techniques of pacemaker implantation and removal. In: Ellenbogen K, Wood M, eds. *Cardiac Pacing and ICDs*. 3rd Edn. Malden, MA: Blackwell Science, Inc.; 2002: 216–284.

3 Ellestad MH, French J. Iliac vein approach to permanent pacemaker implantation. *Pacing Clin Electrophysiol*. 1989; 12(7 Pt 1): 1030–1033.

4 Oude Ophuis AJ, van Doorn DJ, van Ommen VA, den Dulk K, Wellens HJ. Internal balloon compression: a method to achieve hemostasis when removing an inadvertently placed pacemaker lead from the subclavian artery. *Pacing Clin Electrophysiol*. 1998; 21(12): 2673–2676.

5 Hilfiker PR, Razavi MK, Kee ST, Sze DY, Semba CP, Dake MD. Stent-graft therapy for subclavian artery aneurysms and fistulas: single-center mid-term results. *J Vasc Interv Radiol*. 2000; 11(5): 578–584.

6 Rotem CE, Greig JH, Walters MB. Air embolism to the pulmonary artery during insertion of transvenous endocardial pacemaker. *J Thorac Cardiovasc Surg*. 1967; 53(4): 562–565.

7 Finlay DJ, Sanchez LA, Sicard GA. Subclavian artery injury, vertebral artery dissection, and arteriovenous fistulae following attempt at central line placement. *Ann Vasc Surg*. 2002; 16(6): 774–778.

8 Chou TM, Chair KM, Jim MH, Boncutter A, Milechman G. Acute occlusion of left internal mammary artery graft during dual-chamber pacemaker implantation. *Catheter Cardiovasc Interv*. 2000; 51(1): 65–68.

9 Hirschl DA, Jain VR, Spindola-Franco H, Gross JN, Haramati LB. Prevalence and characterization of asymptomatic pacemaker and ICD lead perforation on CT. *Pacing Clin Electrophysiol*. 2007; 30(1): 28–32.

10 Occhetta E, Bortnik M, Marino P. Ventricular capture by anodal pacemaker stimulation. *Europace*. 2006; 8(5): 385–387.

11 Ho WJ, Kuo CT, Lin KH. Right pneumothorax resulting from an endocardial screw-in atrial lead. *Chest*. 1999; 116(4): 1133–1134.

12 Van Gelder BM, Bracke FA, Oto A, Yildirir A, Haas PC, Seger JJ, et al. Diagnosis and management of inadvertently placed pacing and ICD leads in the left ventricle: a multicenter experience and review of the literature. *Pacing Clin Electrophysiol*. 2000; 23(5): 877–883.

13 Sharifi M, Sorkin R, Sharifi V, Lakier JB. Inadvertent malposition of a transvenous-inserted pacing lead in the left ventricular chamber. *Am J Cardiol*. 1995; 76(1): 92–95.

14 Hayes DL, Friedman PA. *Implantation-Related Complications. Cardiac Pacing, Defibrillation and Resynchronization*. 2nd Edn. Chichester, UK: John Wiley & Sons, Ltd; 2008: 202–233

15 Wilkoff BL, Love CJ, Byrd CL, Bongiorni MG, Carrillo RG, Crossley GH 3rd, et al.; Heart Rhythm Society; American Heart Association. Transvenous lead extraction: Heart Rhythm Society expert consensus on facilities, training, indications, and patient management: this document was endorsed by the American Heart Association (AHA). *Heart Rhythm*. 2009 Jul; 6(7): 1085–104.

16 Cabell CH, Heidenreich PA, Chu VH, Moore CM, Stryjewski ME, Corey GR, Fowler VG, Jr., Increasing rates of cardiac device infections among Medicare beneficiaries: 1990–1999. *Am Heart J*. 2004; 147(4): 582–586.

17 Uslan DZ, Sohail MR, St Sauver JL, Friedman PA, Hayes DL, Stoner SM, et al. Permanent pacemaker and implantable cardioverter defibrillator infection: a population-based study. *Arch Intern Med*. 2007; 167(7): 669–675.

18 Sohail MR, Uslan DZ, Khan AH, Friedman PA, Hayes DL, Wilson WR, et al. Infective endocarditis complicating permanent pacemaker and implantable cardioverter-defibrillator infection. *Mayo Clin Proc*. 2008; 83(1): 46–53.

19 Duval X, Selton-Suty C, Alla F, Salvador-Mazenq M, Bernard Y, Weber M, et al. Endocarditis in patients with a permanent pacemaker: a 1-year epidemiological survey on infective endocarditis due to valvular and/or pacemaker infection. *Clin Infect Dis*. 2004; 39(1): 68–74.

20 Baddour LM, Epstein AE, Erickson CC, Knight BP, Levison ME, Lockhart PB, et al. Update on cardiovascular

implantable electronic device infections and their management: a scientific statement from the American Heart Association. *Circulation.* 2010 Jan 26; 121(3): 458–477.

21 Pauletti M, Di Ricco G, Solfanelli S, Marini C, Contini C, Giuntini C. Venous obstruction in permanent pacemaker patients: an isotopic study. *Pacing Clin Electrophysiol.* 1981; 4(1): 36–42.

22 Haghjoo M, Nikoo MH, Fazelifar AF, Alizadeh A, Emkanjoo Z, Sadr-Ameli MA. Predictors of venous obstruction following pacemaker or implantable cardioverter-defibrillator implantation: a contrast venographic study on 100 patients admitted for generator change, lead revision, or device upgrade. *Europace* 2007; 9: 328–332.

23 Pasquariello JL, Hariman RJ, Yudelman IM, Feit A, Gomes JA, El-Sherif N. Recurrent pulmonary embolization following implantation of transvenous pacemaker. *Pacing Clin Electrophysiol.* 1984; 7(5): 790–793.

24 Gula LJ, Ames A, Woodburn A, Matkins J, McCormick M, Bell J, et al. Central venous occlusion is not an obstacle to device upgrade with the assistance of laser extraction. *Pacing Clin Electrophysiol.* 2005; 28(7): 661–666.

25 Fischer A, Love B, Hansalia R, Mehta D. Transfemoral snaring and stabilization of pacemaker and defibrillator leads to maintain vascular access during lead extraction. *Pacing Clin Electrophysiol.* 2009; 32(3): 336–339.

26 Ching CK, Elayi CS, Di Biase L, Barrett CD, Martin DO, Saliba WI, et al. Transiliac ICD implantation: defibrillation vector flexibility produces consistent success. *Heart Rhythm.* 2009; 6(7): 978–983.

27 Kleemann T, Becker T, Doenges K, Vater M, Senges J, Schneider S, et al. Annual rate of transvenous defibrilla-

tion lead defects in implantable cardioverter-defibrillators over a period of >10 years. *Circulation.* 2007; 115: 2474–2480.

28 Maytin M, Love CJ, Fischer A, Carrillo RG, Garisto JD, Bongiorni MG, et al. Multicenter experience with extraction of the Sprint Fidelis implantable cardioverter-defibrillator lead. *J Am Coll Cardiol.* 2010; 56: 646–650.

29 Jenney C, Tan J, Karicherla A, Burke J, Helland J. A new insulation material for cardiac leads with potential for improved performance, HRS 2005, *Heart Rhythm,* 2005; 2: S318–S319.

30 Cooper JM, Stephenson EA, Berul CI, Walsh EP, Epstein LM. Implantable cardioverter defibrillator lead complications and laser extraction in children and young adults with congenital heart disease: implications for implantation and management. *J Cardiovasc Electrophysiol.* 2003; 14: 344–349.

31 Fortescue EB, Berul CI, Cecchin F, Walsh EP, Triedman JK, Alexander ME. Patient, procedural, and hardware factors associated with pacemaker lead failures in pediatrics and congenital heart disease. *Heart Rhythm.* 2004; 1: 150–159.

32 Morrison TB, Rea RF, Hodge DO, Crusan D, Koestler C, Asirvatham SJ, et al. Risk factors for implantable defibrillator lead fracture in a recalled and a nonrecalled lead. *J Cardiovasc Electrophysiol.* 2010; 21: 671–677

33 Cecchin F, Atallah J, Walsh EP, Triedman JK, Alexander ME, Berul CI. Lead extraction in pediatric and congenital heart disease patients. *Circ Arrhythm Electrophysiol.* 2010 Oct; 3(5): 437–444. Epub 2010 Aug 20.

CHAPTER 12

Temporary pacing in children

Anjan S. Batra[1] and Ilana Zeltser[2]

[1] Division Chief and Vice Chair of Pediatrics, University of California, Irvine, Director of Electrophysiology, Children's Hospital of Orange County, Orange, CA, USA

[2] Pediatric Electrophysiologist, Children's Medical Center of Dallas, Associate Professor of Pediatrics, University of Texas Southwestern School of Medicine, Dallas, TX, USA

Introduction

Temporary cardiac pacing (TCP) is a widely adopted technique used in the evaluation and management of a variety of cardiac dysrhythmias in the pediatric population. Its applications range from therapeutic interventions for both brady- and tachyarrhythmias, as well as a means to perform provocative diagnostic cardiac testing in a minimally invasive manner. Over the years, TCP techniques have become increasingly sophisticated allowing for programmable dual chamber modes.

TCP involves electrical cardiac stimulation to treat a tachyarrhythmia or bradyarrhythmia until it resolves or until alternative therapy can be initiated. The goal of temporary pacing is to optimize hemodynamics in patients with clinically significant arrhythmias for a finite period of time (Table 12.1). Symptomatic bradycardia, including conditions such as sinus node dysfunction and heart block, may compromise a patient's cardiac output. Whether used as first line therapy or in situations where the bradyarrhythmia is refractory to medical therapy (i.e., atropine, isuprel), TCP provides a more immediate measure to establish a more appropriate heart rate, henceforth preserving adequate cardiac output. Similarly, many tachyarrhythmias compromise ventricular filling time and result in increased myocardial oxygen demand, leading to myocardial dysfunction and poor cardiac output.

TCP can be accomplished by various techniques including: transcutaneous, transesophageal, endocardial, and epicardial pacing. These modalities vary in their suitability for pacing the atria, the ventricles, or to allow for dual chamber synchronous pacing. In order to determine the best and most appropriate modality for TCP, one must first evaluate the conduction system and determine which chamber/chambers require pacing. For example, in the case of sinus node dysfunction in the immediate post-operative patient, the desired increased heart rate could be achieved by effectively pacing the atrium. However, in situations of complete or third degree heart block, ventricular and often dual chamber pacing is indicated. Additional considerations include: (1) urgency, (2) available personnel and equipment, (3) vascular access, (4) ability to maintain patient stability, and (5) anticipated duration of therapy.

This chapter will describe the various approaches to temporary pacing, focusing on the indications for temporary pacing, the technical aspects of the various TCP modalities, and the advantages/ disadvantages associated with each modality.

Cardiac Pacing and Defibrillation in Pediatric and Congenital Heart Disease, First Edition.
Edited by Maully Shah, Larry Rhodes and Jonathan Kaltman.
© 2017 John Wiley & Sons Ltd. Published 2017 by John Wiley & Sons Ltd.
Companion Website: www.wiley.com/go/shah/cardiac_pacing

Table 12.1 *Indications for temporary pacing in children*

I. Bradycardia

   a. Sinus node dysfunction
   b. Heart transplantation associated with injury to the sinus node/artery
   c. Congenital heart surgery resulting in injury to the sinus or AV node
   d. New onset presentation of second or third degree heart block
   e. Congenital heart block in the newborn period
   f. Long QT syndrome in the setting of significant bradycardia or 2:1 AV conduction
   g. Infection resulting in either sinus or AV nodal dysfunction including Lyme disease, myocarditis, subacute
      bacterial endocarditis with an aortic valve abscess damaging the His–Purkinje system
   h. Cardiac trauma resulting in transient SA or AV nodal injury
   i. Toxic, metabolic, electrolyte and drug-induced causes for bradycardia including hyperkalemia, digoxin toxicity,
      beta-blocker sensitivity or overdose, and anti-arrhythmic drug therapy
   j. Catheter trauma resulting in advanced or complete AV block
   k. Pacemaker malfunction in a dependent patient

II. Treatment of tachycardias

   a. Pace termination of reentrant SVT or VT
   b. Pace termination of atrial reentry tachycardia
   c. Overdrive/suppression of junctional ectopic tachycardia in situations where AV synchrony significantly aug
      ments cardiac output

III. Prophylactic

   a. Cardioversion in the setting of sick sinus syndrome
   b. New AV or bundle branch block with acute endocarditis
   c. Allow pharmacologic treatment with drugs that worsen bradycardia
   d. Suppression of bradycardia dependent ventricular tachyarrhythmias (including torsades de pointes)

IV. Provocative diagnostic cardiac procedures

   a. Risk stratification in patients with Wolff–Parkinson–White syndrome
   b. Assess efficacy of anti-arrhythmic therapy

V. Diagnostic applications of temporary cardiac pacing systems

   a. Determine atrial activity
   b. Provide information with respect to the AV and/or VA relationship

Approaches to temporary pacing

Transcutaneous pacing

Indications

Transcutaneous pacing is a temporary means of pacing a patient's heart during a medical emergency. It is accomplished by delivering pulses of electric current through the patient's chest, which stimulates the heart to contract. The most common indication for transcutaneous pacing is an abnormally slow heart rate or asystole. Transcutaneous patches are readily available in the intensive care units and can be used to initiate asynchronous ventricular pacing in a relatively short period of time. External pacing functions in a VOO mode and is only used for emergent pacing. It should not be relied upon if temporary pacing for a longer period of time is required.

Technical considerations

Large, self-adhesive surface chest wall patches with a high impedance interface are required for external pacing. Pediatric specific patches are recommended for children less than 8 years of age. The cardiac pacing patches are attached to the patient's chest with the anterior (negative) electrode to the left of the sternum, centered close to the point of maximal cardiac impulse and the posterior (positive) patch on the back, to the left of the thoracic spinal column (directly opposite the anterior patch) or over the anterior right chest wall. Sedation or a state of unconsciousness is required to use this approach effectively for more than back-up or emergency pacing.

Generators need to have pacing modes with widely adjustable settings for rate and output, and built in filters to electronically minimize the large pacing artifact stimulus. Generators typically provide longer pulse width to allow for lower pacing thresholds in order to minimize collateral skeletal muscle and cutaneous nerve stimulation. Units typically provide up to 200 mA of current and deliver up to 40 ms of pulse width duration. The pacing rate is usually set at 80 bpm or higher. The pacing current output is increased continuously until the ECG tracing indicates electrical capture (generally characterized by a widened QRS complex and broad T wave after each pacer spike), or there is confirmation of capture as evidenced on the pulse oximetry or arterial line tracing. The output is set 10% higher than the threshold of initial electrical capture as a safety margin. Watch for a change in patient's underlying rhythm. Ventricular fibrillation would necessitate immediate defibrillation.

In most instances, pacing thresholds are typically <80 mA. In order to help reduce pacing thresholds, and optimize pacing efficiency, measures should be taken to assure most adequate delivery of the external impulse to the chest wall. Ideally the patient's skin should be prepped with alcohol and excessive body hair should be shaven. Other factors such as obesity, myocardial ischemia, electrolyte abnormalities and the presence of pneumo/hemo-thorax,

do increase the pacing threshold, and should be taken into account when assessing for adequate capture.[1,2]

Limitations

Transcutaneous pacing has many limitations including patient discomfort, requiring high energies for capture, and is generally not recommended for periods over 24 hours, and it is generally recommended that the pads should be rotated every 4–5 hours to reduce skin trauma.[3] Complications of transcutaneous pacing include failure to recognize VF due to the size of pacing artifact on the ECG screen and induction of other dysrhythmias. Soft tissue discomfort may result from pacing and there is a potential for local cutaneous injury with prolonged periods of pacing.

Transesophageal pacing

Indications

Transesophageal pacing (TEP) is relatively noninvasive, efficient, and free of complications, and valuable in the diagnosis and treatment of various cardiac arrhythmias in children. TEP is effective in situations where it is essential to sense and/or pace the atrium in order to provide essential diagnostic information. Atrial electrograms may be recorded to help distinguish between atrial versus junctional versus ventricular rhythm disturbances (Figure 12.1). Transesophageal pacing can yield important information in many situations where invasive atrial stimulation is frequently done (Table 12.2). [4–11] TEP can also be used for noninvasive evaluation of antegrade

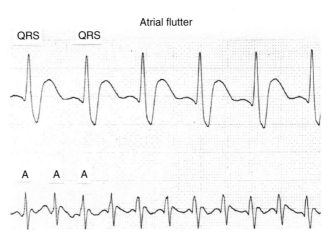

Figure 12.1 *Atrial flutter with 2:1 atrioventricular conduction. While the p-waves are quite difficult to appreciate on the surface lead ECG, the esophageal recording clearly demonstrates the presence of an atrial tachyarrhythmia.*

Table 12.2 *Indications for transesophageal pacing*

- Sinus node evaluation
- Atrioventricular conduction evaluation: permeability, short PR, effects of drugs
- Assessment of Wolff–Parkinson–White syndrome: reciprocating tachycardia inducibility, anterograde refractory period, effect of drugs, ventricular rate during atrial fibrillation
- Assessment of paroxysmal supraventricular tachycardia of unknown origin: mechanism analysis, counselling for radiofrequency ablation, drug evaluation.
- Assessment of palpitations of unknown origin
- Assessment of relationship between atrium and ventricle: differential diagnosis ventricular tachycardia versus supraventricular tachycardia.
- Interruption of supraventricular tachycardia and atrial flutter
- P wave synchronous pacing, evaluation of myocardial ischemia
- Induction of left ventricular fascicular tachycardia

electrophysiological properties of both the sinus and AV node,[12] provide risk-stratification in patients with WPW[13,14] and fascicular ventricular tachycardia[15] and perform anti-arrhythmic drug testing.[16]

TEP is also quite valuable in situations where it is critical to provide atrial pacing in hopes of restoring optimal hemodynamics. TEP can be used for treatment of medically refractory significant sinus or junctional bradycardia, especially in situations of infectious or drug/toxin related bradyarrhythmias. TEP can also be used to provide pace termination of reentry tachyarrhythmias, or provide overdrive suppression of ectopic tachycardias in situations where restoring AV synchrony is crucial. There is limited data to suggest that transesophageal left ventricular pacing and electrogram recording may be play a useful role.[17,18]

Technical considerations

The transesophageal operating system consists of an intraesophageal electrode, a pulse generator, and an ECG recorder. TEP and recording can be done using two different lead types: (1) the pill electrode, connected to a flexible wire that the patient swallows with water. This pill electrode necessitates patient collaboration and hence not used in children: and (2) a flexible catheter that can be used in comatose or intubated patients and the catheter of choice in children.[19] Patients are typically sedated for placement of the electrode and asked to fast for 4 hours before TEP placement.

An intranares insertion of the pacing catheter allows for the most stable positioning (Figure 12.2). The ideal catheter is both soft (given the insertion site) yet somewhat rigid in order to account for passage through the upper airway in patients who cannot cooperate and swallow (Figure 12.3). The

Esophageal Study

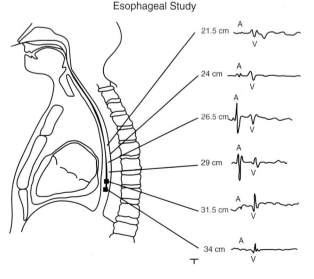

Figure 12.2 *Cartoon demonstrating recommended positioning of the esophageal pacing catheter. Using an intranares approach, the initial depth of insertion is best approximated by using the patient's height/5 + 9 cm. The catheter should be gradually advanced or withdrawn until the maximum p-wave amplitude is obtained. Adapted from instruction manual for Cardio Command, Inc.; Tampa, FL.*

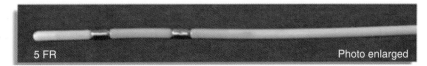

Figure 12.3 *The TAPCATH 205 is a 5 French esophageal bipolar pacing and recording catheter. The intra-electrode spacing is 1–3 cm, and the tip of the catheter is electrode-free.*

ideal intra-electrode spacing is 1–3 cm, and the tip of the catheter is typically electrode-free (to aid through nasal passages). There is an empiric relationship between patient height and insertion depth, and the optimal positioning is where the largest peak-to-peak atrial electrogram is recorded (Figure 12.2). Unipolar electrograms may be recorded using the more traditional precordial ECG lead, and bipolar recordings can be obtained by using the limb leads.[20] Due to the bipolar nature of the lead, pacing and recording cannot be obtained simultaneously.

Most bipolar TEP catheters yield pacing thresholds of 10–15 mA at a pulse width of 10–20 ms. Assuming transesophageal impedances of 700–2600 Ω, generators need to provide outputs of 40–75 V to create currents of 25–30 mA. The pacing generator (Figure 12.4) transmits pacing pulses from the stimulator to the esophageal catheter. Recording is facilitated with preamplifiers to help eliminate background artifact (noise of breathing, swallowing, or peristalsis) and allow for simultaneous recordings of esophageal and surface

lead electrograms. The operator has the ability to customize asynchronous atrial pacing at rates up to 800 ppm, however, rates beyond 400 ppm are rarely used.

Limitations

TEP can be uncomfortable and pacing usually produces a burning chest sensation. When burst pacing in the atrium, there is always the potential of inducing more unstable arrhythmias. In addition, there is no ability to perform demand pacing in the atrium. Inadvertent ventricular pacing occurs when the lead is pushed too deep in the esophagus and high energies are used. Brachial plexus stimulation and phrenic nerve pacing are other potential complications. TEP is also not particularly useful when it is essential to provide ventricular pacing. Finally, there is also the risk of esophageal damage when used for longer periods of pacing at high output.[21] There have been some animal studies where continuous TEP has been shown to be safe and effective for periods of up to 24 hours.[22]

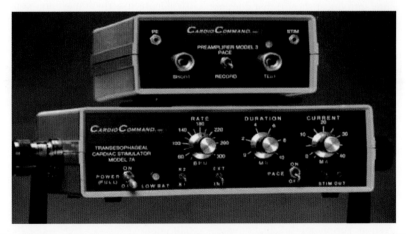

Figure 12.4 *Transesophageal cardiac stimulator (Arzco Medical Electronics). The pacing generator transmits pacing pulses from the stimulator to the esophageal catheter. Recording is facilitated with preamplifiers to help eliminate background artifact and allow for simultaneous recordings of esophageal and surface lead electrograms. Asynchronous atrial pacing at rates up to 800 bpm can be delivered.*

Endocardial Pacing

Indications

In general, endocardial TCP is indicated when a bradyarrhythmia causes severe hemodynamic impairment and when permanent pacing is not immediately indicated, not available, or risky. Endocardial pacing provides the most reliable and consistent means of temporary pacing, but requires the most technical expertise. The main reason for temporary endocardial pacing is the prevention of hemodynamic collapse or severe symptoms. Atrial endocardial leads are indicated when bradycardia alone is the indication for pacing or for pace termination of atrial tachyarrhythmias in children. Pacing within the ventricle allows for management of severe bradyarrhythmias with a more stable ventricular rate but at the expense of AV synchrony.

Technical considerations

Endocardial pacing catheters are typically 2–6 Fr in diameter, use platinum coated electrodes, can be unipolar or bipolar, and come in either passive or active fixation varieties. Catheters are generally stiff; however, adjuncts such as balloon tips or preformed curves can be used to help facilitate insertion. These stiff endocardial leads afford better lead stability over a period of time, but careful positioning, ideally under fluoroscopic guidance, is recommended. A temporary pacemaker lead/electrode placed in the subclavian or right internal jugular that has been inserted in a sheath (or without an indwelling introducer sheath) that does not allow for intravenous infusion can be maintained for as long as 7–10 days without major concern. The ideal vascular insertion site depends on several factors including: urgency, lead stability, anticipated duration of pacing, and the need to avoid specific complications. The best access site for temporary pacing leads in terms of accessibility and stability is via the left subclavian vein or the right internal jugular vein. The subclavian approach permits more freedom of patient motion and might be useful in a patient who requires a long-term temporary pacemaker; however, a permanent pacemaker should be avoided on that side due to the risk of infection. Peripheral (brachial or external jugular vein) routes afford the least bleeding complications or risk of pneumothorax, however,

are more difficult to manipulate. Femoral venous pacing carries the greatest risk of thrombosis and infection; however, venous access is typically most easily accessible in emergent situations.

Generators are powered by commercially available batteries that provide output up to 15 V (or 20 mA of current). Endocardial pacing is usually undertaken with single-chamber external temporary generators or dual chamber temporary external generators programmed as single chamber devices. The Single-Chamber External Pulse Generators (Figure 12.5) are easy to use and can be programmed in the VVI, VOO, AAI, or AOO mode. They also have an increased sensitivity range (0.5–20 mV) to provide more reliable measures of sensing P- and R-wave amplitudes. The pacing mode is classified using the Heart Rhythm Society and British Pacing and Electrophysiology Group generic code.[23]

Limitations

Serious complications of internal pacing are rare, but are important to recognize. There is a need for careful care and proper bandaging of the site of lead placement to prevent infection. There is also a risk of lead dislodgement and ventricular perforation. Complications, including more rare events, of endocardial lead placement are listed in Table 12.3.

Epicardial pacing

Sinus node dysfunction, AV block and supraventricular tachyarrhythmias are common in the post-operative period following CHD surgery and are often poorly tolerated hemodynamically. Accurate and prompt recognition of these dysrhythmias help intensive care unit teams provide better more appropriate post-operative management and treatment. Temporary epicardial atrial or ventricular pacing leads are generally placed at the time of surgery for congenital heart disease or in patients undergoing orthotopic heart transplantation. These wires can serve a useful purpose for both diagnosis and therapy of arrhythmias in the post-operative period.

Indications

Transcatheter epicardial pacing strategies are often useful to aid in the diagnosis and treatment of

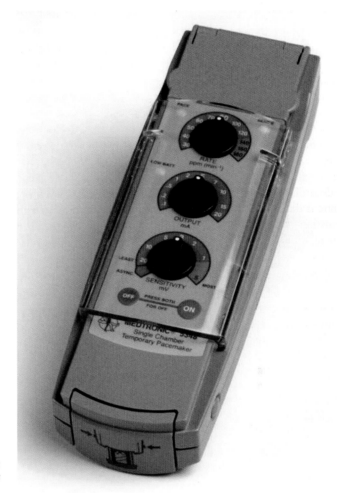

Figure 12.5 *Single chamber temporary pacemaker (Medtronic Model 5348) can pace the atrium or the ventricle at rates of up to 180 bpm.*

Table 12.3 *Complications of temporary endocardial pacing*

- Lead dislodgement and disconnection
- Bleeding
- Pericardial tamponade
- Thrombophlebitis
- Pulmonary embolism
- Catheter knotting
- Air embolism
- Ventricular tachycardia/ventricular fibrillation
- Pneumothorax
- Diaphragmatic stimulation
- Infection
- Perforation
- Asystole

various tachyarrhyhmias. Of particular use is the ability to determine atrial activity in isolation as well as provide information with respect to the AV and/or VA relationship.

The usual method for recording epicardial atrial electrical activity is to connect the standard left and right upper extremity leads to each atrial wire and the standard lower extremity leads to the lower limb. Unipolar signals can be recorded from standard ECG leads II and III and depict moderate atrial activity with a large ventricular deflection. Bipolar signals can be recorded from lead I and contain a large sharp atrial deflection with smaller ventricular activity. Alternatively, the atrial wire can be connected to standard ECG precordial lead V1.

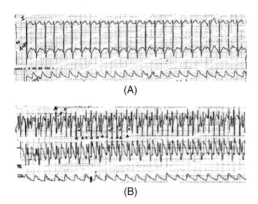

(A)

(B)

Figure 12.6 *(A) Surface ECG of a patient in atrial flutter with 2:1 AV conduction. The P waves are not clearly seen. (B) Atrial ECG of the same patient shows the P waves with 2:1 AV conduction more clearly.*

Diagnostic AEGs are useful when P waves are not clearly visible on a surface ECG. The AV relationship during SVT helps distinguish the underlying mechanism of the tachycardia. For example, identifying AV block or AV dissociation

without the interruption of the atrial rate during tachycardia is highly consistent with the diagnosis of atrial flutter (Figure 12.6). As opposed to sinus tachycardia where the P waves supersede the R waves (Figure 12.7), in junctional tachycardia, the P waves are superimposed/ immediately retrograde or dissociated from the R waves (Figure 12.8).

Sinus node dysfunction, junctional ectopic tachycardia, supraventricular tachycardia (AV nodal reentry, atrio-ventricular reentry, atrial flutter, and sinus node reentry tachycardia), and atrioventricular block are common postoperative arrhythmias.[24] Temporary overdrive pacing can be an effective means of terminating reentry tachycardias such as atrial flutter (Figure 12.9) and paroxysmal supraventricular tachycardia.[25] Pacing for short durations generally takes over the circuit and subsequently terminates the tachycardia. Typically, the pacing rate is set at 10–20 beats faster than the tachycardia rate. Progressively faster rates can be tried with multiple reattempts.

Pacing Wire Study

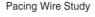

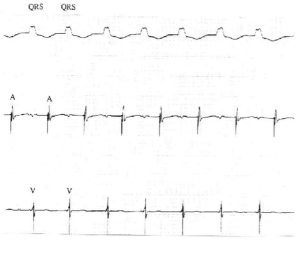

Figure 12.7 *The surface lead ECG demonstrates a wide complex rhythm without identifiable p-waves. The epicardial pacing wires are used to document a simultaneous recording demonstrating clear 1:1 AV relationship translating to the interpretation of this rhythm as an atrially derived rhythm with a bundle branch block aberrancy.*

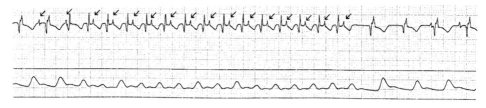

Figure 12.8 *An atrial ECG showing onset and termination of a junctional tachycardia. The P waves are retrograde and marked with arrows.*

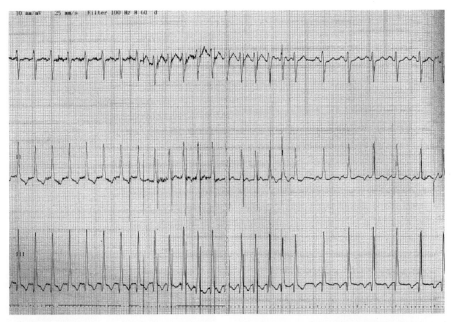

Figure 12.9 *A three-lead ECG: The first part demonstrates a slow atrial tachycardia at a rate of 140 bpm with 1:1 AV conduction, the second part rapid atrial pacing using a temporary pacemaker and the third part sinus rhythm after termination of the tachycardia.*

In patients with atrial or junctional ectopic tachycardia, temporary pacemakers can be used to suppress the arrhythmia and establish AV synchrony by pacing the atrium at rates faster than the tachycardia cycle length. In addition, the ability to provide back up, synchronous dual chamber pacing allows for the more liberal use of certain anti-arrhythmic agents with longer half-lives (i.e., amiodarone), without having to be overly concerned for the negative side-effects on AV nodal conduction.

Sinus node dysfunction and high grade heart block are known complications of surgery for CHD. Over half these patients with conduction abnormalities will recover their conduction system within 10 days from cardiac surgery.[26] Temporary epicardial pacing can be used to bridge this interval between post-operative heart block and either recovery of spontaneous conduction or placement of a permanent pacemaker.

Disturbance of normal AV synchrony and dyssynchronous ventricular contraction may be deleterious in patients with CHD and compromised hemodynamics. Janousek et al. evaluated the effect of optimizing temporary dual chamber pacing

in patients after surgery for congenital heart disease and demonstrated several techniques of individually optimized temporary dual chamber pacing to improve hemodynamics (as measured by a higher systolic arterial blood pressure and lower atrial pressure) by optimizing AV synchrony and/or synchronous ventricular contraction.[27] In extremely low-birth-weight infants with complete heart block, patient size may preclude implantation of a permanent pacemaker. Extrathoracic temporary epicardial pacing may provide support to these patients for up to 3 months at which time permanent, epicardial-pacing leads can be implanted.[28] A unique indication for temporary epicardial pacing is in the management of refractory ventricular arrhythmias in the neonatal long QT syndrome.[29,30]

Technical considerations

Epicardial wires come in two forms: unipolar and bipolar. A unipolar system (Figure 12.10) consists of the negative cathode attached to the epicardium and the positive anode attached to the subcutaneous tissue (Figure 12.11A and B). The pediatric unipolar lead is designed for thinner

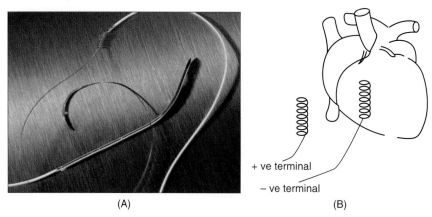

+ ve terminal

− ve terminal

(A)   (B)

Figure 12.10 *Unipolar pediatric temporary pacing lead (Medtronic Model 6491).*

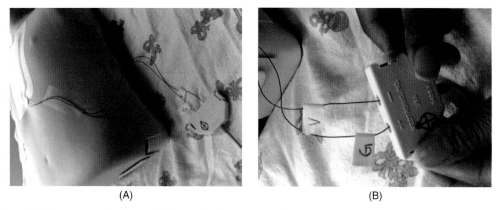

(A)   (B)

Figure 12.11 *Temporary unipolar ventricular pacing in a neonate with post-operative third degree AV block. (A) The ground wire is directly sutured to the skin. (B) The ground wire is always inserted into the positive terminal of the temporary pacemaker cable. A = atrium, V = ventricle, G = ground.*

pediatric and atrial tissue by being smaller and having a curved chest needle for better leverage through small chest cavities. The larger current path in a unipolar system creates a larger pacing spike on the surface ECG. It also has a cost advantage over the bipolar pacing lead. A bipolar system (Figure 12.12) consists of a single wire with both the anode and the cathode on this wire attached to the epicardial surface, or two unipolar wires. The cathode is usually the more distal electrode and the anode is 8 mm proximal to the cathode (the Medtronic bipolar coaxial 6495: Medtronic, Minneapolis, MN). Because of the shorter distance between the two poles in the bipolar lead, the capture threshold is generally lower and the sensing more specific when compared to the unipolar lead. Temporary epicardial pacing leads

are typically placed in the operating room after the cardiac procedure is completed and before chest closure. Epicardial pacing wires were historically placed only on the right ventricle. As patients with congenital heart disease are often dependent on the atrial contraction for better preload and cardiac output, most institutions currently place both atrial and ventricular pacing wires. The atrial wires are placed on the right atrium. By informal convention, wires placed on the right atrium are brought out through the skin on the right of the sternum, and those on the right ventricle are brought out on the left of the sternum. Also, radiographically, typically, ventricular pacing wires are seen on the left side of the sternum; atrial pairs are seen on the right side.

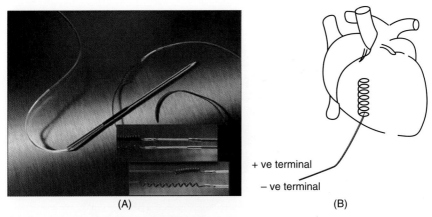

+ ve terminal

− ve terminal

(A)   (B)

Figure 12.12 *Bipolar temporary myocardial pacing lead (Medtronic Bipolar Coaxial 6495). Two discreet electrodes are optimally spaced at 8 mm for consistent pacing and sensing.*

An implanted pacing lead forms a direct current path to the myocardium. As with the case of enodcardial pacing, during pacing lead insertion, and testing, only battery-powered equipment specially designed for this purpose should be used to protect against fibrillation that may be caused by alternating currents. Line-powered equipment used in the vicinity of the patient must be properly grounded. Pacing lead connector pins must be insulated from any leakage currents that may arise from line-powered equipment. Care should be taken to avoid the possibility of unintentional contact between the pacing lead(s), including extension cable, and any equipment used as well as any conductive surface contact. The temporary cardiac pacemakers used for epicardial pacing are the same as those used for temporary endocardial pacing and the programming is also similar. However, because both atrial and ventricular leads are placed, dual chamber external pacemakers allow more extensive and effective programming in these patients. Modern day dual chamber temporary pacemakers (Figure 12.13) allow adjustment of parameters such as mode of pacing, lower and upper rate limits, AV interval, and post ventricular atrial refractory period. The most important of these are rate, atrial output and ventricular output (in most commercially available temporary pacemakers, the duration of the electrical impulse, namely the pulse width is fixed and cannot be programmed by the physician). Making appropriate adjustments of these three parameters will provide effective pacing in most clinical situations. Changing the pacing rate automatically adjusts other dual-chamber temporary pacing parameters. Pediatric patients may need a pacing rate up to 200 ppm. A patient's high stimulation threshold may require a ventricular output of 25 mA. For managing atrial tachyarrhythmias, a rapid atrial pacing rate up to 800 ppm is possible but rates beyond 400/min are rarely used.

The optimal sensing and pacing parameters need to be adjusted based on the thresholds. The capture threshold is the minimum pacemaker output (current intensity measured as voltage or amperage) required to stimulate an action potential in the myocardium. Only the current amplitude (volts/amperes) is altered in measuring threshold since temporary pacemakers come with a fixed current duration (also termed pulse width). This should be checked on a daily basis especially in patients who are dependent on the temporary pacing. Typically, the outputs are set at twice threshold in both atrium and ventricle to allow for a margin of safety. This however may not be possible if the capture threshold is >10 mA. The sensing threshold is the minimum voltage the pacemaker is able to sense. It is generally recommended to set the sensitivity at half the minimum voltage sensed. If sensing is set too high (insensitive) the pacemaker will fail to sense intrinsic events, thereby converting it from a demand to a fixed-rate pacemaker. Setting the sensitivity too low (over-sensitive) will make the pacemaker potentially sense muscle noise, and

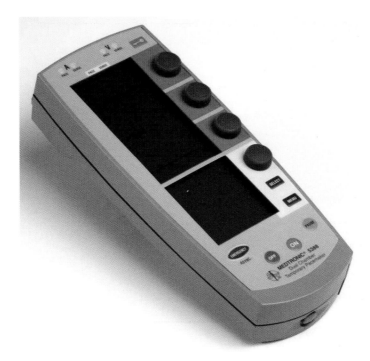

Figure 12.13 *Dual chamber temporary pacemaker (Medtronic Model 5388). The dual chamber model can be used where short-term demand (synchronous) or asynchronous pacing is indicated for therapeutic, prophylactic, or diagnostic purposes. The device paces up to 200 ppm, allows ventricular output to 25 mA for high stimulation thresholds and rapid atrial pacing rates up to 800 ppm for managing atrial tachyarrhythmias.*

other ambient events common to the intensive care situation (such as ventilators, intravenous pumps, etc.) as intrinsic events leading to inappropriate loss of pacing. The upper and lower rate limits and AV intervals vary with age and should be set to maximize cardiac output within the range of age appropriate physiological parameters. In general, the AV delay is set between 100–140 ms in most children.

Newer applications of temporary pacemakers include their use for the simultaneous pacing of both ventricles. Both ventricles can be simultaneously paced by placing a right and a left ventricular lead at implant and connecting both wires to the same output terminal of the pulse generator. There is evidence to show that biventricular pacing can augment cardiac performance in patients after repair of CHD and that this form of pacing may be better than conventional RV pacing in patients with normal interventricular conduction.[31–33] On a practical note, it is important to check the threshold for each ventricle and set the ventricular

output above the higher of the two thresholds so that both ventricles can be successfully paced.

Although both atrial and ventricular temporary epicardial leads are reliable for short-term use, their function deteriorates on a daily basis. Increases in stimulation thresholds typically occur after 4 days in both the atrial and ventricular wires.[34] The reason for increasing thresholds is believed to be secondary to inflammation around the surface of the myocardium where the wire is attached. As bipolar electrodes require less energy for capture, they have a greater longevity for pacing when compared to a unipolar system.[35,36] In a patient with post-operative heart block, permanent pacemaker implantation is indicated if the need for a temporary pacemaker persists longer than 10–14 days post-operatively.[37]

Limitations

There is a small but definite risk of epicardial pacing. Complications of epicardial wires include infection, myocardial damage, ventricular arrhythmias, perforation, and tamponade.[38,39] While temporary pacing leads can be removed by gentle traction, monitoring of the rhythm should be undertaken while pacing wires are being removed and the patient should be observed for a few hours after lead removal because of the risk of tamponade. Leaving the lead implanted for longer than 7 days may result in difficulty or inability to extract the lead, increased risk of bleeding, and increased risk of mediastinitis.

The use of MRI is currently not recommended in patients who are dependent on temporary epicardial pacing because of the potential risk of precipitating an arrhythmia[40] or causing injury from excessive heat at the electrode tip.[41] An MRI may, however, be safely performed in a patient with retained epicardial wires that have been cut off at the skin because of the absence of an antennae effect capable of concentrating the energy from the MRI.[42]

Conclusion

There are numerous applications for the use of TCP in the pediatric population. Depending on the modality chosen, TCP can provide treatment for medically refractory, symptomatic bradycardia, treatment for various tachycardias, and provide essential diagnostic information. TCP can be performed effectively and safely in the pediatric population. When determining the appropriate TCP strategy, one must take into account variables including: (1) the integrity of underlying conduction system, (2) urgency, (3) availability of personnel and equipment, (4) vascular access, and (5) anticipated duration of therapy.

References

1 Ceresnak SR, Pass RH, Starc TJ et al. Predictors for hemodynamic improvement with temporary pacing after pediatric surgery. *J Thorac Cardiovasc Surg* 2011; 141 (1): 183–187.

2 Zoll PM, Zoll RH, Falk RH, Clinton JE, Eitel DR, Antman EM. External noninvasive temporary cardiac pacing: clinical trials. *Circulation*. May 1985; 71(5): 937–944.

3 Falk RH, Zoll PM, Zoll RH. Safety and efficacy of noninvasive cardiac pacing. A preliminary report. *N Engl J Med*. Nov 10 1983; 309(19): 1166–1168.

4 Fenici R, Ruggieri MP, di Lillo M, Fenici P. Reproducibility of transesophageal pacing in patients with Wolff–Parkinson–White syndrome. *Pacing Clin Electrophysiol*. 1996 Nov; 19(11 Pt 2): 1951–1957.

5 Gallagher JJ, Smith WM, Kerr, CR, et al. Esophageal pacing: a diagnostic and therapeutic tool. *Circulation* 1982; 65: 336–341.

6 Critelli G, Grassi G, Perticone F, et al. Transesophageal pacing for prognostic evaluation of preexcitation syndrome and assessment of protective therapy. *Am J Cardiol* 1983; 5(1): 513–518.

7 Gallagher JJ, Smith WM, Kasell J, et al. The use of the esophageal lead in the diagnosis of mechanisms of reciprocating supraventricular tachycardia. *PACE* 1980; 3: 440–451.

8 Falk RH, Werner M. Transesophageal atrial pacing using a pill electrode for the termination of atrial flutter. *Chest* 1987; 92: 110–114.

9 Benson DW, Dunnigan A, Sterba R, et al. Atrial pacing from the esophagus in the diagnosis and management of tachycardia and palpitations. *J Pediatr* 1983; 102: 40–46.

10 Burack B, Furman S. Transesophageal cardiac pacing. *Am J Cardiol* 1969; 23: 469–472.

11 Lubell DL. Cardiac pacing from the esophagus. *Am J Cardiol* 1971; 27: 641–664.

12 Pietrucha AZ, Wnuk M, Wojewódka-Zak E, Wegrzynowska M. Evaluation of sinus and atrioventricular nodes function in patients with vasovagal syncope. *Pacing Clin Electrophysiol*. 2009 Mar; 32 Suppl 1: S158–S162.

13 Brembilla-Perrot B, Chometon F, Groben L. Interest of non-invasive and semi-invasive testings in asymptomatic children with pre-excitation syndrome. *Europace*. 2007; 9: 837–843.

14 Pappone C, Santinelli V, Rosanio S, Vicedomini G, Nardi S, Pappone A, et al. Usefulness of invasive electrophysiologic testing to stratify the risk of arrhythmic events in asymptomatic patients with Wolff–Parkinson–White pattern: results from a large prospective long-term follow-up study. *J Am Coll Cardiol*. 2003; 41: 239–244.

15 Williams CS 4th,, Khatib S, Dorotan-Guevara MM, Snyder CS. Induction of left ventricular fascicular tachycardia with transesophageal pacing in a toddler. *Congenit Heart Dis*. 2010; 5: 312–315.

16 Fenici R, Ruggieri MP, di Lillo M, Fenici P. Reproducibility of transesophageal pacing in patients with Wolff–Parkinson–White syndrome. *Pacing Clin Electrophysiol*. 1996 Nov; 19(11 Pt 2): 1951–1957.

17 Heinke M, Ismer B, Kühnert H, Figulla HR. Transesophageal left ventricular electrogram-recording and temporary pacing to improve patient selection for

cardiac resynchronization. *Med Biol Eng Comput.* 2011; 49: 851–858.

18 Yamanaka A, Kitahata H, Tanaka K, Kawahito S, Oshita S. Intraoperative transesophageal ventricular pacing in pediatric patients. *J Cardiothorac Vasc Anesth.* 2008 Feb; 22(1): 92–94. Epub 2006 Dec 8.

19 Verbeet T, Castro J, Decoodt P. Transesophageal pacing: a versatile diagnostic and therapeutic tool. *Indian Pacing Electrophysiol J.* 2003; 3: 202–209.

20 Hammill SC, Pritchett ELC: Simplified esophageal electrocardiography using bipolar recording, leads. *Ann Intern Med* 1981; 95: 14–18.

21 Köhler H, Zink S, Scharf J, Koch A. Severe esophageal burn after transesophageal pacing. *Endoscopy.* 2007; 39: E300.

22 Green H, Sanders R, Ramos-Vera J, Hogan D, Batra AS. Safety of transesophageal pacing for 24 hours in a canine model. *Pacing Clin Electrophysiol.* 2009 Jul; 32(7): 888–893.

23 Bernstein AD, Daubert JC, Fletcher RD, et al. The revised NASPE/BPEG generic code for antibradycardia, adaptive-rate, and multisite pacing. North American Society of Pacing and Electrophysiology/British Pacing and Electrophysiology Group. *Pacing Clin Electrophysiol* 2002; 25: 260–264.

24 Rekawek J, Kansy A, Miszczak-Knecht M, et al. Risk factors for cardiac arrhythmias in children with congenital heart disease after surgical intervention in the early postoperative period. *J Thorac Cardiovasc Surg.* 2007; 133: 900–904.

25 Brockmeier K, Ulmer HE, Hessling G. Termination of atrial reentrant tachycardias by using transesophageal atrial pacing. *J Electrocardiol.* 2002; 35 Suppl: 159–163.

26 Gross GJ, Chiu CC, Hamilton RM, Kirsh JA, Stephenson EA. Natural history of postoperative heart block in congenital heart disease: implications for pacing intervention. *Heart Rhythm.* 2006; 3: 601–604.

27 Janousek J, Vojtovic P, Chaloupecký V, et al. Hemodynamically optimized temporary cardiac pacing after surgery for congenital heart defects. *Pacing Clin Electrophysiol.* 2000; 23: 1250–1259.

28 Filippi L, Vangi V, Murzi B, Moschetti R, Colella A. Temporary epicardial pacing in an extremely low-birth-weight infant with congenital atrioventricular block. *Congenit Heart Dis.* 2007; 2: 199–202.

29 Tanel RE1, Triedman JK, Walsh EP, Epstein MR, DeLucca JM, Mayer JE Jr, et al. High-rate atrial pacing as an innovative bridging therapy in a neonate with congenital long QT syndrome. *J Cardiovasc Electrophysiol.* 1997; 8: 812–817.

30 Aziz PF1, Shah MJ. Efficacy of ventricular pacing in the treatment of an arrhythmic storm associated with a congenital long QT mutation. *Congenit Heart Dis.* 2013; 8: E165–E167.

31 Pham PP, Balaji S, Shen I, Ungerleider R, Li X, Sahn DJ. Impact of conventional versus biventricular pacing on hemodynamics and tissue Doppler imaging indexes of resynchronization postoperatively in children with congenital heart disease. *Journal of the American College of Cardiology* 2005; 46: 2284–2289.

32 Zimmerman FJ, Starr JP, Koenig PR, Smith P, Hijazi ZM, Bacha EA. Acute hemodynamic benefit of multisite ventricular pacing after congenital heart surgery. *Ann Thorac Surg* 2003; 75: 1775–1780.

33 Janousek J, Vojtovic P, Hucin B, et al. Resynchronization pacing is a useful adjunct to the management of acute heart failure after surgery for congenital heart defects. *Am J Cardiol* 2001; 88: 145–152.

34 Elmi F, Tullo NG, Khalighi K. Natural history and predictors of temporary epicardial pacemaker wire function in patients after open heart surgery. *Cardiology* 2002; 98: 175–180.

35 Wirtz S, Schulte HD, Winter J, Godehardt E, Kunert J. Reliability of different temporary myocardial pacing leads. *Thoracic and Cardiovascular Surgeon* 1989; 37: 163–168.

36 Yiu P, Tansley P, Pepper JR. Improved reliability of post-operative ventricular pacing by use of bipolar temporary pacing leads. *Cardiovascular Surgery* 2001; 9: 391–395.

37 Driscoll DJ, Gillette PC, Hallman GL, Cooley DA, McNamara DG. Management of surgical complete atrioventricular block in children. *Am J Cardiol.* 1979; 43: 1175–1180.

38 Carroll KC, Reeves LM, Anderson G, et al. Risks associated with removal of ventricular epicardial pacing wires after cardiac surgery. *American Journal of Critical Care* 1998; 7: 444–449.

39 Reade MC. Temporary epicardial pacing after cardiac surgery: a practical review: part 1: general considerations in the management of epicardial pacing. *Anaesthesia.* 2007; 62: 264–271.

40 Peden CJ, Collins AG, Butson PC, Whitwam JG, Young IR. Induction of microcurrents in critically ill patients in magnetic resonance systems. *Critical Care Medicine* 1993; 21: 1923–1928.

41 Luechinger R, Zeijlemaker VA, Pedersen EM, et al. In vivo heating of pacemaker leads during magnetic resonance imaging. *European Heart Journal* 2005; 26: 376–383

42 Hartnell GG, Spence L, Hughes LA, Cohen MC, Saouaf R, Buff B. Safety of MR imaging in patients who have retained metallic materials after cardiac surgery. *American Journal of Roentgenology* 1997; 168: 1157–1159.

PART 4

Device Programming and Follow-Up

CHAPTER 13

Pacemaker and ICD programming in congenital heart disease

Jonathan Kaltman[1] and Jeffrey Moak[2]

[1]Chief, Heart Development and Structural Disease Branch, Division of Cardiovascular Sciences, National Heart, Lung, and Blood Institute, NIH, Bethesda, MD, USA

[2]Director, Electrophysiology and Pacing, Children's National Health System, Professor, Pediatrics George Washington University, Washington, DC, USA

Programming a pacemaker or ICD in a patient with congenital heart disease is not dissimilar from doing so in a patient with a structurally normal heart. The underlying arrhythmia mechanism(s) are the same. However, consideration of additional factors, such as patient size, anatomy, and hemodynamic status, may affect programming decisions. This chapter will review special issues related to pacemaker and ICD programming in patients with congenital heart disease.

Pacemaker programming

The overall goals of programming a pacemaker are to correct the underlying rhythm defect, maintain appropriate hemodynamics, and reproduce normal physiological functions as closely as possible. In patients with congenital heart disease, additional consideration must be given to patient size and cardiac anatomy as these will determine how many leads the heart can accommodate. Whether a single chamber or dual chamber pacemaker system is implanted will ultimately determine how the system can be programmed.

Pacemakers typically address two rhythm abnormalities: sinus node dysfunction and disturbances in atrioventricular conduction (AV block). These abnormalities may exist individually or in combination. Sinus node dysfunction is defined as abnormal sinus node impulse formation (or propagation) resulting in sinus bradycardia, sinus pauses, or absence of sinus impulses with slow escape rhythms originating below the sinus node. AV block is defined as impairment of electrical impulse conduction across the AV junction from atrium to ventricle (AV block may be in the AV node or in the His-Purkinje conduction system). Third degree AV block occurs when no atrial impulses reach the ventricle and there is typically a slow junctional or ventricular escape rhythm.

Both of these rhythm abnormalities are characterized by abnormally slow heart rates. Therefore, the basic function of the pacemaker is to provide appropriate rate support. With junctional or ventricular escape rhythms, synchrony of atrial and ventricular contraction is lost. Dual chamber pacemakers can reproduce AV synchrony by either

Cardiac Pacing and Defibrillation in Pediatric and Congenital Heart Disease, First Edition.
Edited by Maully Shah, Larry Rhodes and Jonathan Kaltman.
© 2017 John Wiley & Sons Ltd. Published 2017 by John Wiley & Sons Ltd.
Companion Website: www.wiley.com/go/shah/cardiac_pacing

pacing the atrium and the ventricle with an appropriately timed AV pacing delay (mimicking the PR interval) or by sensing intrinsic atrial activation which then triggers ventricular pacing after an appropriately timed AV delay. In patients with sinus node dysfunction, there is an inadequate chronotropic response to exercise. To address this issue, a rate adaptive pacing mode can be enabled.

Sinus node dysfunction

Sinus node dysfunction is a common complication of congenital heart disease and typically results from surgical injury to the sinus node itself, its arterial supply, or its autonomic innervations. Sinus node dysfunction occurs frequently after atrial switch surgery for d-transposition of the great arteries, Fontan palliation for single ventricle physiology and complete repair of anomalous pulmonary venous connection and sinus venosus atrial septal defects. However, sinus node dysfunction can be found after nearly any type of surgical repair of congenital heart disease.

Atrial pacing in the AAI mode is commonly used to treat sinus node dysfunction. It mimics physiologic function by providing rate support during periods of sinus pauses or sinus bradycardia. Impulse formation in the atrium maintains AV synchrony with conduction through the AV node and normal ventricular activation through the His–Purkinje system. The main parameter programmed in AAI pacing is the lower pacing rate. If the device senses an intrinsic atrial event at a rate greater than the lower rate, device output is inhibited. If there is no sensed event, the device will pace the atrium at the lower rate.

Patients with chronotropic incompetence can be programmed in a rate adaptive mode, AAIR. Depending upon the sensor used, the rate response mode will enable an increase in the heart rate (decrease in the cycle length) with progressive increase in the patient's level of exertion up to a programmed upper rate limit. The most widely used rate adaptive sensors respond to patient activity by detecting vibration of the device (piezo-electric crystal or accelerometer); or changes in intrathoracic impedance (minute ventilation). Parameters that can be altered when programming the rate response mode include the threshold of activity required to trigger the increased heart rate and the slope of the heart rate response.

Sinus node dysfunction and accelerated junctional rhythm occurs relatively commonly in post-op CHD patients. Single chamber atrial pacing (and dual chamber pacing) is often difficult in these patients. The junctional rhythm may compete with the lower pacing rate shortening the PR interval or even causing atrial and ventricular contraction to occur simultaneously. Also, retrograde P waves, if they exist, may inhibit atrial pacing altogether. If the P waves are not sensed and the junctional rhythm is close to the atrial paced rhythm, isorhythmic dissociation between the atrial paced rhythm and the intrinsic junctional rhythm may occur. Various atrial overdrive pacing algorithms typically used to suppress atrial arrhythmias have been used to maintain effective atrial pacing in the setting of accelerated junctional rhythm.[1] These algorithms (atrial preference pacing (Medtronic) and dynamic atrial overdrive algorithm (St. Jude)) work by setting the pacing rate just above the sensed intrinsic rhythm.

In specific situations, access to the atrium for lead placement can be anatomically limited. The very small hearts and thin walled atria of infants and small children may only support the placement of a single ventricular lead. Alternatively, the atria of patients who have undergone a Mustand/Senning procedure for d-TGA or a Fontan operation for a single ventricle may be so scarred that adequate sensing and stimulation thresholds cannot be achieved. In these situations, ventricular pacing may have to suffice using either a VVI or VVIR mode. The downside to ventricular pacing in this situation is the lack of AV synchrony and the abnormal ventricular activation caused by the impulse originating from outside of the His-Purkinje system. VVI pacing occurs in a similar fashion to AAI pacing with the main difference that pacing and sensing occur from the ventricle.

If AV node conduction is unreliable in the setting of sinus node dysfunction, the pacemaker must provide adequate rate support as well as ventricular back up pacing in case AV conduction fails. AAI and AAIR pacing are inadequate for this situation. In a patient with only a ventricular pacing system, this can be accomplished with VVI or VVIR pacing mode. A more ideal pacing solution to such a problem is to have a dual chamber pacemaker with both an atrial and ventricular lead, which can be programmed in the DDD (pacing and sensing from both the atrium and ventricle). With DDD mode, rate support is provided by atrial pacing. With normal AV conduction, ventricular pacing is inhibited allowing for ventricular activation through the intrinsic AV node. The AV delay can be lengthened to encourage intrinsic conduction in patients with mild to moderate first degree AV block. When AV conduction fails, DDD mode allows for both atrial and ventricular pacing. DDDR can be programmed in patients with chronotropic incompetence.

AV node dysfunction

In patients with congenital heart disease, AV node dysfunction may be associated with the structural heart disease or may result as a complication of surgery. Structural defects associated with spontaneous development of heart block include L-transposition of the great arteries, AV discordance, and polysplenia with AV canal defect. Repairs where the surgeon is operating close to the AV node may result in surgical induced AV block and include ventricular septal defect closures and repair of tetralogy of Fallot.

AV block results in bradycardia and loss of AV synchrony. Ventricular pacing in VVI mode can prevent bradycardia or prolonged pauses. VVIR pacing allows for rate adaptation to exercise. Single chamber ventricular pacing for AV block is used typically in infants and small children. The downside to VVI/VVIR pacing is that it does not allow for AV synchrony.

Pacemaker syndrome is a constellation of symptoms resulting from loss of AV synchrony after pacemaker implantation. It may occur with VVI/VVIR pacing but may also occur with any pacing mode in which there is suboptimal AV synchrony. The loss of the atrial kick reduces cardiac output which can produce symptoms of elevated pulmonary venous pressure or low cardiac output. These symptoms may include dizziness, near syncope, fatigue, weakness, dyspnea, orthopnea, and mental status changes. Atrial contraction against a closed AV valve can result in pulsations in the neck or abdomen, headache, cough, or jaw pain. The contribution of atrial kick to overall cardiac output is much smaller in infants and young adults. This

may partly explain why VVI/VVIR pacing is so well tolerated in this age group.

DDD pacing for AV block provides rate support while maintaining AV synchrony. In a patient with normal sinus node function, DDD pacing mode will allow for atrial sensed and ventricular paced rhythm such that the intrinsic sinus node rate drives the ventricular pacing rate. In a patient with sinus node dysfunction, DDD mode enables atrial paced and ventricular paced rhythm or AV sequential pacing. In a patient with chronotropic incompetence, DDDR can be set to adapt the pacing rate to the patient's activity. The parameters programmed in the DDD mode include the lower pacing rate, the upper pacing rate for AV sequential pacing, the upper tracking rate for atrial sensed, ventricular pacing, and the AV delay for AV sequential pacing and atrial sensed, ventricular pacing.

Optimizing the AV delay is important for obtaining ideal hemodynamics. If the AV delay is too short, ventricular filling may be abbreviated and atrial contraction may occur against a closed AV valve. If the AV delay is too long, diastolic AV regurgitation may occur. A very prolonged AV delay may cut short ventricular filling. A sensed AV interval begins at the moment the atrial impulse is sensed. A paced AV interval begins at the moment the atrial output pulse is delivered. Typically, the sensed event occurs later than the paced pulse. To keep these two AV interval physiologically similar, the sensed AV interval is typically programmed 20–30 ms shorter than the paced AV interval.

Atrial synchronous ventricular pacemakers (VDD) can be used for patients with normal sinus node function and AV node conduction disease. In these systems, sensing occurs in both chambers with pacing only in the ventricle. Ventricular activation tracks atrial activation and is inhibited by intrinsic ventricular activity. The VDD mode is available in a single transvenous lead pacing system. The tip of the lead senses and paces the ventricle and a remote electrode situated in the atrium senses atrial activity.

Reducing unnecessary ventricular pacing

Numerous studies in adult and children with pacemakers have shown that chronic ventricular pacing reduces cardiac function. Deterioration in cardiac performance is thought to be related to the dyssy-chronous contraction that results from ventricular pacing. Several novel pacing modes and parameters have been developed to reduce unnecessary ventricular pacing. Unnecessary pacing might occur in the context of a patient with a dual chamber ICD who has normal AV conduction or in a patient with sinus node dysfunction who has a dual chamber device, when programmed to the DDD mode.

Managed Ventricular Pacing (MVP) is an atrial based pacing mode (ADI/R) with back up ventricular pacing at times of AV block. The MVP algorithm defines AV block as the loss of ventricular sensing between two out of four atrial to atrial depolarization intervals. When AV block is detected, the device switches from AAI/R to DDD/R mode. The device then checks for return of AV conduction at pre-specified time intervals. Once AV conduction resumes, the device returns to pacing in AAI/R mode. MVP has been shown to significantly reduce the percentage of ventricular pacing in adult patients.[2] MVP significantly reduces the percentage of ventricular pacing in patients with congenital heart disease with normal AV conduction.[3] Care must be used in using MVP as it may be pro-arrhythmic in certain cases.[4]

Another approach to reducing unnecessary pacing is to encourage intrinsic conduction by lengthening the AV interval. Various proprietary algorithms from different companies accomplish this task: Search AV+ (Medtronic), and AV Search Hysteresis (Boston Scientific). These algorithms function in the DDD/R mode. The paced AV and sensed AV delay are automatically increased up to a programmed maximum AV delay to allow for intrinsic AV conduction. If ventricular sensing occurs, the AV delay will remain extended. Continuous surveillance for intrinsic conduction occurs. If lost, the AV interval will shorten to preprogrammed values. These algorithms have been shown to reduce ventricular pacing in adult patients[5] but have not been rigorously evaluated in patients with congenital heart disease.

Antitachycardia pacing for atrial arrhythmias

Atrial arrhythmias are a significant source of morbidity and mortality for patients with congenital heart disease. Arrhythmias are a common complication of atrial switch for d-TGA and Fontan palliation surgeries but can also be seen following repair of tetralogy of Fallot and atrial septal defect. Typical observed atrial arrhythmias following surgical repair of congenital heart disease include atrial tachycardia and intra-atrial reentrant tachycardia (IART). IART is distinct from typical atrial flutter seen in structurally normal hearts, relying on scars and suture lines to establish the reentrant circuit. Medical therapy is often inadequate for these arrhythmias. However, atrial overdrive pacing is often successful at terminating IART.

Various antitachycardia pacing algorithms have been incorporated into pacing systems to detect and treat atrial arrhythmias. These modes have been developed to target typical atrial flutter (and to a lesser extent, atrial fibrillation) seen in adult patients. However, antitachycardia algorithms have demonstrated efficacy in treating atrial arrhythmias found in patients with congenital heart disease.[6]

The antitachycardia pacing algorithm must correctly identify and classify a treatable atrial arrhythmia from sinus tachycardias and ventricular arrhythmias. Various criteria are used to correctly detect the targeted arrhythmia. These include atrial cycle length, ratio of P to R events, rate onset, and cycle length regularity. These features can be optimized to meet the needs of individual patients. Prior history of arrhythmia characteristics from clinical experience or noninvasive or invasive programmed stimulation should be used to inform programming. Under-detection is not uncommon in patients with congenital heart disease and rapid AV node conduction due to 1-to-1 conduction of the atrial tachycardia. Currently available pacemakers cannot detect and treat 1-to-1 atrial tachycardias. Customized software can be obtained at times on a compassionate-use basis from the FDA.

Once an atrial arrhythmia is detected, the device will automatically deliver pacing therapy. Various pacing protocols are used for therapy. The ramp protocol is a decremental drive of a programmed number of pulses. The first cycle length is generally a certain percentage of the measured cycle length of the arrhythmia. Subsequent cycle lengths are reduced by a pre-specified amount. A burst protocol uses a constant cycle length for a certain number of pulses. A burst + protocol uses a constant cycle length drive train followed by two extrastimuli.

Care must be used with antitachycardia pacing. This is especially true in patients with rapid AV conduction. Sudden death has been documented when the antitachycardia pacing accelerated the tachycardia cycle length. A rapid ventricular response eventually deteriorated into ventricular tachycardia and fibrillation.

While not an antitachycardia algorithm, automatic mode switching is an algorithm developed to ameliorate the negative hemodynamic consequences of atrial tachycardia in the presence of a dual chamber pacemaker. Depending upon the atrial tachycardia rate and upper tracking rate of the device, rapid ventricular tracking of an atrial tachycardia may occur in the DDD/R mode. Mode switching algorithms detect atrial tachycardia based upon sensed atrial rate and then automatically change the pacing mode from DDD/R to DDI/DDIR to prevent rapid ventricular tracking of an atrial tachycardia. Algorithms differ in the criteria used to trigger a mode switch as well as the criteria used to revert to the baseline pacing mode.

Automatic adjustments to lead parameters

Changes in capture and sensitivity thresholds can occur due to alterations in physiology, disease conditions, and maturation of the lead/tissue interface. Enabling automatic tracking and adjustment of these parameters can improve the safety and efficiency of a device. Various algorithms can be programmed on pacemakers that automatically track and/or adjust specific lead parameters. The most commonly used algorithms affect capture threshold and sensitivity.

Automatic tracking of capture threshold (Capture Management, Medtronic; Autocapture, St. Jude Medical; Automatic Capture, Boston Scientific) requires accurate detection of the capture threshold. This is typically accomplished by detection of evoked responses following a test pace at a specific pacing amplitude. Other methods, especially to detect atrial capture threshold, may be used.[7] Once capture threshold has been determined, the algorithm automatically adjusts the

operating amplitude to a target amplitude that represents a programmable safety margin above the measured amplitude threshold. Typically, a minimum amplitude is also programmed. Various algorithms have been shown to work reliably in pediatric patients and patients with congenital heart disease.[7, 8] Importantly, these algorithms have been shown to work with both endocardial and unipolar epicardial leads. Significant energy savings may potentially be derived from the use of these algorithms.[8]

Management of the sensitivity setting (Sensing Assurance, Medtronic; Automatic Sensitivity Control, St. Jude; AutoSense, Boston Scientific) occurs by automatically increasing or decreasing the sensitivity to maintain an adequate sensing margin in response to monitoring. The device monitors nonrefractory sensed events in the atrium or ventricle and measures the peak amplitude of the P or R wave. The algorithm compares the peak amplitude to a reference (the operating sensitivity setting or the measured noise level) and adjusts the sensitivity setting accordingly (to maintain a nonprogrammable sensitivity margin or to achieve a prespecified percentage of the difference between the amplitude of sensed events and the measured noise level, respectively).

ICD programming

Implantable cardioverter defibrillators (ICDs) are highly sophisticated medical devices that regulate the heart rhythm using a combination of low energy stimulation (≤ 8 V) to prevent bradycardia and treat rapid and regular heart rhythms and a high energy shock (>200 V) to correct abnormally rapid and irregular heart rhythms. Burns et al. characterized the growing trend of ICD use in the United States in patients younger than 18 years of age, with the average age of implantation decreasing from 13.6 to 12.2 years.[9]

While designed in general to be a combination pacemaker and defibrillator, ICDs vary significantly among manufacturers in the types of cardiac arrhythmias that can be treated and the algorithms incorporated within the device software to detect and treat slow, as well as fast heart rates. While capable of most basic functions performed by a stand-alone pacemaker used to treat bradycardia or correct AV conduction disturbances within physiology heart rates, the pacemaker function of an ICD is limited in some functional elements from what was described earlier in this chapter.

On the other hand, ICDs are potent therapeutic tools to correct tachyarrhythmias. Some devices are capable of treating atrial and ventricular arrhythmias; others are limited to treating abnormal ventricular rhythms only. Treatment of ventricular tachycardia and ventricular fibrillation through ICD technology is remarkably successful and highly sensitive. ICD devices on rare occasion need to reprogrammed or surgically modified to enable *effective* energy delivery to the heart. The extent and type of available options for non-invasive programmability varies amongst devices (shock vector, wave form polarity, and waveform shape/duration). The weakest facet of ICD technology continues to be its ability to avoid inappropriate treatment of fast atrial heart rhythms, resulting in inappropriate shocks, the false positive treatment of an atrial arrhythmia. Software options that facilitate discrimination of atrial from ventricular arrhythmias are one of the programmable feature sets that differentiate device manufacturers, and further depend on whether the ICD is a single or dual chamber device.

The increasing prevalence of dilated cardiomyopathy and congestive heart failure in the population, in conjunction with the development of interest in using medical devices to treat congestive heart failure, for example biventricular pacemakers, has encouraged interest in the development of features within ICDs to monitor and alert health care providers of impending heart failure.

In the following sections of this chapter, we will detail the importance of learning and performance of meticulous ICD device programming. Programming the ICD will be divided into its fundamentals of arrhythmia detection, arrhythmia treatment and arrhythmia re-detection. We will highlight some of the limitations of the pacemaker element of the ICD, and innovations for heart failure detection.

Arrhythmia detection

ICD implantation seems to be very effective in prevention of future sudden death events in the pediatric and young age group. Subsequent to ICD implantation, appropriate ICD shocks have been reported to occur in a highly variable range (26–75%) of children and young adults,[10, 11] with most ICD shocks occurring in the first 5 years. Korte et al. noted an average time to first appropriate ICD therapy at 16 ± 18 months.[11] Seven percent of ICD implants did not receive therapy until after receiving their second ICD (average 5.5 years).[11] ICD therapy was more common in secondary prevention patients (32%) than primary prevention (18%) patients. Older patients (age greater than 18 years, 33%) are more likely to have appropriate shocks compared to children and adolescents less than 18 years old (23%).[10] No difference in the occurrence of ICD therapy was noted by Berul et al.[10] between different arrhythmia substrates (primary electrical disease, congenital heart disease, or cardiomyopathy).

Inappropriate ICD therapy is almost as common in the pediatric population as is appropriate therapy, and ranges in occurrence between 3 and 50%.[11, 12] Inappropriate therapy can be caused by supraventricular tachycardias (SVT), T wave oversensing, and ICD lead failures, with rapid atrial arrhythmias being the most prevalent culprit (15–40%).[11, 13] Little data exists comparing different strategies of ICD programming to minimize inappropriate shock in the pediatric age group. Concern for under-detection and failure to treat hemodynamically significant ventricular arrhythmias is often voiced as the justification for accepting a "high" inappropriate ICD shock rate. The PREPARE investigators tested a more aggressive arrhythmia detection algorithm in adult primary ICD recipients and were able to show a lower inappropriate ICD shock rate (9 vs 17%), and no difference in the incidence of untreated ventricular tachycardia (VT) and arrhythmic syncope compared to a control cohort.[14] VT/ventricular fibrillation detection rates were programmed ≥182 bpm for at least 30 of 40 beats. Antitachycardia pacing was programmed as the first therapy for regular ventricular rhythms with rates between 183 to 250 bpm, and SVT discriminators were used for rhythms ≤ 200 bpm. First shocks were programmed to high-output (30–35 J). In a small series of 33 "pediatric" patients, Botsch et al. reported using a concomitant approach of ICD programming along the lines of the PREPARE study and incorporating an aggressive strategy of arrhythmia treatment using ablation and anti-arrhythmic medication administration. These investigators observed one of lowest reported inappropriate ICD shock rate in the pediatric population (3%).[12]

Programming of ICDs is frequently complicated by differences in nomenclature used by different device manufacturers and differences in algorithms incorporated into the device software. Proprietary differences in arrhythmia discrimination algorithms are often protected information. Toward the goal of increasing awareness of these differences and to help the health care provider not familiar with differences amongst the varying vendors, we have endeavored to highlight these differences in Tables 13.1–13.4 (Table 13.1 = Medtronic, Table 13.2 = Boston Scientific, Table 13.3 = St. Jude, and Table 13.4 = BIOTRONIK). Less clear is whether arrhythmia discrimination software features in devices between manufactures truly result in differences in inappropriate shocks for SVT.

Some programming features differ quite dramatically, for example algorithms and programming options for handling T wave oversensing and lead "noise."

While still a matter of contention, dual chamber ICDs do not seem to decrease the incidence of inappropriate ICD shocks in children and young adults. Implantation of dual chamber devices is mainly justified for bradycardia rhythm management in those patients with AV conduction disturbances.[15]

We, along with other investigators, perform exercise testing before hospital discharge to determine the appropriate lower limit of the high rate zone for that specific individual, and look for intermittent T wave oversensing. If the treatment plan includes a beta-blocker or calcium channel blocker medication, we adjust the dosage to obtain a blunted heart rate response to exercise (70% of the max predicted heart rate) Longer detection times for arrhythmia recognition are programmed if there is no evidence for a time-dependent rapid increase in the defibrillation threshold during testing in the lab. To prevent this situation from

Table 13.1 *Medtronic ICD – key programmable features*

(1) Arrhythmia Detection:

Single Chamber Device:

- Ventricular rate is given highest priority

NID (Detection counter, number of intervals to detect)

Fixed number of intervals for ventricular tachycardia detection

Probabilistic % (75%) for ventricular fibrillation

Algorithms for SVT – VT Discrimination

- Electrogram Morphology (Wavelet): Can be programmed to on/off/monitor.

Can program % wavelet match and vector for morphology comparison (far field: can to RV coil or SVC coil to RV coil)

Template morphology can be programmed to update (on, off, monitor)

- Rate Onset (% difference): on/off/monitor

- Rate Stability (ms): on/off.

(If one of the discriminators suggests the arrhythmia is SVT, device will withhold Rx)

SVT limit (Can program to what cycle length the device with attempt to discriminate SVT from VT): 240 ms

Dual Chamber Device:

Algorithms for SVT – VT Discrimination

PR Logic is the SVT Discriminator used, can be programmed on/off

AF/AFL: on/off

Sinus tach: on/off

Other 1:1 SVTs (junctional or AVNRT): on/off

(continued)

Table 13.1 *(Continued)*

Programmable Features:
Detection Rate: programmable up to 3 zones
Wavelet: on/off/monitor
Onset: on/off/monitor
Stability: ms, on/off

SVT Discrimination Timer:
VF Time Out: Program time interval between 15–300 s, off
General Time Out (for VT): 30 s to 30 min, off
If after time-out limit is reach, the device will deliver zone appropriate therapy

Detection of Lead Problems:
Lead Impedance Monitoring: can be programmed low limit (200–500 Ω) and upper limits (1000–3000 Ω);
High voltage impedance: can program low limit (20–50 Ω) and upper limits (100–200 Ω)
Lead Integrity Alert: on/off
RV Lead Noise Discriminator Alert: On/off
RV Lead noise off/on + programmable time out.
T wave Oversensing: on/off

Arrhythmia Zones: max = 3 ventricular arrhythmia zones, and 2 atrial arrhythmia zones

(2) Arrhythmia Treatment:
Ventricular Arrhythmia Treatment:
-ATP: Burst, Ramp, Burst+
Smart Mode: on/off. Will program ATP off if unsuccessful after 4 consecutive attempts
ChargeSaver: on/off. Monitors ATP performance and will switch to ATP before charge if successful on a pro-
    grammable number of intervals.

-Shock
Programmable Shock Features: polarity, vector, waveform characteristics
Number of Programmable Shocks: 6 shocks, program polarity – reverse, standard
Shock Pathways (RV to Can, RV to Can+SVC, RV +SVC to can). Can program can or SVC off.
Programming of Waveform: NA

Max Energy Stored: 39 J
Max Energy Delivered: 35 J

Atrial Arrhythmia Treatment:
ATP: A-Burst +, A-Ramp
50 Hz:
Cardioversion: auto/patient activated

Confirmation +: on/off
Charge can be aborted when initial detection criteria no longer met (60 ms less than detection interval)

Capacity Reformation: auto, # of desired months

(3) Arrhythmia Re-Detection:
Programmable features:
SVT Discriminator – not used
Stability – used, if on
T wave oversensing - used if on
NID: programmable, not greater than initial detection NID

Table 13.1 *(Continued)*

(4) Heart Failure Detection:
Optivol: always on
Optivol CareAlert (via Carelink) is programmable on/off
Impedance monitoring: Programmable reference line (reset), and threshold
SDNN variable
Heart rate – night/daytime HR
Patient activity

(5) Pacemaker Features:
Lower Rate: max lower rate = 150 bpm
Upper Rate: max upper rate = 175 bpm
Rate Response: accelerometer.
Max Sensor Rate: 175 bpm
Sleep Rate: available, program time of onset/offset
Scan for Intrinsic Rate: Rate hysteresis for single chamber pacing. Can program rate
AV intervals: rate responsive AV delay. Program start/stop rate, minimum, and paced AV interval
Features to limit ventricular pacing:
MVP: on/off
AV interval search: NA
Voltage Output: max output of 8.0 V at 1.5 ms
Ventricular capture management in ventricle with single or dual chamber devices.
Atrial capture management
Program frequency of capture management: every 24 h
Programmability in Sensing:
Atrial Refractory Periods: partial, partial +, absolute blanking
RV sensing: bipolar/integrated bipolar
Atrial and ventricular sensitivity:
Atrium 0.15–4.0 mV
Ventricular: 0.15–1.2 mV
PMT: On/off
PVARP: (125–500 ms), auto
PVARP after PVC (PVARP = 400 ms), off
Competitive atrial pacing: on/off, programmable atrial pacing extension interval
Safety Pacing (110 ms); on/off
Post shock pause: can program separate atrial and ventricular outputs, pacing rate, and overdrive duration
Specialized atrial pacing algorithms:
    Atrial preference pacing
    Atrial rate stabilization
    Post atrial mode switch overdrive pacing
High Atrial Rate Detection: rate 133–400 bpm. More As than Vs
Atrial Mode Switch: non-programmable # of atrial intervals prior to mode switch. Can program atrial rate for
    mode switch

being a clinical issue, we usually program energy delivery to maximum device output. To prevent T wave oversensing, we commonly program higher ventricular sensitivities. For patients with rapid polymorphic VT, two detection zones are programmed: (1) for heart rates ≥ 220 bpm and (2) a VT monitor zone to observe for previously unknown slower VTs.

Arrhythmia treatment

Programming of ICD therapy must balance the need to treat "malignant" ventricular arrhythmias

Table 13.2 *Boston Scientific ICD – key programmable features*

(1) Arrhythmia Detection:

Single Chamber Device:

Available zones: 1–3.

VF zone cannot be programmed above 220 if single zone is selected.

Detection: Arrhythmia is declared when rate threshold is exceeded for 8/10 intervals, which is a fixed parameter. BSC does not program NID but rather adds DURATION parameter.

Duration-interval count starts once event is declared, i.e., 8/10 fast intervals has occurred. The rate must remain above the rate cutoff for a running 6/10 intervals. If less than 6 intervals are fast, the event is considered terminated and initial detection must again be met.

Initial Detection:

VT-1 zone (three zone configuration); 1–60 s

VT zone (two or three zone configuration); 1–30 s

VF zone (one, two, or three zone configuration); 1–15 s

SVT vs VT Discriminators:

Rhythm ID: template matching algorithm that requires 94% correlation to sinus template. This template will update automatically every 2 h, off.

The device can be programmed to periodically decrease Lower Rate Limit (LRL) in an attempt to acquire an updated template.

Onset: can be used to discriminate sinus tachycardia.

Stability: can be used to discriminate atrial fibrillation

Onset and Stability can be used together, in which case, both must agree, or independently.

All 3 discriminators have a Sustained Rate Duration parameter that will override the discriminators if rate remains above cutoff for a programmable time, nominally 3 minutes.

These discriminators are available for both VT-1 and VT zone or just for VT-1 zone, i.e., only applicable for a selected rate range.

Dual Chamber Device:

Available zones: 1–3

SVT vs. VT Discriminators:

Rhythm ID: template matching algorithm that requires 94% correlation to sinus template.

Atrial Tachyarrhythmia Discriminator looks to see if V rate is greater than A rate: on, off.

Atrial Fibrillation Rate Threshold: on, off; program detect rate

If Rhythm template does not match stored template, the device then looks at:

Stability: +

Onset: +

Onset and Stability: +

Sustained Rate Duration: on/off, nominally "ON" at 3 min (10 s – 60 min)

Detection of Lead Problems:

Lead Impedance Monitoring: alert through Latitude only, not programmable.

Lower limit (<200 Ω) and upper limits (2000 Ω);

High voltage impedance: program low limit (<20 Ω) and upper limits (125 Ω)

RV Lead noise: NA

T wave Oversensing: NA.

(2) Arrhythmia Treatment:

- ATP: There are two independently programmable ATP schemes available in each VT zone, i.e., a three-zone device with VT-1 zone and VT zone will allow four different ATP schemes. Parameters include: Bursts, Pulses per Burst, Incremental Additional Pulses per Burst, Coupling Interval, Burst Interval, Ramp Decrement, Scan Decrement, and Minimum Interval.

ATP in the VF zone (Quick Convert) is nominally on. It will attempt one burst for any VF detected with a rate of less than 250 bpm. Device does not charge unless burst is unsuccessful.

Table 13.2 (*Continued*)

- Shock Therapy

High voltage therapy is an option in the lowest zone of any two- or three-zone configuration, i.e., device may be programmed to deliver ATP only.

Shocks Delivered: 5 in lowest zone of three-zone configuration, VT-1 zone

6 in lowest zone of two-zone configuration, VT zone

8 in VF zone

Energy programmable: 0.1 to 41.0 J stored

Shock Waveform: Non-programmable. Biphasic, Fixed Tilt, 60% first phase, 50% second phase

Vectors: RV to Can/SVC, RV to SVC, RV to Can.

Polarity reversible in all vectors

Shock Polarity Reversal-is automatic in last programmed shock in any zone.

Atrial Therapies: NA.

Capacitor Maintenance: non-programmable, every 90 days until 6 months remaining on battery, then every 30 days.

(3) Arrhythmia *Redetection*:

Redetection Duration-applied after therapy is delivered (ATP), or if shock is diverted during charge

VT-1 zone; 1–15 s

VT zone; 1–15 s

VF zone; fixed at 1 s

Post Shock Duration-applied after shock is delivered

VT-1 zone; 1–60 s

VT zone; 1–30 s

VF zone; fixed at 1 s

For Post Shock Detection, the algorithm uses Stability only since morphology will be altered by shock.

(4) *Heart Failure Detection*:

SDNN variable – new devices

Heart rate – night/daytime HR

Patient activity

Blue tooth enabled – BP and weight

(5) *Pacemaker Features*:

Modes: off, AAI, VVI, VDD, DDI, DDD plus rate response for all

Rate Range:

LRL: 30–185

MTR: 185

MSR: 185

Rate response: Accelerometer based

Rate Enhancements:

Rate Hysteresis: available with or without Search, not available in Rate Response Modes

Rate Hysteresis Search Frequency-programmable in number of intervals, 256–4096, device will pace at hysteresis rate for 8 cycles to encourage intrinsic rhythm

Rate Smoothing Up: maximum percentage decrease beat-to-beat in ventricular rate during atrial tracking, 3–25%

Rate Smoothing Down: maximum interval-to-interval lengthening, 3–25%

Ventricular Rate Regulation: Low, Medium or High provides elevated rates keyed off of intrinsic activity to regulate RVR in ICD device

(*continued*)

Table 13.2 (*Continued*)

Blanking:

A Blank after V-Pace

A Blank after V-Sense

RV Blank after A-Pace

PVARP After PVC – 0–500 ms

AV Delay
 Dynamic or Fixed, Program minimum and maximum

   Paced and Sensed AV delays are independently programmable

AV Delay Range

Paced AV: 30–400 for ICD

Sensed AV: 65–400 ms for ICD

AV Search Hysteresis:

Extend AV up to maximum 400 ms during search

Search Frequency is programmable – 32–1024 intervals

Search Duration is fixed, eight cycles at extended value before returning to programmed AV

Rhythmiq: AAI with VVI backup at 15 beats below programmed LRL, mode switch to DDD if conduction block
 detected

Pacing Outputs:

Voltage
 Atrium: 0.1–5.0 V

  Right Ventricle: 0.1–7.5 V

Pulse Width – 0.05–2.00 ms, all chambers

Sensing
 Atrium and Right Ventricle, 0.15–1.5 mV

Refractory
 Dynamic or Fixed for RA and RV, range 150–500 ms

ATR (Atrial Tachy Respons – Mode Switch) Parameters

 Trigger Rate – 100–300

 Entry Count – # of atrial events of trigger rate, 1–8

 Duration – # of ventricular events that must occur once entry count is met

 Exit Count – # of slow intervals required before return to tracking, 1–8

 Fallback Mode – VDI, DDI, VDIR, DDIR

 ATR Lower Rate-independently programmable for device lower rate, it may be set less than programmed
  lower rate limit of device

 Fallback Time – 0 s – 2 min, this is time device will use to linearly reduce rate from max achieved prior to ATR,
  to the programmed ATR rate

Atrial Flutter Response – 100–300 ms.

PMT Termination – on, off

Post Shock Pacing Therapy – Outputs and Lower Rate are independent from permanent values and can be
 applied for 15–60 post shock period.

to prevent syncope or sudden cardiac arrest; and avoid ICD shocks that may result in morbidity (pain, adverse psychological sequelae and heart failure following multiple ICD shocks).[16] Recent studies have suggested that many VT episodes may self-terminate prior to therapy delivery if allowed enough time to spontaneously end. Inherent in ICD programming, as traditionally practiced, are two assumptions: (1) the physician knows the best treatment strategy and (2) patient-specific customization of ICD programming will result in the most optimal outcome. The EMPIRIC trial performed in adult ICD recipients compared empiric ICD programming (specific algorithm) with physician-tailored programming options in a group of adult subjects with a mix of primary and secondary indications for ICD implantation.[17] Using Empiric ICD programming, time to first shock was non-inferior. No significant differences were noted in total mortality, or syncope between

Table 13.3 *St. Jude ICD – key programmable features*

---

(1) Arrhythmia Detection:

Single Chamber Device:

Ventricular Rate: given highest priority

Algorithms for SVT – VT Discrimination

Discriminator (on/off/passive)

- Electrogram Morphology: + template

Can program % match with template, in addition to programming the ratio of matches needed. Template morphology can be programmed to update automatically (8 h, 1, 3, 7, 14, 30 days, on demand in clinic, off)

- Rate Onset: + (ms or % difference) on/off/passive*

Rate Stability: on, on with SIH, off. Sinus interval history counter (SIH) – programmable count of sinus beats (1–8), on/off/passive. Used to discriminate atrial fibrillation with rapid AV conduction from VT

Program number of criteria need to be meet for therapy: 1/1, 1/2, 2/2, 1/3, 2/3, 3/3

NID: Detection counters – NID only. Fixed number of intervals for VT and VF

*On: Discriminator will make diagnosis, and diagnosis will affect therapy delivery

Passive: Discriminator will make diagnosis, but diagnosis will not affect therapy delivery. (When viewing an episode, Passive discriminators will report their diagnosis.)

Off: Discriminator will not make diagnosis.

Dual Chamber Device:

Algorithms for SVT – VT Discrimination

Arrhythmia Logic:

Rate: +

Rate Branch: On/off

Morphology: +

Stability: +

Onset: +

Rate Branch: V < A, V = A, V > A

Programmed: on/off. Off- ventricular only.

- If V > A = treatment

- If V = A:

Assess changes in AV interval relationship;

AV interval delta: on or off. Programmable: on/off, 30–150 ms

If AV interval delta > TH, device will give VT therapy (Looks at second longest and shortest intervals)

Onset and/or morphology

1/1, 1/2, or 2/2

- If A>V:

–Stability: on, on with AVA, off. AV Association Delta: Programmable: on/off, 30–150 ms

- Morphology: +

1/1, 1/2, 2/2

SVT Discriminator Time Out: Programmable time interval between 20 s to 60 min, off

Atrial Rate Detection: rate 110–300 bpm.

Needs to be at least 20 bpm > max track rate

Atrial Mode Switch: (Filtered Atrial Rate Interval, FARI), non-programmable

Atrial Flutter Search: NA

(continued)

Table 13.3 *(Continued)*

Features for Detection of Lead Problems:

Lead Monitoring impedance: Can be programmed to lower limit (100–500 Ω) or

(750 - > 3000 Ω)

High voltage impedance: can be programmed to lower limit (20–80 Ω) and upper limit (40–125 Ω)

Lead Integrity Alert: NA

RV Lead Noise Discriminator Alert: NA

RV Lead noise: NA

T wave Over-Sensing: T wave attention filter: on/off

(2) Arrhythmia Treatment

- ATP: Burst, Ramp, Burst +. For ventricular rates in the VF zone – 1 ATP prior to or during charging

VT Time out for all VT therapies (takes therapy to VF zone): 10–300 s, or off. Can program either for use with VT 1 and VT 2 zones or just VT 2 zone.

- Shock

Programmable Shock Features: polarity, vector, waveform characteristics

Number of Programmable Shocks: 6

Shock polarity – reverse, or standard

Shock Pathways (RV to Can, RV to Can + SVC). Can cannot be programmed off.

Waveform:

Fixed Tilt: 42/50/60/65%

Fixed pulse width: Pulse 1: 3–12 ms, Pulse 2:1.2–12 ms (Pulse 2 cannot be longer than Pulse 1.)

Monophasic/biphasic waveforms

PC Shock – ICD shock on command (0.1–40 J)

Max Energy Stored: 40.5, 45 stored (second shock)

Max Energy Delivered: 36 J, 40 J (second shock)

Max number of Ventricular Arrhythmia Zones: 3 zones

Atrial Arrhythmia Zones: Device counts number of mode switch events above Atrial Tachycardia Detection Rate (ATDR). Cannot program separate rate bins

Treatment of Atrial Arrhythmias: NA

ATP: NA

50 Hz: NA

Cardioversion: NA

Confirmation: always on

Charge can be aborted when device has detected return to sinus

Treatment Success:

5 (default): Number of sinus totals not interrupted by tachycardia intervals (VT or VF). Can program to 3, 5, 7 intervals.

Capacity Reformation: 4, 5, 6 months

(3) Arrhythmia Re-Detection

Programmable features:

SVT Discriminator – not used

Rate: Programmable

NID: 6–20 intervals. Not greater than initial detection

VT Zone: Boundaries can be modified within an episode

Table 13.3 (*Continued*)

---

(4) Heart Failure Detection
Heart rate
Patient activity %

(5) Pacemaker Features
Lower Rate: max 100
Upper Rate: max 150
Rate Response: accelerometer.
Max Sensor Rate: 150 bpm
Sleep Rate: +, based or activity
Scan for Intrinsic Rate: Yes
AV intervals: Customizable slope (low, medium, high) of PR interval shortening as HR increases. Can programmable floor of how short PR interval can become.
Features to limit ventricular pacing:
Ventricular Intrinsic Preference
VIP Extension: AV interval Delay max AV delay of 450 ms.
Search Interval: 30 s – 30 min
Search Cycles: 1–3 beats
Voltage Output: Auto-capture in ventricular with single or dual chamber device.
Atrial capture – ACapConfirm
Program frequency of looking: 8/24 h
Max 7.5 V at 1.5 ms
Sensing: SenseAbility
Threshold: 50, 62.5, 75%
Decay Delay: 0, 30, 60, 95, 125, 160, 190, and 220 ms
Sensing Refractory Periods: 125, 157 ms
Sensing can be changed differently for post-paced and post-sensed intervals (threshold start and decay delay)
Atrial and ventricular sensitivity:
Atrium 0.2–1.0 mV
Ventricular: 0.3–2.0 mV
Atrial and ventricular sensitivity for bradycardia pacing can be programmed separate from defibrillator sensitivity, but not lower
PMT: on/off
PVARP: 125–500 ms
PVARP after PVC: PVARP = 450 ms
Atrial Upper Rate: No competitive atrial pacing feature
Safety Pacing: 120 ms
Post shock pause: 1–7 s
Post shock pacing mode: +
Duration of post shock pacing mode: +
Separate Programmability atrial and ventricular output post shock: +

---

the two treatment arms, thereby suggesting that a more "generic" approach may be just as effective as a customized ICD treatment programming approach. Whether this data is applicable in the pediatric and young adult age ICD group has not yet been studied.

PainFREE RX and PainFREE Rx II were two multicenter clinical trials in adult ICD subjects testing the safety and utility of ATP treatment of VT at different rates. ATP successfully treated 72% of VTs with CL $\geq$ 260 ms.[18, 19] ATP was less successful for VT with a cycle length $\leq$ 240 ms.

Table 13.4 *BIOTRONIK ICD – key programmable features*

(1) Arrhythmia Detection:

Single Chamber Device:

Ventricular rate is given highest priority

SVT vs VT Discrimination:

- Electrogram Morphology: NA
- Rate Onset: +
- Rate Stability: +

VT Detection counters- the number of intervals required to declare VT

VT1 = 10–60

VT2 = 10–40

VF Detection- Can program minimal and maximum number of intervals to detect. The X/Y intervals for VF detection, if X out of the most recent Y intervals fall within the VF zone, then VF detection is declared.

X = 6–30

Y = 8–31

Dual Chamber Device

Differentiation of Atrial vs. Ventricular Arrhythmias - SMART Algorithm

Stability: off, 8–48%

Multiplicity: if average ventricular rate is found to be a multiple of average atrial rate

AV trend

Rate

PR regularity: is half of whatever the stability criterion is programmed to

OnseT: off, 4–20%

VT Time Out: Program time interval between 30 s and 30 min. Redetection occurs w/ no detection enhancements (i.e., rate only). The therapy supplied will be that programmed in the zone redetection occurs in.

Forced Termination (if SMART algorithm programmed on): 1–15 min, off. Forces the device to declare the episode as terminated and restart detection algorithm.

Detection of Lead Problems:

Monitor lead impedance: programmable lower limit (<200–) Ω or upper limit (- > 2000 Ω).

Mobile Cellular Home Monitoring System: Lead Impedance, Sensing alerts and Episode information with alert triggered EGMs can be remotely followed

Lead Integrity Alert: NA

RV Lead Noise Discriminator Alert: NA

RV Lead noise: NA.

T wave Oversensing: offer Enhance T-wave Suppression sensitivity setting

(2) Arrhythmia Treatment:

- ATP (Delivered at max output): Burst, Ramp, Burst + PES, ATP One Shot (ATP in VF zone)

ATP: rule of rate stability. If RR variability > 12%, skips ATP, and goes directly to shock Rx if rate is in the VF zone

ATP Optimization: on/off

ATP Time Out: off, 15–300 s.

- Shock

Programmable Shock Features: polarity, vector, waveform characteristics

Number of Programmable Shocks: 8 shocks per zone (VT-1, VT-2, and VF) - the first 2 are programmable, the only programmability of the last N shocks is how many you want delivered.

Table 13.4 *(Continued)*

Shock polarity: reverse, standard, alternating

Lumax 540: Shock Pathways: RV to Can, RV to SVC, RV to Can + SVC.

Lumax 340 is always RV to SVC + Can

Shock Waveforms: 2 options – standard biphasic (60/50 tilt) and biphasic 2 (Phase 1 has a tilt of 60% and 2nd Phase is truncated to 2 ms)

Lumax 540 and 340: Max energy stored: 40 J. Max energy delivered: 35 J

Lumax 300: Max energy stored 30 J

Ventricular Arrhythmia Zones: Max number of zones – 3 (VT1, VT2, VF). Without programmed therapies in VT1, VT1 becomes a functional monitoring zone

Atrial Arrhythmia Zones for Detection Only: Max number of zones 2 (SVT, AT/AF zone)

Treatment of Atrial Arrhythmias:

ATP: NA

50 Hz: NA

Cardioversion: Can be done in clinic via manual shock

Confirmation: on/off. Charge can be aborted when 3 out of the last 4 ventricular intervals are "slow" (either Vp, sensed outside of a detection zone, or fall in a VT1 monitoring zone) Charge can be aborted when initial detection criteria are no longer met.

Capacity reformation: Quarterly automatic reformation and cap reform can be manually executed as well.

(3) Arrhythmia Re-Detection:

Programmable features:

Smart Detection: on/off

VT Detection counters: the number of intervals required to declare VT can be programmed differently from initial detect criteria

VT1 = 10–30

VT2 = 10–30

Rate of each zone is non-programmable and equal to initial rate of zone

VF redetection criteria = same as initial detection X out of Y interval values

(4) Heart Failure Detection

Heart rate

SDNN

Patient activity %

(5) Pacemaker Features

Lower Rate: 30–160/min

Upper Rate: 90–160/min

Max Sensor Rate: 160 bpm

Rate Response: accelerometer. No CLS available yet.

Sleep Rate: rate, program time onset and offset

Rate Hysteresis: off, programmed rate, repetitive and scan

AV intervals: Customizable slope (low, medium, high) of PR interval shortening as HR increases

Features to limit ventricular pacing: **Intrinsic Optimization**, a specialized form of the AV Hysteresis feature, to maximize AV conduction, up to 400 ms. Can program AV hysteresis AVD out to 450 ms.

Voltage Output: 0.2–7.5 V. Can monitor capture TH in the RV. No capture control in Lumax.

Sensing: Automatic Sensitivity Control (ASC) Two stage step down algorithm with flexible programmability: floor of minimum sensitivity, upper sensitivity, duration of upper sensitivity, lower sensitivity and band pass filters and rectification.

(continued)

Table 13.4 *(Continued)*

Filter Settings: Can change band pass filters (20–40 Hz) and rectification (positive, negative or automatic)

There are three programmable options for Right Ventricle Sensitivity Settings: Standard, Enhanced T wave suppression, Enhanced VF sensitivity

Atrial and ventricular minimum sensitivity:

Atrium: 0.2–2.0 mV

Ventricular: 0.5–2.5 mV

PMT: on/off. VA Criteria: 250–500 ms

PVARP: auto, 175–600 ms

PVARP after PVC: PVARP + 225 ms

Far-field Protection Parameters: after Ventricular pacing (50–225 ms) or Ventricular sensing (25–225 ms)

Atrial Upper Rate: (240 bpm) – limits pacing after AR sensed event

Safety Pacing: 100 ms

Atrial Rate Detection: rate 100–250 bpm

Atrial Mode Switch: separate programmable activation and deactivation – X out of 8 intervals.

Can program pacing mode, rate, post mode switch rate and duration, rate smoothing (change of rate)

Post shock: can program pacing mode, pacing rate and duration, AV delay, and rate hysteresis

The incidence of acceleration of VT was low, and occurred at a similar frequency in the ATP group (1%) and the ICD shock arm (2%). The limited data available for the pediatric age group has suggested that ATP in this age / disease group may have limited efficacy (only in the range of 4–5%).[11, 20] ATP is less effective for polymorphic ventricular tachycardia, which more commonly occurs in the disease substrates dealt with in the pediatric age group. Most investigators will program a VT monitor zone to observe slower monomorphic VTs that are more amenable to ATP therapy. ATP can be pro-arrhythmic in the setting of sinus tachycardia or SVT, and should be avoided if the patient has only exhibited polymorphic VT or VF in the past.

Arrhythmia re-detection

Following therapy delivery (ATP or shock), the ICD device reassesses whether the targeted arrhythmia has been successfully treated (either returned to sinus rhythm or to bradycardia requiring bradycardia pacing support); persisted, or transitioned to another arrhythmia, therefore requiring continued tachycardia intervention. Each manufacturer's device provides limited programming options to allow the use of the SVT discriminator algorithm during redetection (total or subcomponents of the algorithm), define new rate boundaries for the VT and VF zones and number of interval required

for detection (NID). The programmable options offered vary amongst the different manufacturer's ICD devices (see Tables 13.1–13.4 – Re-detection).

Heart failure detection

In addition to providing therapy for tachy- and bradyarrhythmias, most ICD devices provide for patient diagnostic monitoring. The chronically monitored diagnostic parameters vary amongst different manufacturers and their various ICD devices but generally include heart rate (both daytime and nighttime), heart rate variability (time dependent parameters of heart rate), patient daily activity, and atrial and ventricular tachyarrhythmia frequency and duration (see Tables 13.1–13.4, Heart Failure Detection).

Changing trends in these parameters can provide indirect evidence for improving cardiovascular health or, on the contrary, deterioration in the patient's health status and possible congestive heart failure. However, measurement of intrathoracic impedance more directly indicates changes in lung water content, which can be more specifically associated with increasing pulmonary edema and the development of congestive heart failure. Currently, Medtronic ICDs have the capability to trend daily impedance measurements, and compare the daily impedance measurement with a running daily "reference" impedance that represents the expected trend in the daily impedance for the subject that day. Differences between the reference impedance and the measured daily impedance can be tracked to create the OptiVol fluid index. The OptiVol fluid index contains two pieces of information: (1) the magnitude of the impedance difference (reduction) with regard to the reference impedance (measured in ohms) and (2) the sustainability of that reduction (measured in days). An OptiVol threshold can be programmed to indicate a level that might be of potential clinical significance for that patient. This threshold is nominally programmed to 60 Ω-days, but can be adjusted between 30 and 180 Ω-days based on the fluid tolerance level that the clinician determines is best for that patient. Multiple other factors can alter intrathoracic impedance measurements resulting in false positive OptiVol threshold crossings. These factors include intrathoracic processes such as pneumonia or pleural effusion, changes in air volume in the lung such as occurs with obstructive pulmonary disease, and total body fluid accumulation, such as occurs in patients on dialysis, pre-menstruating female patients, or dietary and pharmacologic nonadherence.

Monitoring of intrathoracic impedance has been shown to be of clinical use in older adult subjects, with a sensitivity in the high 70% range.[21] Little to no data regarding the utility of this parameter in children and adolescent is currently published.

Pacemaker function

The functionality of the pacemaker component of most ICD devices has some limitations in comparison to high-end dedicated pacemaker models manufactured by the same company, for example a lower upper tracking rates in the DDD pacing mode, lower atrial/ventricular pacing outputs, reduced functionality of capture threshold management, and limited programmability of individual chamber-specific sensitivity (see Tables 13.1–13.4 – Pacemaker Function). Despite these minor limitations, the pacemaker element is very clinically useful. For guidance in programming the pacemaker component of the ICD, the reader will be referred to earlier sections of this chapter.

References

1 Orem RC, Ahmad S, Siudyla P. A novel approach to the management of symptomatic junctional and ectopic atrial rhythms. *J Interv Card Electrophysiol.* 2003; 9(3): 353–356.

2 Sweeney MO, Ellenbogen KA, Casavant D, Betzold R, Sheldon T, Tang F, et al. Multicenter, prospective, randomized safety and efficacy study of a new atrial-based managed ventricular pacing mode (MVP) in dual chamber ICDs. *J Cardiovasc Electrophysiol.* 2005; 16(8): 811–817.

3 Kaltman JR, Ro PS, Zimmerman F, Moak JP, Epstein M, Zeltser IJ, et al. Managed ventricular pacing in pediatric patients and patients with congenital heart disease. *Am J Cardiol.* 2008; 102(7): 875–878.

4 Gow RM, Snider K, Chiu-Man C. Atrial fibrillation in a LQTS patient with an ICD programmed for managed ventricular pacing: what is the cause? *Pacing Clin Electrophysiol.* 2012 Mar; 35(3): 357–359.

5 Olshansky B, Day J, McGuire M, Hahn S, Brown S, Lerew DR. Reduction of right ventricular pacing in patients with dual-chamber ICDs. *Pacing Clin Electrophysiol.* 2006; 29(3): 237–243.

6 Stephenson EA, Casavant D, Tuzi J, Alexander ME, Law I, Serwer G, et al. Efficacy of atrial antitachycardia pacing using the Medtronic AT500 pacemaker in patients with congenital heart disease. *Am J Cardiol.* 2003; 92(7): 871–876.

7 Hiippala A, Serwer GA, Clausson E, Davenport L, Brand T, Happonen JM. Automatic atrial threshold measurement and adjustment in pediatric patients. *Pacing Clin Electrophysiol.* 2010; 33(3): 309–313.

8 Cohen MI, Buck K, Tanel RE, Vetter VL, Rhodes LA, Cox J, et al. Capture management efficacy in children and young adults with endocardial and unipolar epicardial systems. *Europace.* 2004; 6(3): 248–255.

9 Burns KM, Evans F, Kaltman JR. Pediatric ICD utilization in the United States from 1997 to 2006. *Heart Rhythm.* 2011; 8(1): 23–28.

10 Berul CI, Van Hare GF, Kertesz NJ, Dubin AM, Cecchin F, Collins KK, et al. Results of a multicenter retrospective implantable cardioverter-defibrillator registry of pediatric and congenital heart disease patients. *J Am Coll Cardiol.* 2008; 51(17): 1685–1691.

11 Korte T, Koditz H, Niehaus M, Paul T, Tebbenjohanns J. High incidence of appropriate and inappropriate ICD therapies in children and adolescents with implantable cardioverter defibrillator. *Pacing Clin Electrophysiol.* 2004; 27(7): 924–932.

12 Botsch MP, Franzbach B, Opgen-Rhein B, Berger F, Will JC. ICD therapy in children and young adults: low incidence of inappropriate shock delivery. *Pacing Clin Electrophysiol.* 2010; 33(6): 734–741.

13 Love BA, Barrett KS, Alexander ME, Bevilacqua LM, Epstein MR, Triedman JK, et al. Supraventricular arrhythmias in children and young adults with implantable cardioverter defibrillators. *J Cardiovasc Electrophysiol.* 2001; 12(10): 1097–1101.

14 Wilkoff BL, Williamson BD, Stern RS, Moore SL, Lu F, Lee SW, et al. Strategic programming of detection and therapy parameters in implantable cardioverter-defibrillators reduces shocks in primary prevention patients: results from the PREPARE (Primary Prevention Parameters Evaluation) study. *J Am Coll Cardiol.* 2008; 52(7): 541–550.

15 Lawrence D, Von Bergen N, Law IH, Bradley DJ, Dick M, 2nd,, Frias PA, et al. Inappropriate ICD discharges in single-chamber versus dual-chamber devices in the pediatric and young adult population. *J Cardiovasc Electrophysiol.* 2009; 20(3): 287–290.

16 Larsen GK, Evans J, Lambert WE, Chen Y, Raitt M. Shocks burden and increased mortality in implantable cardioverter-defibrillator patients. *Heart Rhythm* 2011 Dec; 8(12): 1881–1886.

17 Wilkoff BL, Ousdigian KT, Sterns LD, Wang ZJ, Wilson RD, Morgan JM. A comparison of empiric to physician-tailored programming of implantable cardioverter-defibrillators: results from the prospective randomized multicenter EMPIRIC trial. *J Am Coll Cardiol.* 2006; 48(2): 330–339.

18 Wathen MS, Sweeney MO, DeGroot PJ, Stark AJ, Koehler JL, Chisner MB, et al. Shock reduction using antitachycardia pacing for spontaneous rapid ventricular tachycardia in patients with coronary artery disease. *Circulation.* 2001; 104(7): 796–801.

19 Wathen MS, DeGroot PJ, Sweeney MO, Stark AJ, Otterness MF, Adkisson WO, et al. Prospective randomized multicenter trial of empirical antitachycardia pacing versus shocks for spontaneous rapid ventricular tachycardia in patients with implantable cardioverter-defibrillators: Pacing Fast Ventricular Tachycardia Reduces Shock Therapies (PainFREE Rx II) trial results. *Circulation.* 2004; 110(17): 2591–2596.

20 Lewandowski M, Sterlinski M, Maciag A, Syska P, Kowalik I, Szwed H, et al. Long-term follow-up of children and young adults treated with implantable cardioverter-defibrillator: the authors' own experience with optimal implantable cardioverter-defibrillator programming. *Europace.* 2013; 12(9): 1245–1250.

21 Sarkar S, Hettrick DA, Koehler J, Rogers T, Grinberg Y, Yu CM, et al. Improved algorithm to detect fluid accumulation via intrathoracic impedance monitoring in heart failure patients with implantable devices. *J Card Fail.* 2011; 17(7): 569–576.

CHAPTER 14

Pacemaker troubleshooting and follow-up

Ronn E. Tanel[1] and Frank Zimmerman[2]

[1]Director, Pediatric and Congenital Arrhythmia Service, University of California-San Francisco Benioff Children's Hospital, Professor of Clinical Pediatrics, University of California-San F School of Medicine, San Francisco, CA, USA

[2]Co-Director, Pediatric Electrophysiology Service, Advocate Children's Hospital, Clinical Associate Professor, University of Chicago, Oak Lawn, IL, USA

Chronic follow-up of the pediatric pacemaker patient requires attention to both the common problems that occur in any paced patient and the unique issues specific to the pediatric population. The purpose of this chapter is to identify those issues and describe their relevance to young pacemaker patients, as well as pacemaker patients of all ages who have had surgery for congenital heart disease.

Pacemaker programming for unique conditions

Not only do children and adolescents require special consideration with regard to programming of the permanent pacemaker, but specific diagnoses often require attention to certain programmable parameters.

Long QT syndrome

Long QT syndrome (LQTS) is a genetic condition that results in abnormal cardiac repolarization and a prolonged QT interval on the surface electrocardiogram. The abnormality of repolarization is associated with ventricular arrhythmias, specifically torsades de pointes. The ventricular arrhythmias may cause syncope, seizures, and sudden death. There is also an increased incidence of bradycardia in patients with long QT syndrome, and bradycardia has been shown to be an independent risk factor for sudden death, aborted sudden death, and syncope.[1] This is partly due to the pause-dependent nature of ventricular arrhythmias in some patients with LQTS. The prevention of bradycardia, specifically significant sinus pauses, has been described as helping to prevent the associated ventricular arrhythmias.[2] A specific programmed lower rate limit that provides significant benefit has not been validated, but rates faster than those programmed for other children and adolescents of the same age appear to be appropriate.

The mainstay of medical therapy for children and adolescents with LQTS continues to be chronic beta blocker therapy. Of course, beta blocker therapy alone may result in significantly lower heart rates in the pediatric patient, and medication-induced bradycardia may be so severe that a permanent pacemaker may be necessary to prevent symptoms. In general, permanent pacemaker implantation is indicated in patients with LQTS and pause-dependent QT prolongation

Cardiac Pacing and Defibrillation in Pediatric and Congenital Heart Disease, First Edition.
Edited by Maully Shah, Larry Rhodes and Jonathan Kaltman.
© 2017 John Wiley & Sons Ltd. Published 2017 by John Wiley & Sons Ltd.
Companion Website: www.wiley.com/go/shah/cardiac_pacing

resulting in torsades de pointes, inherent sinus bradycardia, or bradycardia due to beta blocker therapy.

These recommendations are supported by data from the International Long QT Syndrome registry, which described patients who underwent pacemaker implantation for recurrent syncope or aborted sudden death.[3] Beneficial effects of pacing in high-risk LQTS patients were thought to be related to the prevention of bradycardia and pauses, and shortening of prolonged QT intervals, all factors that are known to help trigger arrhythmias. Permanent cardiac pacing reduced the rate of recurrent syncope in these patients, but was not completely protective.

The neonatal presentation of long QT syndrome is rare, and sometimes accompanied by 2:1 atrioventricular (AV) block and lethal ventricular arrhythmias. Historically, beta blocker therapy with permanent ventricular pacing was the standard therapy, but sudden death was still reported.[4, 5] Chronic therapy with medication and a permanent pacemaker also showed disappointing long-term outcomes during early studies with a mortality rate > 50%.[6] In patients with the longest QT intervals, VVI and DDD pacing are often difficult to achieve and sometimes completely unsuccessful due to pacing before the completion of prolonged ventricular repolarization and proarrhythmia in the presence of a relatively rapid age-dependent sinus rhythm rate. When ventricular pacing is possible, pacing at relatively fast heart rates can result in physiologic shortening of the QT interval and reduction of pauses responsible for ventricular arrhythmias.

High-rate atrial pacing to produce intentional 2:1 AV block as a method of achieving the greatest rhythm stability through constant ventricular rates and QT intervals has been reported (Figure 14.1).[7] When this approach to pacing is used, there must be close follow-up since QT intervals may decrease over time, and may result in 1:1 AV conduction at high ventricular rates. Shortening of the QT interval over time may also allow for stable dual-chamber pacing with 1:1 AV conduction. This approach has the potential to serve as a bridge for the child to reach a size more appropriate for implantable cardioverter-defibrillator implantation.

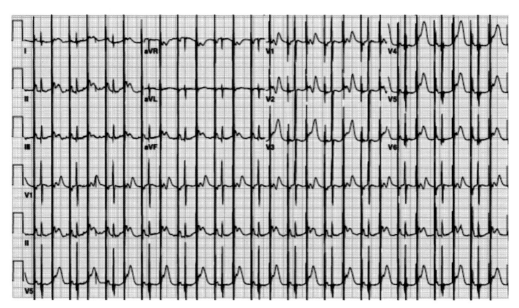

Figure 14.1 *High-rate atrial pacing produces intentional 2:1 AV block, achieving rhythm stability through constant ventricular rates and QT intervals. There is atrial capture with each atrial pacing stimulus, but every other P wave does not conduct to the ventricle because the P wave occurs well before completion of the T wave and ventricular refractoriness.*

Hypertrophic cardiomyopathy

Hypertrophic cardiomyopathy is characterized by concentric or asymmetric left ventricular hypertrophy that is often associated with left ventricular outflow tract obstruction. There is an increased risk of sudden death due to ventricular arrhythmias. Although dual-chamber pacing has been effective in reduction of the left ventricular outflow tract gradient and symptoms, this therapy has not been accepted universally since pacing has not been shown to improve survival compared to other therapies.[8] Pacing of the right ventricular apex reduces the left ventricular outflow tract gradient by reversing ventricular activation with subsequent late activation of the septum. Dual-chamber pacing in patients with hypertrophic cardiomyopathy requires optimization of the AV pacing parameters to achieve complete capture of the ventricle and determine the optimal AV delay. Dual-chamber pacing has been shown to be an effective therapy in selected pediatric patients, but relatively rapid atrial rates and intrinsically shorter AV conduction times must be taken into consideration.[9] Some patients require drug therapy or AV node ablation in order to achieve optimal pacing conditions. The use of a rate-adaptive AV interval function with short AV interval options may allow for customization to assure complete ventricular capture.

Neurocardiogenic syncope

Neurocardiogenic syncope results from inappropriate bradycardia and vasodilation in the setting of reduced venous return and arterial blood pressure causing cerebral hypoperfusion. Older model pacemakers only allowed for prevention of bradycardia with a programmed lower heart rate limit that maintained the heart rate above a predetermined specified rate. The introduction of a "rate-drop sensing" feature allows the pacemaker to sense an abrupt non-physiologic drop in heart rate and respond with a programmed pacing rate above the lower rate limit for a specified period of time (Figure 14.2). As a result, the pacemaker augments the cardiac output with an increased heart rate. If the cardioinhibitory component of the event is the predominant cause of symptoms, then the pacemaker may be very effective in preventing symptoms. However, if the vasodepressor response due to vasodilation predominates, the patient is unlikely to benefit very much from pacing therapy since the cause of the event is not addressed.

Pallid breathholding

Breathholding spells are relatively common events in young children. Although they are generally considered to be benign, they can be particularly distressing to parents and other observers. Fortunately, these episodes usually resolve spontaneously without any permanent adverse effects. However, on occasion, the events can be more prolonged, severe, and result in significant intervention, including cardiopulmonary resuscitation. Pallid breathholding spells are usually more severe than cyanotic breathholding spells, are triggered by pain, have a rapid onset of symptoms, and are the result of profound bradycardia and periods of asystole (Figure 14.3).[10] The mechanism that causes bradycardia and syncope is autonomic nervous system dysfunction that alters vagus nerve control of the heart rate.[11] Since these episodes are primarily a cardioinhibitory event, back-up ventricular pacing is a reasonable option for the most severely affected. The goal of ventricular pacing is to prevent personal injury, relieve parent anxiety, and to avoid preventable and inappropriate therapies, such as cardiopulmonary resuscitation and anticonvulsants. Clinical reports of pacing for pallid breathholding spells have justified the indication, safety, and efficacy of the therapy.[12] Since the patient population is young, epicardial pacing is often performed in order to avoid vascular injury or occlusion. A simple single-chamber ventricular device is all that may be necessary since the goal of pacing is to prevent infrequent and brief events. As such, it is expected that the rhythm will only be paced for a small percentage of the time.

Complex congenital heart disease

Improved survival of patients with congenital heart disease has increased the need for long-term pacing in some of the most complex pediatric cardiac patients. The pediatric patient with complex congenital heart disease often poses difficult management issues with regard to pacemaker programming. Specific anatomic and physiologic circumstances each require special attention. A detailed list of issues relevant to each type of complex congenital heart disease is beyond the

Rate Drop Response Detail Overview – Ventricular Collected – 03/15/09 10:12 PM

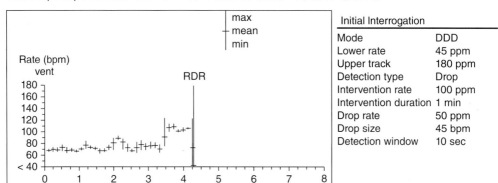

(A)

Rate Drop Response Detail Zoom – Ventricular Collected – 03/15/09 10:12 PM

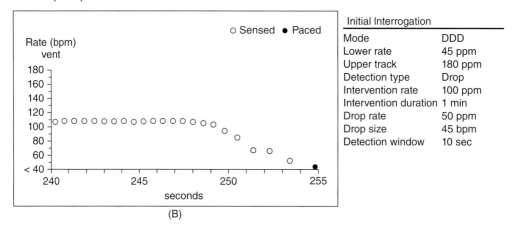

(B)

Figure 14.2 *Heart rate graphic trends over time as recorded by the rate-drop sensing feature. The heart rate trends are illustrated over a longer period of time (A), as well as in a more detailed, higher magnification, over a shorter period of time (B). There is an abrupt heart rate-drop that meets criteria limits for activation of pacing. The rate-drop criteria are defined in the text to the right of each graph. In (B), the open circles on the graph represent sensed heart rates, and the last circle, which is black, represents the onset of pacing.*

scope of this chapter, but some examples are worth reviewing.

Patients with single ventricle physiology who have had a modification of the Fontan operation may require pacing for either bradyarrhythmias or tachyarrhythmias. They often develop accelerated junctional rhythm, which results in a loss of AV synchrony. In order to restore AV synchrony, atrial pacing at a rate faster than the junctional rhythm is necessary. However, sometimes the junctional rhythm rate fluctuates, and exceeds the rate of atrial pacing. Careful attention to ambulatory cardiac monitoring data and heart rate histograms stored

by the device will help to determine the optimal pacing rate for these patients.

The patient with repaired congenital heart disease often has unusual and distorted anatomy that must be understood in order to achieve lead fixation at an appropriate site. Avoidance of scars, patches, and the phrenic nerve is important for optimal long-term lead function. High-output testing, especially of the atrial lead, should be routinely performed in order to avoid phrenic nerve stimulation. This is particularly important in the patient with transposition of the great arteries who has had a Mustard or Senning procedure. In this situation, the transvenous atrial lead passes through the superior limb of the Mustard or Senning baffle and is typically secured to the superior aspect of the left atrium. The left phrenic nerve can be stimulated easily from this location and measures must be taken to avoid this outcome.

Sensing issues

Undersensing occurs in either chamber when an intrinsic atrial (P wave) or ventricular (R wave) event is not appropriately sensed. As a result, there is a paced event in that chamber that occurs earlier than would otherwise be expected. It is important to recognize and address undersensing, since this type of inappropriate pacemaker behavior has the potential for proarrhythmia. If inappropriate pacing occurs in the atrium with critical timing, atrial flutter or atrial fibrillation could be induced. If this were to occur in the ventricle, ventricular tachycardia or ventricular fibrillation could be induced. If there does not appear to be any sensing, it is important to confirm whether the pacemaker is programmed in an asynchronous mode (AOO, VOO, DOO). Otherwise, undersensing occurs when the P or R wave amplitude is less than programmed sensitivity, which may occur with an

acute lead dislodgment or with lead maturation. Sometimes this can be addressed by reprogramming the lead sensitivity to a more sensitive setting (lower value). For the acute lead, waiting for stabilization of the electrode-tissue interface may result in an intrinsic P or R wave with greater amplitude. If there is an insulation break or lead fracture resulting in undersensing, the lead may need to be replaced. A particularly important and unique situation involving atrial undersensing is single-lead VDD pacing, in which there is a tip electrode for ventricular sensing and pacing in addition to floating atrial electrodes for P wave sensing. There has been concern that long-term stability of atrial sensing for this lead is not as reliable as for DDD systems. Although atrial sensing may appear adequate during implant testing, VDD lead function under real-life conditions may result in variable atrial sensing.[13] During atrial undersensing, the VDD system is functionally in a VVI mode. Despite this concern, there have been several studies that have demonstrated adequate atrial sensing during long-term follow-up in this configuration.[14, 15] An often unrecognized cause of undersensing is the effect of quiet timer blanking intervals that are triggered due to high signal amplitudes or large post pace polarization (Figure 14.4).

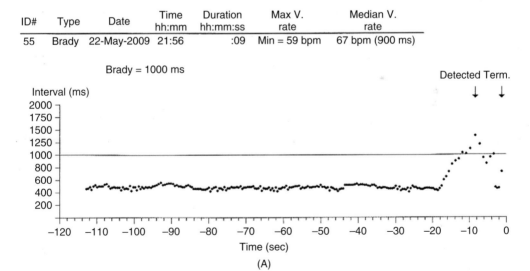

ID#	Type	Date	Time hh:mm	Duration hh:mm:ss	Max V. rate	Median V. rate
55	Brady	22-May-2009	21:56	:09	Min = 59 bpm	67 bpm (900 ms)

(A)

Figure 14.3 (A) Heart rate dot plot from an implantable loop recorder shows a heart rate just over 100 bpm that rapidly drops over a few seconds. The solid line on the graph illustrates the programmed detection limit for bradycardia. The episode lasted for 9 s, resulted in a minimum heart rate of 59 bpm, and was associated with a fit of anger that progressed to pallor and near-syncope. In panel (B), representative electrograms from an implantable loop recorder during a clinical event show abrupt slowing, ventricular asystole, and tremor artifact.

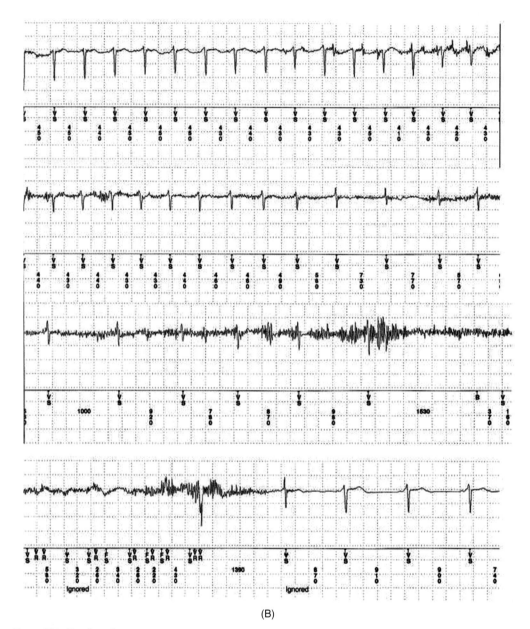

(B)

Figure 14.3 *(Continued)*

Oversensing occurs when the pacemaker senses activity without a corresponding cardiac depolarization from that chamber. Oversensing may occur as a result of a lead fracture. A lead fracture may be intermittent or incomplete, resulting in intermittent oversensing. Generally, an intermittent lead fracture would be expected to progress to a complete lead fracture and more frequent oversensing. Sensing of electromagnetic interference or myopotentials may cause oversensing in a completely intact lead. The source of electromagnetic interference may be difficult to determine, especially in young, active children and adolescents. However, a thorough and investigative history may be revealing. Oversensing of myopotentials is more commonly observed with unipolar

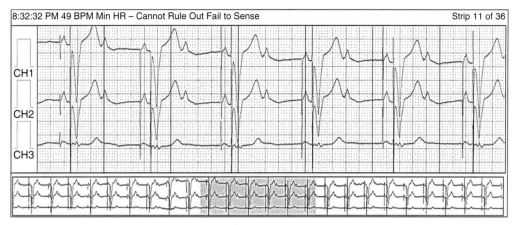

Figure 14.4 *A Holter recording demonstrating atrial undersensing in a 14-year-old girl s/p a dual chamber epicardial pacemaker for complete heart block after surgical repair of a ventricular septal defect. The programmed pacemaker parameters at the time of the Holter were as follows: Pacing mode: DDD, lower rate: 50 bpm, upper rate: 160 bpm. AV delay (paced and sensed): 160 ms, PVARP: 180 ms, ventricular refractory period: 200 ms, ventricular blanking period: 28 ms, Atrial output: 2 V and 0.4 ms, ventricular output 7.5 V and 1 ms, programmed atrial sensitivity 0.7 mV, programmed ventricular sensitivity 2.8 mV. Atrial and ventricular lead polarity is unipolar. Sensing assurance was on. The patient's sensed P waves were 2.8 mV and there were no R waves to sense as patient is pacemaker dependent. The patient had an elevated ventricular stimulation threshold requiring a high ventricular output for adequate capture and to provide a 2× safety margin. The measured waves were 2.8 mV with the atrial sensing channel set to 0.7 mV, and the PVARP was 180 ms indicating that the P wave is of adequate amplitude and outside the refractory period. This suggests that there is another reason for atrial undersensing. Quiet timer blanking intervals occur after any paced event or large enough intrinsic signal deflection and allow the sense amplifier circuit response, known as "ringing," to die down before bringing the sense amplifier back online. Thus, if large and/or wide signals and/or high levels of postpace polarization are sensed, as in this case with high ventricular pacing outputs, quiet timer blanking periods are initiated and may cover the entire intra-ventricular atrial sensing window resulting in undersensing of P waves.*

leads, but an insulation break in either a unipolar or bipolar lead may also result in oversensing of myopotentials. Electromagenitc interference and myopotential sensing can sometimes be dealt with by decreasing the sensitivity (higher value). Finally, a programmed sensitivity that is too sensitive may result in oversensing. In this case, simply reprogramming the device to a decreased sensitivity (higher value) may be enough to correct the problem. For oversensing due to an insulation break, lead fracture, or myopotential sensing on a unipolar lead, it may be necessary to replace the lead.

Maladaptive pacemaker function in the young patient or patient with repaired congenital heart disease

Remarkable progress has been made over the last decades in pacemaker generator and lead design and implementation. However, in general, these progressive functions are proposed for patients with a structurally normal heart and adequate size. Advanced pulse generators with automatic threshold determination are becoming a standard feature. This battery-saving feature has functioned very well in children with transvenous leads, but appears to be less suitable for epicardial systems.[16, 17]

Stimulation of the phrenic nerve, diaphragm, and other extacardiac skeletal muscles is a significant problem, and children with or without repaired congenital heart disease may be at risk. The relative small size of some pediatric pacemaker patients, along with the requisite proximity of pacing leads to other extracardiac structures that makes direct stimulation more likely. For example, a transvenous lead at the right ventricular apex is a few millimeters from the diaphragm, separated only by the thin right ventricular wall. Thus, direct stimulation of the diaphragm during cardiac pacing is quite feasible. In the post-operative patient with repaired congenital heart disease, scarring and fibrosis makes phrenic nerve stimulation easier to achieve. Especially during implantation of transvenous leads, it is always important to perform high-output pacing at the implant site in order to be certain that there is no phrenic nerve capture. Finally, very young pediatric patients and patients with single ventricle physiology or residual right-to-left shunts often receive an epicardial pacing system. Unipolar leads may be easier to implant, but extracardiac skeletal muscle stimulation is a significant problem in this situation. Even when care is taken during implantation to avoid capture of skeletal muscle, fibrosis and positional changes after the patient has recovered from surgery may result in compromised lead function.

Loss of capture issues

Capture of myocardial tissue with pacing is usually easy to appreciate in the ventricle, but may be more difficult to determine in the atrium. In patients with congenital heart disease, who frequently have sinus node dysfunction, atrial capture may be particularly difficult to assess. In those cases, a 12-lead electrocardiogram should be performed in order to more confidently assess atrial capture. For patients with intact AV conduction, loss of atrial capture may be easiest to recognize when there is a pause or decrease in the ventricular rate during atrial pacing. Finally, during atrial capture threshold testing, there will be atrial sensed events if normal sinus node activity occurs when the capture threshold is established.

Loss of capture on the atrial or ventricular leads is generally due to similar etiologies. When the programmed atrial or ventricular lead output is subthreshold, reprogramming of the amplitude or pulse width may be all that is necessary. Lead dislodgment is another cause of loss of capture, but there are usually other findings aside from loss of capture (P or R wave amplitude changes, impedance changes, and ectopy) that indicate a lead dislodgement. Exit block may occur with lead maturation, and manifests as increased pacing thresholds. Exit block occurs with a higher incidence in epicardial leads, presumably due to increased scar and fibrosis.[18] Improved epicardial leads, specifically steroid-eluting designs, have been successful in improving this problem. Long-term performance data suggest that these leads maintain low capture thresholds over time in growing children and outperform older non-steroid lead varieties.[19] Some anti-arrhythmic medications are known to affect pacing lead capture thresholds. For example, amiodarone can increase capture thresholds significantly. Finally, insulation breaks may result in loss of capture and are usually associated with a decrease in the lead impedance.

Upper rate behaviors

Upper rate behaviors are designed for safe and effective pacemaker function over a range of rates. In general, tracking occurs in order for the atrium to be able to influence the events of the ventricle. This allows the P wave to be conducted to the ventricle via the pacemaker. As a result, the ventricular rate can adjust according to the native atrial activity. The maximum tracking rate is the fastest rate at which the atrial rhythm can be tracked by ventricular pacing. The maximum sensor rate is the fastest rate at which the atrium and ventricle can be paced, based on the device's sensor and response to the sensor. The programmed upper rate depends on several variables, including the age of the patient, the expected activity level of the patient, the cardiac diagnosis, and the physiologic tolerance of high ventricular rates. For example, younger patients and more active patients may require programmed upper rates that are higher than for other patients. For patients with diagnoses that would benefit from slower rates, the programmed upper rate should be limited. For example, patients with long QT syndrome and hypertrophic cardiomyopathy should have a limited upper rate limit (URL) for different reasons. Some patients with long QT syndrome have a higher incidence of arrhythmias at higher ventricular rates. Patients with hypertrophic cardiomyopathy benefit from slower rates due to the resultant increased diastolic filling time. Patients with single ventricle physiology and a Fontan operation may also benefit from limiting the maximum possible heart rate.

If the P-wave rate is higher than the maximum tracking rate, several responses can occur. All of these responses result in a paced ventricular rate that does not exceed the programmed upper rate. A fixed ratio block is when there are two, three, or more P waves for every paced ventricular complex. This is a function of the programmed total atrial refractory period [AV interval + post-ventricular atrial refractory period (PVARP)]. There is normal tracking of the P wave until the P wave rate reaches the 2:1 rate, at which time the ventricular rate will suddenly drop to half of the atrial rate. This results in a constant P-to-paced QRS interval. However, the patient may become quite symptomatic due to the abrupt drop in the ventricular rate. As the atrial rate first exceeds the programmed upper rate, the pacemaker begins Wenckebach-like behavior (Figure 14.5). Successive A-V intervals are prolonged until a P wave occurs during the PVARP,

is not sensed, and fails to initiate an AV interval. When this occurs, the pacemaker synchronizes its ventricular output to the next sensed P wave. Therefore, the ventricular paced intervals are at the upper rate, except for the interval in which the P wave occurs during the PVARP. This results in an overall ventricular rate that is less than the programmed rate. This Wenckebach-like behavior provides a more gradual transition between 1:1 tracking and 2:1 AV block. Without such a sudden drop in the ventricular pacing rate and with AV synchrony, the patient often notices fewer symptoms with this type of upper rate behavior. In order for pacemaker Wenckebach to occur,

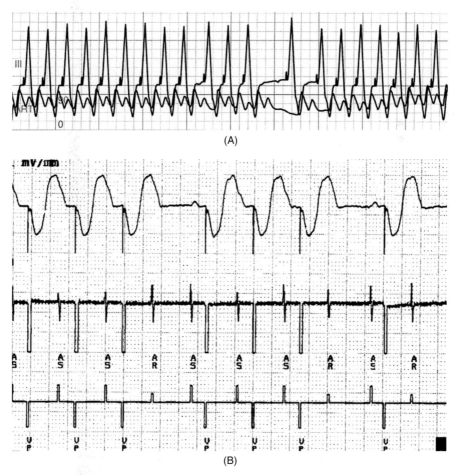

Figure 14.5 *In panel (A), pacemaker Wenckebach occurs during an atrial sensed-ventricular paced rhythm as the atrial rate just exceeds the upper tracking rate of the pacemaker, which is 150 ppm in this case. The P wave is difficult to identify on the bedside monitor recording at such a rapid rate. In panel (B), marker channels are shown to illustrate the atrial sensed-ventricular paced rhythm at a rate that just exceeds the upper tracking rate of the pacemaker. Successive A-V intervals are prolonged until a P wave occurs during the PVARP (AR), is not sensed, and fails to initiate an AV interval.*

the maximum tracking rate must be less than the total atrial refractory period. As the P wave rate increases, there will be 2:1 pacemaker block when the P wave rate exceeds the total atrial refractory period. Pacemaker Wenckbach occurs with a variable P-to-paced QRS interval and some variability in the ventricular rate. As the atrial rate increases further, fewer P waves will be sensed because more will fall into the PVARP. Depending on the P-P coupling interval, the paced rhythm may go to 2:1 or 3:1 sensing block.

Automatic mode switch algorithms

Mode switching is an upper rate behavior that allows an algorithm to smooth the paced upper rate during an atrial arrhythmia. Some devices have the capability of being programmed for a higher mode switch rate than the lower rate during dual chamber programming. This feature helps to compensate for the loss of AV synchrony during the atrial arrhythmia.

Pacemaker mediated tachycardia

Pacemaker mediated tachycardia (PMT) is an inappropriate rapid pacing rate that involves active participation of the pacemaker. There are many forms of PMT that may occur in clinical practice. Historically, a runaway pacemaker was a concern as a cause of PMT. This occurred when internal components of the pacemaker generator failed

and the pacemaker produced an inappropriate rapid rate. Modern devices protect against runaway pacemaker by limiting the URL to 180–210 bpm. Another cause of PMT is far-field sensing on the atrial lead. Atrial lead oversensing of far-field ventricular activity may result in rapid pacing rates (Figure 14.6). Far-field ventricular signals seen on the atrial electrogram should be assessed during pacemaker lead implantation. The atrial lead can be repositioned or the PVARP or post-ventricular atrial blanking period can be extended to prevent oversensing of far-field electrograms. PMT can result in patients with dual chamber pacemaker systems that develop atrial tachycardia. Atrial tracking of the tachycardia can result in ventricular pacing at or near the maximum tracking rate. Mode switch algorithms to identify atrial tachycardias are available and can prevent this form of PMT.

The classic form of PMT is known as endless loop tachycardia (ELT). The most common trigger of ELT occurs when a ventricular paced beat or PVC is conducted retrograde through the AV node to the atrium. This results in an atrial sensed event leading to a ventricular paced beat, which in turn conducts retrograde through the AV node thus continuing the "reentry" loop tachycardia (Figure 14.7). In order to develop ELT, one must have a dual chamber pacemaker system with atrial tracking, in addition to intrinsic retrograde AV node conduction. The rate of ELT is most often at the URL, but certain conditions may result in a sustained PMT slower than the URL ("balanced

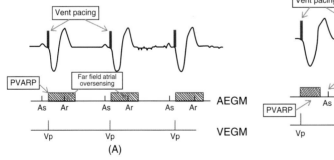
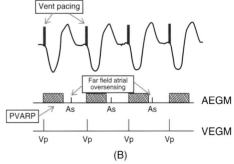

Figure 14.6 *Atrial sensing of far-field T wave. In panel A, there is an atrial sensed rhythm with ventricular pacing. There is far-field oversensing of the T wave seen on the atrial sensing channel. The post-ventricular atrial refractory period (PVARP) is appropriately set so that the far-field T wave signal is seen as an atrial refractory (Ar) event. In panel B, the PVARP was programmed too short so now the far-field T wave is seen on the atrial sensing channel as an atrial sensed (As) event. This results in tracking of the far-field T wave and inappropriate rapid pacing. AEGM: atrial electrogram, Vp: ventricular paced event, VEGM: ventricular electrogram, Vent Pacing: ventricular pacing.*

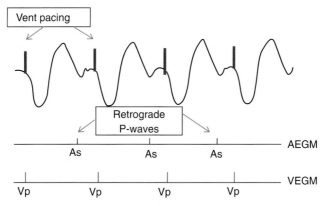

Figure 14.7 *Endless loop tachycardia. Ventricular pacing (Vp) is followed by a retrograde P wave which is seen on the atrial sensing channel as an atrial sensed event (As). This triggers a ventricular paced beat and results in inappropriate rapid pacing (endless loop tachycardia). AEGM: atrial electrogram, PVARP: post-ventricular atrial refractory period, VEGM: ventricular electrogram.*

ELT"). If ELT is suspected, placing a magnet over the device will either terminate the tachycardia (ELT) or unmask intrinsic sinus tachycardia or atrial tachycardia.

Other triggers that may promote ELT include a premature atrial complex falling in the refractory period (PVARP), followed by a ventricular paced beat and retrograde conduction, or atrial oversensing or undersensing resulting in a ventricular paced beat with retrograde conduction. During pacemaker implantation or follow-up device testing, one can check for susceptibility to ELT by performing one of two tests; (1) pacing in the VVI mode at a rate faster than the intrinsic atrial rate, and assessing the atrial electrogram for retrograde atrial conduction (Figure 14.8A) or (2) pacing in the DDD mode at a rate faster than the intrinsic atrial rate, then decreasing the atrial output to sub-threshold (atrial non-capture) and shortening the PVARP to assess if ELT is initiated by a retrograde P-wave (Figure 14.8B).

There are various pacemaker algorithms used to detect and terminate ELT. One algorithm is based on assessment of the number of ventricular paced beats at the URL. If a pre-determined number of consecutive ventricular paced beats occur at the URL (or a fixed rate below the URL), then either a single ventricular paced beat is withheld, PVARP is extended, or DVI mode is initiated for one beat (Figure 14.9A). A second algorithm is based on the finding of a short ventricular paced-atrial

sensed (VA) interval. If the interval between a ventricular paced beat to the following atrial sensed event is shorter than a pre-determined value (e.g., 400 ms) for consecutive beats, then the PVARP is extended to that value (e.g., 400 ms) for one beat (Figure 14.9B). A third algorithm is based on assessment of the stability of the VA interval. If the VA interval remains fixed for a number of consecutive beats, the sensed AV interval is lengthened for one beat. A fixed VA interval indicates ELT, and the next ventricular paced beat is withheld or the PVARP is increased in order to terminate ELT (Figure 14.9C). Finally, a premature ventricular complex response algorithm can be programmed to prevent the development of PMT. If a ventricular sensed event meets pacemaker criteria for a premature ventricular complex, the PVARP is automatically extended to avoid sensing of a retrograde P-wave (Figure 14.9D).

A less common form of PMT is known as repetitive nonreentrant ventriculoatrial synchronous rhythm. This is a phenomenon due to intrinsic retrograde AV node conduction similar to ELT, but it does not result in tachycardia. In this situation, a ventricular paced beat is followed by a retrograde atrial beat. This depolarizes the atrium, but unlike ELT, this beat falls within the PVARP and is not sensed. If the lower rate limit is sufficiently high, an atrial paced event occurs but finds the atrium refractory (functional atrial non-capture). This is then followed by a ventricular paced beat, and a

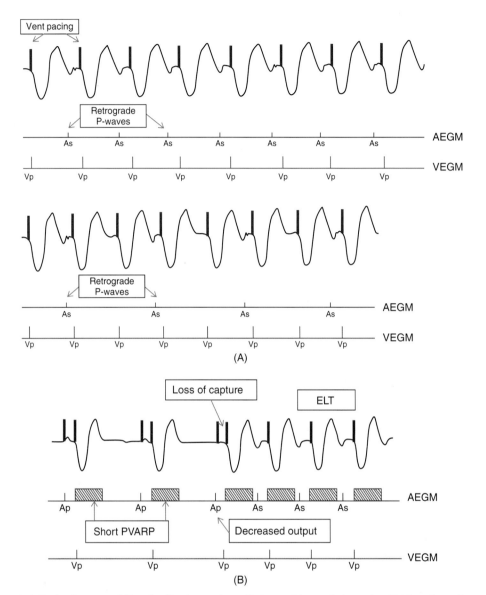

Figure 14.8 *Testing for susceptibility of endless loop tachycardia. In panel A, ventricular pacing (Vp) is performed at a rate faster than the intrinsic atrial rate. Intact ventriculoatrial (VA) conduction would lead to susceptibility of endless loop tachycardia. VA dissociation or 2:1 VA conduction (shown in the lower tracing) would indicate that the risk for endless loop tachycardia is low or not possible. In panel B, dual chamber pacing is performed to assure an atrial paced (Ap) and ventricular paced (Vp) rhythm. The atrial output is then decreased until there is loss of atrial capture. This results in a ventricular paced event followed by retrograde conduction to the atrium (As). The atrium is no longer refractory because of the loss of atrial capture on the previous beat. The pattern can lead to endless loop tachycardia (ELT) if the post-ventricular atrial refractory period (PVARP) is set short enough to allow for the retrograde beat to fall outside of the refractory period. AEGM: atrial electrogram, VEGM: ventricular electrogram.*

retrograde atrial beat that falls within the PVARP. The entire process is then repeated. The resultant rhythm of ventricular pacing with retrograde atrial activation can lead to symptoms of pacemaker syndrome. This problem can be resolved by slowing the programmed lower rate or shortening the AV delay, allowing for recovery of the atrial tissue following a retrograde atrial depolarization.

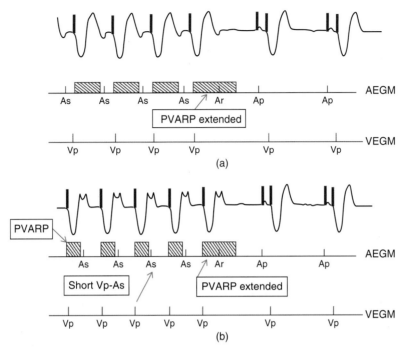

Figure 14.9 *Algorithms to detect and treat endless loop tachycardia. In panel (**A**), a predetermined number of atrial sensed-ventricular paced beats have occurred triggering an algorithm to extend the post- ventricular atrial refractory period (PVARP). The following atrial event falls in the refractory period (Ar) and is not tracked. In this case of endless loop tachycardia (ELT), the pattern is disrupted and an atrial paced (Ap) –ventricular paced (Vp) rhythm commences. In panel B, there is an atrial sensed (As) –ventricular paced (Vp) rhythm at a rapid rate. This results in a "short" Vp-As interval (which is predetermined) and triggers an algorithm to extend the PVARP. The following atrial event falls in the refractory period disrupting the ELT cycle and an atrial paced-ventricular paced rhythm commences. In panel (**C**), a rapid atrial sensed-ventricular paced rhythm results in a "fixed" Vp-As interval. This triggers an algorithm to extend the AV (As-Vp) interval. The following Vp-As interval is assessed. If it remains "fixed," ELT is indicated and the PVARP is extended, disrupting the ELT cycle and an atrial paced- ventricular paced rhythm commences. If the Vp-As interval does not remain "fixed" after extending the AV interval, a sinus or atrial rhythm is indicated and there is no further intervention. In panel (**D**), there is an atrial sensed- ventricular paced rhythm. A premature ventricular complex (PVC) occurs and is detected by the pacemaker. This triggers an algorithm to extend the PVARP. The retrograde P wave that follows the PVC falls within the atrial refractory period and is not tracked. This algorithm prevents ELT initiation from a PVC with retrograde conduction. AEGM: atrial electrogram, VEGM: ventricular electrogram.*

Pacemaker crosstalk

Pacemaker crosstalk occurs when a paced event in one chamber is inappropriately sensed in the other chamber, leading to inhibition of pacing. It occurs most commonly in dual chamber pacing systems when the device is programmed for atrial pacing and ventricular sensing and pacing. The most concerning consequence of crosstalk is when an atrial paced event is sensed by the ventricular lead, causing inhibition of ventricular pacing (Figure 14.10A). Pacemaker crosstalk is more likely to occur if atrial pacing outputs are high, especially in the unipolar mode. It may also occur

if the ventricular lead is programmed with high sensitivity (lower value), or if there is an insulation breach on the atrial lead. Crosstalk may also occur within the pacemaker circuitry.

Prevention of crosstalk can be accomplished by avoiding high-output atrial lead pacing and atrial pacing in the unipolar mode. There are two programming features that are available to help avoid the consequences of crosstalk. The ventricular blanking period begins immediately after an atrial paced event and lasts for a programmable duration in most devices. During this time, ventricular sensing in disabled, thus preventing inhibition of pacing if crosstalk occurs (Figure 14.10B). The

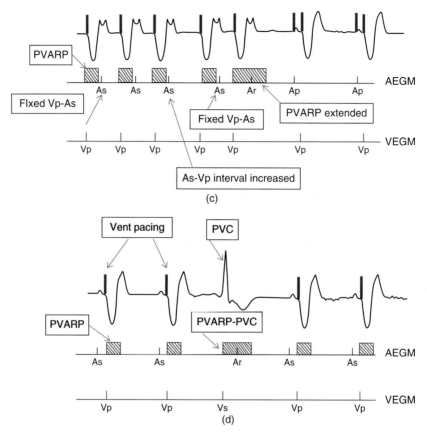

Figure 14.9 *(Continued)*

problem with setting a long ventricular blanking period is that a late-coupled premature ventricular complex or premature junctional complex would not be sensed. If the AV interval is long enough, a ventricular paced beat could occur shortly after the premature ventricular complex and induce a ventricular arrhythmia. A second feature that is helpful in preventing crosstalk is ventricular safety pacing. Safety pacing allows for programming a short ventricular blanking period, but still protects against the consequences of crosstalk. If a ventricular sensed event occurs within a short time following an atrial paced event, the AV interval is shortened and a ventricular paced beat is delivered (Figure 14.11). If the ventricular sensed event is crosstalk, this will prevent inhibition of pacing. If the ventricular sensed event is a premature ventricular complex, the ventricular pacing stimulus will fall harmlessly in the refractory period of the ventricle. Ventricular safety pacing will result in a shorter AV interval than is programmed, and may also result in pacing at a rate higher than the lower rate limit in ventricular paced systems.

Noise reversion

Noise reversion is an operation that occurs if there are continuous sensed events noted during atrial or ventricular refractory periods. The sensed events may occur as a result of exposure to electromagnetic interference, low sensing thresholds, or high-output pacing settings (Figure 14.12). During noise reversion, pacing will continue at the sensor-driven rate or the lower rate limit. Therefore, pacing is not inhibited. Noise reversion can be avoided by removing the exposure to electromagnetic interference, decreasing pacing outputs, or increasing the sensing threshold.

Pacemaker reset may occur if there is exposure to a high level of electromagnetic interference, such as with direct X-ray exposure, electrocautery,

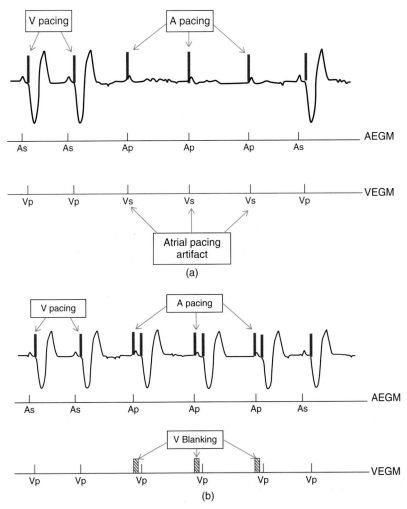

Figure 14.10 *Atrial pacing artifact seen on the ventricular sensing channel. In panel (A), there is initially an atrial sensed (As)-ventricular paced (Vp) rhythm. Atrial pacing (Ap) then occurs at the lower rate limit. The atrial pacing causes artifact on the ventricular sensing channel and is seen as a ventricular sensed event (Vs). This inhibits ventricular pacing (inappropriately) and results in asystole. In panel (B), ventricular blanking is programmed to occur after an atrial paced event inhibiting ventricular sensing. The atrial pacing artifact previously seen on the ventricular sensing channel now falls in the blanking period and does not cause inhibition of ventricular pacing. AEGM: atrial electrogram, A Pacing: atrial pacing, V Pacing: ventricular pacing, VEGM: ventricular electrogram.*

or defibrillation shock. This may cause loss of the programmable pacemaker settings (RAM), resulting in the pacemaker reverting to a preset safety mode (ROM). The pacemaker settings can be reprogrammed if this occurs.

Pacemakers and MRI

The management of patients with pacemakers requiring magnetic resonance imaging (MRI) is becoming an increasingly important issue. The prevalence of comorbidities in those with pacemakers requiring an MRI increases with age. Currently, about 3% of patients with pacemakers have undergone an MRI and it is estimated that 50–70% will need an MRI over the lifetime of one's device.[20] The use of MRI in patients with congenital heart disease is also becoming an important diagnostic tool.

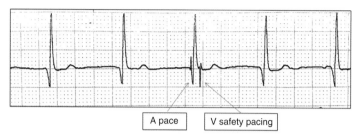

Figure 14.11 *Ventricular safety pacing. The rhythm shown is junctional rhythm in a patient with a dual chamber pacemaker. An atrial pacing spike occurs at the lower rate limit. A junctional beat follows the atrial pacing spike with a short atrial paced-ventricular sensed interval. This triggers the ventricular safety pacing algorithm, and a ventricular pacing stimulus occurs with a short atrial paced-ventricular paced interval. The ventricular pacing stimulus in this case falls harmlessly in the ventricular refractory period. A Pace: atrial paced event, V Safety Pacing: ventricular safety pacing.*

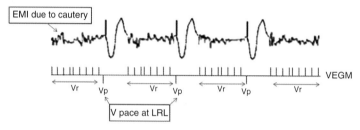

Figure 14.12 *EMI causing noise reversion. A patient with a ventricular pacemaker is noted to have noise on the ventricular sensing channel from Bovie cautery during surgery. This results in many rapid ventricular refractory events (Vr) and triggers the noise reversion algorithm. The pacemaker reverts to ventricular pacing (Vp) at the lower rate limit (V Pace at LRL) to avoid potential inappropriate inhibition of pacing. EMI: electromagnetic interference, VEGM: ventricular electrogram.*

Table 14.1 *Potential risks to a device from exposure to MRI*

Potential Pacemaker/MRI Interactions
1. Pulse generator heating
2. Force and torque
3. Vibration
4. Device interactions
5. Lead heating
6. Myocardial stimulation

The potential risks to the device and the patient undergoing an MRI are listed in Table 14.1.[21] Adverse interactions with the pacemaker and leads occur due to three electromagnetic fields generated by MRI: static, gradient, and radiofrequency energy. An especially important problem is lead tip heating from the radiofrequency energy field, which can cause damage to the myocardium and result in increased pacing thresholds.[22] This seems to be more severe with abandoned pacing leads that are no longer attached to a pulse generator. Another serious potential problem is overstimulation of the tissue, leading to the induction of ventricular fibrillation.[23] This is due to both radiofrequency energy and gradient fields generated during MRI. Retained epicardial leads that have been cut at the skin do not appear to pose a significant risk for heating or arrhythmia induction in patients undergoing MRI.[24]

The frequency of adverse events in pacemaker patients undergoing MRI is unclear. Several large studies of adults with transvenous pacemakers undergoing MRI showed minimal changes in battery voltage and pacing thresholds.[21] A smaller study in young patients with congenital heart disease and epicardial pacing systems showed similar results with MRI.[25] Because of the uncertainty of these risks, the American Heart Association guidelines state that "an MRI should only be considered in cases in which the potential benefit to the patient clearly outweighs the risks ... "[26]

Recent modifications in specific pacemaker systems have resulted in products that may avoid some of the unwanted interactions of MRI. Changes in the pacemaker generator include isolation of the circuit board and reduction of ferromagnetic material. Lead conductor design changes can help to reduce heating of myocardial tissue. Finally, new programming features can avoid inappropriate oversensing and allow for safe pacing modes.[21]

These newer pacing systems have been designated as "MRI conditional" devices, indicating that there are no known hazards or risks under specific conditions of use.[27] These conditions include using a 1.5 Tesla static magnetic field, limiting the whole body specific absorption rate, and avoiding the isocenter being positioned directly over the device. Specific device requirements include an implant date greater than 6 weeks prior, adequate pacing thresholds and lead impedances, pectoral implant, no additional hardware, and the use of the MRI conditional pacemaker generator connected to MRI conditional atrial and ventricular leads.[21]

Follow-up

Protocols for pacemaker follow-up have evolved over time, especially with the availability of more detailed information from transtelephonic monitoring. Current pacemaker follow-up guidelines are published by the Heart Rhythm Society (Table 14.2).[28] Transtelephonic monitoring in the past contained limited data on pacemaker function. Overall assessment of battery status, limited threshold data, and functioning of the programmed settings were available (Figure 14.13). Current devices have the ability to transmit full interrogations, either automatically or patient-directed.

Table 14.2 *Frequency of pacemaker monitoring*

Minimum Frequency of Pacemaker Monitoring (In Person or Remote)	
1. Within 72 h of implantation	in person
2. 2–12 weeks post implantation	in person
3. Every 3–12 months	in person or remote
4. Annually until battery depletion	in person
5. Every 1–3 months at signs of battery depletion	in person or remote

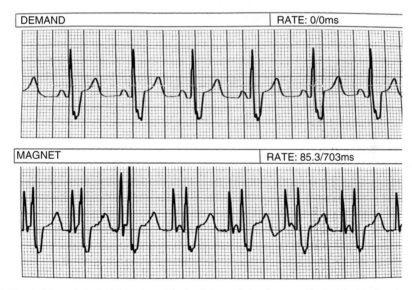

Figure 14.13 *Threshold margin test. This is a transtelephonic transmission from a patient with a Medtronic pacemaker. The top panel shows that the presenting rhythm (demand mode) is an atrial sensed-ventricular paced rhythm. The bottom panel is recorded when a magnet is placed over the pacemaker. The magnet mode triggers a threshold margin test, which performs DOO pacing at 100 ppm for three beats. The pulse width is reduced by 25% on the third beat. Loss of capture on this beat would indicate an inadequate safety margin for the programmed pacing output. The following rhythm is DOO at 85 ppm (battery at beginning of life). Pacing in the DOO mode at 65 ppm would indicate battery depletion (elective replacement indicator).*

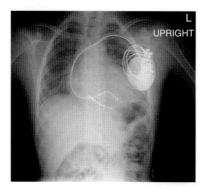 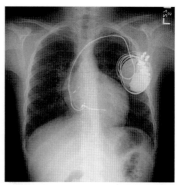

Initial post-procedure CXR   Follow-up post-procedure CXR

(A)

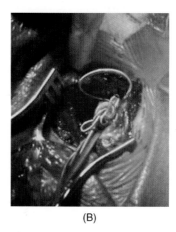

(B)

Figure 14.14 *Twiddler syndrome. The post-implant CXR of an 11-year-old male who underwent placement of a biventricular ICD placed in a subpectoral pocket (A, left panel). Several weeks later, pacing thresholds were found to be elevated and a follow-up post-procedure CXR was obtained (A, right panel). The patient was brought back to the operating room and the leads were found twisted in the pocket due to Twiddler syndrome (B).*

The office evaluation allows for patient evaluation, device evaluation, and use of ancillary tests.

Patient evaluation

Patients should be evaluated for symptoms of palpitations, discomfort at the pacemaker generator pocket site, exercise tolerance, and overall symptom status since having the pacemaker placed. Exam should focus on the pacemaker generator pocket site for signs of infection, erosion, or necrosis. Excessive mobility of the pacemaker may indicate "twiddler syndrome" (Figure 14.14). Edema or engorgement of superficial veins of the ipsilateral upper extremity may indicate venous obstruction.

Pacemaker device evaluation

The interrogation of the pacemaker should assess diagnostic data such as heart rate histograms, percent of atrial and ventricular pacing (and biventricular pacing), and arrhythmias or mode-switch episodes. Battery status can be assessed by voltage and impedance (which rises with battery depletion). Lead impedance issues can be detected by looking for any change $> 200–300 \ \Omega$, low impedance ($<200 \ \Omega$) suggesting insulation breach, or high impedance alerts suggesting a lead fracture. If this is suspected, assessment of lead impedance during maneuvers involving isometric tension can be performed to reproduce an abnormal change in impedance (Figure 14.15). Pacing thresholds are

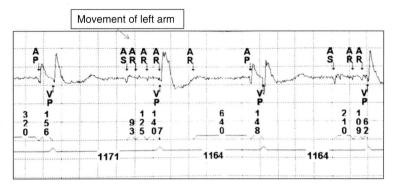

Figure 14.15 *Noise on atrial sensing channel reproduced with arm movements. Pacemaker tracing of a patient with a dual chamber transvenous pacemaker. The initial rhythm is atrial paced (Ap)-ventricular paced (Vp) but movement of the left arm results in noise on the atrial sensing channel (As, Ar). This noise inhibits atrial pacing and results in loss of atrioventricular synchrony. The noise seen on the atrial sensing channel was due to a fracture of the atrial lead.*

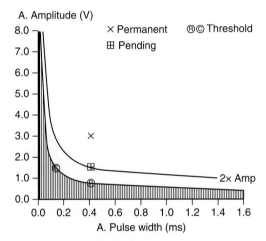

Figure 14.16 *Pacing threshold curve. The pacing threshold curve is obtained from a Medtronic pacemaker using the automated threshold program. The threshold curve is marked with the dark line. A 2× safety margin curve (2× amp) is automatically generated and optimal pacing outputs are plotted (pending). The current pacing outputs are also shown on the graph (permanent).*

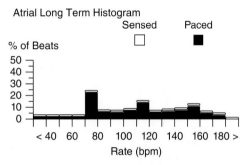

Figure 14.17 *Oversensitive rate response histogram. The rate histogram shown is from a Medtronic pacemaker programmed in the AAIR mode for a 16-year-old patient with sinus node dysfunction. The heart rate profile demonstrates that there is atrial pacing at high heart rates, which are not physiologic for this age. This was due to an oversensitive rate response setting and was corrected when the setting was made to be less responsive.*

assessed and outputs can be decreased to chronic settings at 6–8 weeks after implant. A 2:1 voltage safety margin is usually programmed at this time to preserve battery life while maintaining an adequate safety margin (Figure 14.16). Use of an autocapture feature may also be effective for extending battery life in a safe fashion. Sensing thresholds are performed, and a 2:1 safety margin for sensing is usually programmed. During the pacemaker evaluation, determination of pacemaker dependency

and assessment of retrograde AV node conduction may be performed. In patients with chronotropic incompetence, assessment of rate-response pacing includes evaluation of the heart rate histograms, assessment of patient symptoms and exercise tolerance, and evaluation of automatic optimization of rate-response parameters. Over-sensitive rate response pacing may occur in sensor-driven pacemakers when the rate response settings are too sensitive to non-physiologic activity (such as vibrations from driving in a car, exposure to loud noise or music, pressure on the pacemaker generator, or use of vibrating tools) (Figure 14.17). Hyperventilation or use of electrocautery may cause high pacing rates in devices with minute ventilation based rate-response sensors. Knowledge of normal heart rate histograms for children and adults are helpful for determination of appropriate rate-response settings. A limited exercise (or walk) test may be performed in the office to help optimize rate-response parameters.

Ancillary testing

Supplemental testing such as an electrocardiogram, ambulatory cardiac monitor, chest radiograph, or exercise stress test may be performed based on the clinical situation. An echocardiogram to assess ventricular function in the setting of chronic ventricular pacing should be performed on a regular basis.

Database

A method for tracking pacemaker patients is important to assure proper patient follow-up testing and communication regarding device alerts. There are commercially available pacemaker databases that directly communicate with and download both in-person and transtelephonic pacemaker interrogations.

References

1 Moss AJ, Schwartz PJ, Crampton RS, Tzivoni D, Locati EH, MacCluer J, et al. The long QT syndrome: Prospective longitudinal study of 328 families. *Circulation* 1991; 84: 1136–1144.

2 Kay GN, Plumb VJ, Arciniegas JG, Henthorn RW, Waldo AL. Torsade de pointes: the long-short initiating sequence and other clinical features: observations in 32 patients. *J Am Coll Cardiol* 1983; 2: 806–817.

3 Moss AJ, Liu JE, Gottlieb S, Locati EH, Schwartz PJ, Robinson JL. Efficacy of permanent pacing in the management of high-risk patients with long QT syndrome. *Circulation* 1991; 84: 1524–1529.

4 Villain E, Levy M, Kachaner J, Garson A Jr., Prolonged QT interval in neonates: Benign, transient, or prolonged risk of sudden death. *Am Heart J* 1992; 124: 194–197.

5 Weintraub RG, Gow RM, Wilkinson JL. The congenital long QT syndromes in childhood. *J Am Coll Cardiol* 1990; 16: 674–680.

6 Trippel DL, Parsons MK, Gillette PC. Infants with long-QT syndrome and 2:1 atrioventricular block. *Am Heart J* 1995; 130: 1130–1134.

7 Tanel RE, Triedman JK, Walsh EP, Epstein MR, DeLucca JM, Mayer JE, et al. High-rate atrial pacing as an innovative bridge therapy in a neonate with congenital

long QT syndrome. *J Cardiovasc Electrophysiol* 1997; 8: 812–817.

8 Nishimura RA, Symanski JD, Hurrell DG, Trusty JM, Hayes DL, Tajik AJ. Dual-chamber pacing for cardiomyopathies: A 1996 clinical perspective. *Mayo Clin Proc* 1996; 71: 1077–1087.

9 Nishimura RA, Hayes DL, Ilstrup DM, Holmes DR Jr, Tajik AJ. Effect of dual-chamber pacing on systolic and diastolic function in patients with hypertrophic cardiomyopathy. Acute Doppler echocardiographic and catheterization hemodynamic study. *J Am Coll Cardiol* 1996; 27: 421–430.

10 Lombroso CT, Lerman P. Breathholding spells (cyanotic and pallid infantile syncope). *Pediatrics* 1967; 39: 563–581.

11 DiMario FJ Jr, Chee CM, Berman PH. Pallid breath-holding spells. Evaluation of the autonomic nervous system. *Clin Pediatr* 1990; 29: 17–24.

12 Kelly AM, Porter CJ, McGoon MD, Espinosa RE, Osborn MJ, Hayes DL. Breath-holding spells associated with significant bradycardia: successful treatment with permanent pacemaker implantation. *Pediatrics* 2001; 108: 698–702.

13 Hunziker P, Buser P, Pfisterer M, Burkart F, Osswald S. Predictors of loss of atrioventricular synchrony in single lead VDD pacing. *Heart* 1998; 80: 390–392.

14 Naegeli B, Osswald S, Pfisterer M, Burkart F. VDD(R) pacing: short- and long-term stability of atrial sensing with a single lead system. *Pacing Clin Electrophysiol* 1996; 19: 455–464.

15 Santini M, Ricci R, Pignalberi C, Auriti A, Pepe M, Assale R, Caporicci D. Immediate and long-term atrial sensing stability in single-lead VDD pacing depends on right atrial dimensions. *Europace* 2001; 3: 324–331.

16 Nurnberg JH, Adbul-Khaliq H, Ewert P, Lange PE. Antibradycardia pacing in patients with congenital heart disease: experience with automatic threshold determination and output regulation (Autocapture). *Europace* 2003; 5: 199–205.

17 Kucukosmanoglu O, Celiker A, Ozer S, Karagoz, T. Compatibility of automatic threshold tracking pacemakers with previously implanted pacing leads in children. *Pacing Clin Electrophysiol* 2002; 25: 1624–1627.

18 Villafane J, Austin E. Cardiac pacing problems in infants and children: Results of a 4-year prospective study. *South Med J* 1993; 86; 784–788.

19 Horenstein MS, Hakimi M, Walters H 3rd, Karpawich PP. Chronic performance of steroid-eluting epicardial leads in a growing pediatric population: a 10-year comparison. *Pacing Clin Electrophysiol* 2003; 26: 1467–1471.

20 Kalin R, Stanton MS, Current clinical issues for MRI scanning of pacemaker and defibrillator patients. *Pacing Clin Electrophysiol* 2005; 28(4): 326–328.

21 Shinbane JS, Colletti PM, Shellock FG, Magnetic resonance imaging in patients with cardiac pacemakers: era of "MR Conditional" designs. *J Cardiovasc Magn Reson* 2011; 13: 63.

22 Pictet J, Meuli R, Wicky S, van der Klink JJ, Radiofrequency heating effects around resonant lengths of wire in MRI. *Phys Med Biol* 2002; 47(16): 2973–2985.

23 Fontaine JM, Mohamed FB, Gottlieb C, Callans DJ, Marchlinski, FE. Rapid ventricular pacing in a pacemaker patient undergoing magnetic resonance imaging. *Pacing Clin Electrophysiol*, 1998; 21(6): 1336–1339.

24 Hartnell GG, Spence L, Hughes LA, Cohen MC, Saouaf R, Buff B. Safety of MR imaging in patients who have retained metallic materials after cardiac surgery. *AJR Am J Roentgenol* 1997; 168(5): 1157–1159.

25 Pulver AF, Puchalski MD, Bradley DJ, Minich LL, Su JT, Saarel EV, Whitaker P, Etheridge SP. Safety and imaging quality of MRI in pediatric and adult congenital heart disease patients with pacemakers. *Pacing Clin Electrophysiol* 2009; 32(4): 450–456.

26 Levine GN1, Gomes AS, Arai AE, Bluemke DA, Flamm SD, Kanal E, and American Heart Association Committee on Diagnostic and Interventional Cardiac Catheterization; American Heart Association Council on Clinical Cardiology; American Heart Association Council on Cardiovascular Radiology and Intervention. Safety of magnetic resonance imaging in patients with cardiovascular devices: An American Heart Association scientific statement from the Committee on Diagnostic and Interventional Cardiac Catheterization, Council on Clinical Cardiology, and the Council on Cardiovascular Radiology and Intervention: endorsed by the American College of Cardiology Foundation, the North American Society for Cardiac Imaging, and the Society for Cardiovascular Magnetic Resonance. *Circulation* 2007; 116(24): 2878–2891.

27 Shellock FG, Woods TO, Crues JV. MR labeling information for implants and devices: explanation of terminology. *Radiology*, 2009; 253(1): 26–30.

28 Wilkoff BL, Auricchio A, Brugada J, Cowie M, Ellenbogen KA, Gillis AM, et al. HRS/EHRA expert consensus on the monitoring of cardiovascular implantable electronic devices (CIEDs): description of techniques, indications, personnel, frequency and ethical considerations. *Heart Rhythm* 2008; 5(6): 907–925.

CHAPTER 15

ICD troubleshooting and follow-up

Steven Fishberger[1] and Maully Shah[2]

[1]Nicklaus Children's Hospital, Miami, FL, USA
[2]Perelman School of Medicine, University of Pennsylvania, The Children's Hospital of Philadelphia, Philadelphia, PA, USA

Introduction

The implantable cardioverter-defibrillator (ICD) has been demonstrated to be the superior treatment for patients at risk for life-threatening ventricular arrhythmias. However, ICD therapy may be associated with a variety of problems including lead dislodgement or fracture, device malfunction, and inappropriate therapy. The unique features of the pediatric population including increased activity, diminutive size, and potential for somatic growth put them at greater risk for many of these problems. Troubleshooting an ICD requires a thorough understanding of its features, how it is programmed, and the patient population. This chapter describes how to recognize and treat complications associated with ICD therapy.

Implantable cardioverter defibrillators have become the treatment of choice for primary and secondary prevention of sudden cardiac death.[1] The superiority of ICDs in reducing all-cause mortality compared with antiarrhythmic therapy has been established in high-risk patients with ischemic and non-ischemic cardiomyopathy.[2,3] This strategy has been applied to the pediatric population at risk for sudden cardiac death, though indications often differ from the adult population. Pediatric indications include primary electrical disease, structural congenital heart disease, hypertrophic cardiomyopathy, and dilated cardiomyopathy.[4,5] Pediatric patients represent <1% of all patients with ICDs, however ICD use in the pediatric population has increased significantly, in part due to technological advancements, including smaller devices and the introduction of transvenous leads.[6] Increased identification of primary electrical diseases that may result in cardiac arrest in the pediatric population including long QT syndrome (LQT), Brugada syndrome, and catecholaminergic polymorphic ventricular tachycardia (CPVT) has further increased the application of ICD implant.

ICD therapy may be associated with a variety of problems or perceived problems. While troubleshooting is defined as fixing a problem, an initial assessment is required to determine if there is a problem. Troubleshooting an ICD requires a thorough understanding of its features, how it is programmed, and the patient population. Complications associated with ICDs in the pediatric and congenital heart population mirror those that occur in their adult counterparts including lead dislodgement, lead failure/fracture, device failure/malfunction, and inappropriate

Cardiac Pacing and Defibrillation in Pediatric and Congenital Heart Disease, First Edition.
Edited by Maully Shah, Larry Rhodes and Jonathan Kaltman.
© 2017 John Wiley & Sons Ltd. Published 2017 by John Wiley & Sons Ltd.
Companion Website: www.wiley.com/go/shah/cardiac_pacing

therapy. The unique features of the pediatric population including a higher level of activity, diminutive size, and potential for somatic growth put them at increased risk for many of these problems.[7] The pediatric cohort tends to be healthier and more active, resulting in more wear and tear on the ICD leads and a greater risk of lead fracture.

While there are some variations among device manufacturers, the majority of features are common to all ICDs. Often the differences are a matter of semantics, as each manufacturer attempts to brand their device functions. They all contain detailed comprehensive data storage capabilities that greatly enhance the clinician's ability to troubleshoot device malfunction. These include stored electrograms, telemetered marker annotations, discriminators for supraventricular versus ventricular tachycardia, and automatic measurements of capture thresholds, sensed electrograms, and lead impedances. When there is an abnormal measurement or deviation from previous measurements, it is highlighted as an alert on the programming screen upon interrogation. Patient alarms, manifested as audible tones when there is an abnormal measurement, alerts the patient to have the device interrogated by the clinician. The development of home monitors that perform and transmit extensive device information routinely and when an event occurs has revolutionized the care of patients with ICDs.[8] Another important advance that was introduced in the late 1990s was the expansion of the ICD from a single-purpose "shock box" to a device that incorporated bradycardia pacing. This has eliminated the problem of interactions between ICDs and separate pacemakers, which principally was the delay or prevention of ICD therapy due to oversensing of high-amplitude pacemaker stimulus artifact.[9]

ICD therapy

The purpose of an ICD is to prevent sudden cardiac death in the event of a ventricular arrhythmia. An ICD is programmed to deliver a shock if there is a detected rapid ventricular arrhythmia. Alternatively, the initial therapy particularly for a less rapid ventricular arrhythmia may be anti-tachycardia pacing (ATP). ICD therapy delivered for a reason other than a potentially life-threatening ventricular arrhythmia is categorized as inappropriate. Pediatric patients and patients with congenital heart disease have a relatively high rate of this complication, with approximately 20% of patients receiving an inappropriate shock.[10, 11] Inappropriate shocks are painful and have been associated with psychosocial morbidity and increased mortality.[8, 9] Whether a shock or ATP, it is important to determine the appropriateness of any delivered ICD therapy.

Therapy is delivered when the ICD categorizes a rhythm as ventricular tachycardia and the programmed rate and duration criteria have been met. ICD detected ventricular tachycardia (VT) or ventricular fibrillation (VF) may represent true ventricular arrhythmia, supraventricular tachycardia (SVT), or sensing of nonarrhythmic electrical signals. Stored ICD electrograms along with corresponding annotated markers from detected SVT, VT, or VF episodes provide the essential data for interpreting the causes and outcomes of ICD therapy.

Inappropriate therapy occurs in the absence of a ventricular arrhythmia (VT or VF) due to nonphysiologic or physiologic signals that are sensed and determined to be ventricular in origin. Analysis of sensing begins with recording ICD electrograms (EGM). The sensing EGM records a near field ventricular signal between the RV tip electrode and the RV ring electrode or right RV coil and the timing of the sensed EGMs is indicated by the marker channels. Therefore, the sensing EGM is used in tachycardia detection. The shock EGM records a far field ventricular signal between widely separated electrodes, commonly the RV coil and ICD Can. The shock EGM is utilized to determine morphology for SVT-VT discrimination and not for tachycardia detection.

Oversensing may represent sensing of an event, typically nonventricular, which is erroneously incorporated into the tachycardia detection algorithm. Oversensing in the ventricular channel may also result in inappropriate inhibition of ventricular pacing in a patient with AV block and cause

Table 15.1 *Differential diagnosis of extracardiac "noise" signals*

	Signal Characteristics	EGM Source
Conductor/Connector problem	Intermittent, postural, variable amplitude, frequency and morphology	Sensing EGM more common
Insulation breach (inside-out)	Spikes	Simultaneous spikes on multiple sources
Insulation breach (in pocket)	Variable amplitude, high frequency, occurs with pectoral muscle exercise	Sensing EGM
EMI	Continuous, high frequency	Signal amplitude on shock EGM > Signal amplitude on near field sensing EGM
Pectoral myopotentials	Variable amplitude, high frequency, occurs with pectoral muscle exercise	Far field EGM that includes can more common
Diaphragmatic myopotentials	Low amplitude, high frequency, occurs after ventricular paced events or long diastolic intervals	Near field sensing EGM

Table 15.2 *ICD oversensing: potential causes and solutions*

Oversensing Causes	Possible Solutions
Physiological Signals	
• P wave oversensing	↓ ventricular sensitivity, forced atrial pacing, ↑ ventricular blanking after atrial event
• R wave double counting	↑ ventricular blanking period
• T wave oversensing	↓ ventricular sensitivity, adjusting dynamic sensitivity (manufacturer specific), algorithmic rejection of T waves, changing from dedicated to integrated bipolar sensing, add new pace-sense lead or re-position lead
• Diaphragmatic myopotentials	↓ ventricular sensitivity, manufacture specific noise rejection algorithm, lead replacement or repositioning
Nonphysiological Signals	
• Loose set screw	Surgical intervention
• Pace-sense conductor fracture	Replace or add new lead
• High voltage component fracture	Replace lead
• Insulation breach	Replace lead
• Lead-lead interaction	Reposition new lead if identified at implant, remove old lead if possible or remove new lead and replace at a different position
• Implanted electronic devices (nerve stimulators, gastric pacemakers, etc.)	Depends on individual risk /benefit of implanted electronic device with ICD

syncope or pre-syncope. Physiologic signals may be intracardiac (P, R, or T waves) or extracardiac (myopotentials). Nonphysiologic signals can be due to a lead or connector problem or from electromagnetic interference (EMI) (Tables 15.1 and 15.2).

Nonphysiologic oversensing

Electromagnetic interference (EMI) can result in inappropriate tachycardia detection and therapy.[12] Interrogation of the ICD reveals characteristic high-frequency electrical signals that do not have a constant relationship to the cardiac cycle. EMI can arise from normally functioning equipment such as electronic article surveillance systems, arc welders, electrolysis, internal combustion engines, and electrocautery.[13] It can also arise from alternating current leak from improperly grounded electronic equipment including a washing machine, swimming pool, or fish pond cleaning equipment (Figure 15.1A and B).[12, 14] The source of EMI is not always readily apparent and in the event of an inappropriate shock or the identification of high-frequency signals during interrogation, may require some detective work. The availability of the date and time of the stored event frequently aids in the investigation.

Lead or connector problems are additional sources of nonphysiologic oversensing that may cause inappropriate ICD therapy. ICD lead fracture is an important concern in children due to their level of activity and growth (Figures 15.2 and 15.3). A loose set screw at the lead's attachment to the generator results in electrical noise generated from the collision of the lead's connecting pin with the set screw. These conditions can be detected by

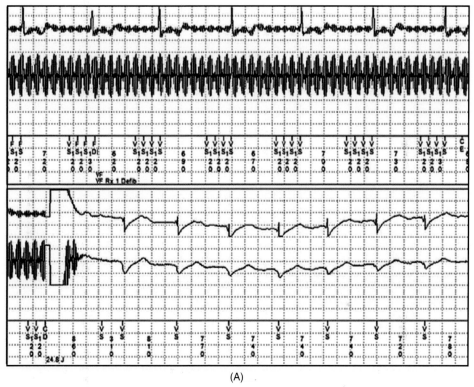

(A)

Figure 15.1 *Noise caused by alternating current leak presumably from an improperly grounded swimming pool in two patients. The noise is on both near field (RVtip-RVring) EGM (Top channel) and far field (RVcoil-Can) EGM (bottom channel), which is characteristic of EMI coming from an external source. (A) EMI noise resulted in an inappropriate ICD shock. (B) In another patient, remote monitoring transmission shows similar findings with date and time stamp correlating with swimming, however, no ICD shock was administered. This is because the shock was aborted as insufficient number of ventricular intervals were detected between capacitor charging and ending of charge cycle, that is the reconfirmation period. Even though "noise" is apparent on the near and far field EGMs, it intermittently diminishes in the near field EGM and this results in the device not "seeing" it as it is below the sensitivity cut off. Note that after an inherent QRS, the "noise" signal diminishes. This is the function of the auto-adjusting sensitivity threshold. After sensed ventricular events, Medtronic ICDs reset the sensing threshold to 8–10× the time programmed sensitivity, up to a maximum of 75% of sensed the R wave. The value of auto-adjusting sensitivity then decays exponentially from the end of the (sense) blanking period with a time constant of 450 ms until it reaches the programmed (maximum) sensitivity. From top to bottom, near field EGM, far field EGM, and marker channels.*

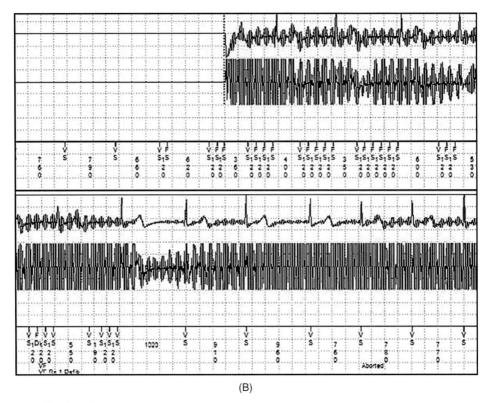

(B)

Figure 15.1 *(Continued)*

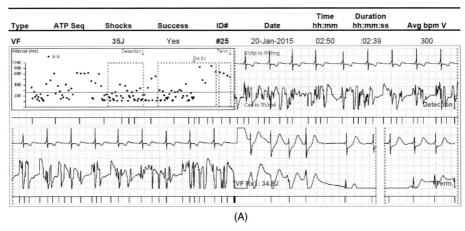

(A)

Figure 15.2 *Remote monitoring transmission showing inappropriate ICD shock secondary to lead fracture in a 10-year-old boy with Tetralogy of Fallot. (A) The top and bottom channels show EGMs from RV tip to RV ring and Can to RV coil, respectively. High amplitude noise is seen on the bottom channel but not on the RV tip to RV ring tracing, suggesting involvement of the RV coil. (B) RV pacing impedance trend shows no abrupt changes. (C) RV defibrillation impedance shows an isolated but abrupt increase to 72 Ω. Analysis of the extracted lead showed a fracture of the RV defibrillation conductor.*

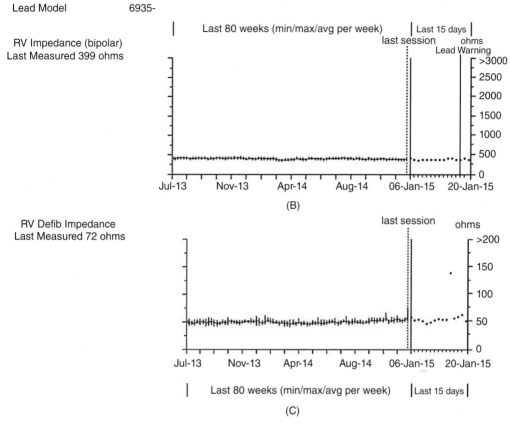

Figure 15.2 *(Continued)*

measurement of the lead impedance (Table 15.3) or the presence of extremely short nonphysiologic sensed intervals, though this may be intermittent and may require generator pocket manipulation or patient motion (Figure 15.4).

Physiologic oversensing

Extracardiac signals
Myopotential oversensing occurs when electronic signals from skeletal muscle are detected. ICD leads use bipolar sensing and as a result, pectoral myopotential oversensing is a rare event. However, oversensing of myopotentials arising from the diaphragm is possible. This occurs with devices programmed to extremely high sensitivity settings and may result in inappropriate ICD shocks.[15] Oversensing occurs after long diastolic intervals or after ventricular paced events when amplifier sensitivity or gain is maximized by devices with automatic gain control. It is most common in

patients who have an integrated bipolar lead (tip to distal high voltage coil) rather than dedicated bipolar lead (tip to ring electrode) in the RV apex (Table 15.1). It can often be reproduced with the Valsalva maneuver while recording real-time EGMs and rectified by decreasing the sensitivity.

Intracardiac
Ventricular oversensing of intracardiac signals results in two detected ventricular electrograms for each cardiac cycle (double counting). If the heart rate is rapid enough, this will be inappropriately detected as VT or VF. The oversensing of intracardiac signals are due to depolarization of the atria or ventricle (P or R waves), or repolarization of the ventricle (T waves). While monomorphic VT has a pattern of equally spaced intervals between sensed electrograms, oversensing of intracardiac signals is typically characterized by paired signals that give the appearance of alternating ventricular cycle

Alert Events Report		Page 1
03-May-2012 14:50:36	*RV Lead Integrity warning: -2 or more VT-NS episodes < 220 ms. -Sensing Integrity Counter >= 30 in 3 days.	
16-Mar-2012 21:39:43	*RV Lead Integrity warning: -2 or more VT-NS episodes < 220 ms. -Sensing Integrity Counter >= 30 in 3 days.	

Battery Voltage (RRT=2.63V)		3.05 V
Last Full Charge		9.9 sec
	Atrial(3830)	RV(0180)
Pacing Impedance	551 ohms	475 ohms
Defibrillation Impedance		RV=48 ohms
Programmed Amplitude/Pulse Width	2.00 V/0.40 ms	2.50 V/0.40 ms
Measured P/R Wave	2.9 mV	>20 mV
Programmed Sensitivity	0.30 mV	0.60 mV

Left arm "resistance"

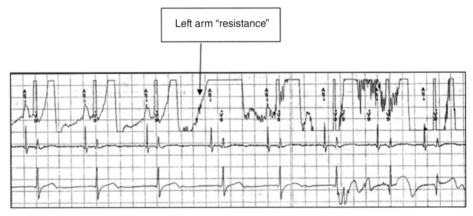

Figure 15.3 *Multiple episodes of nonsustained VT on ICD interrogation. (A) RV pacing and defibrillation impedances are within normal range. Pacing and Impedance trends recorded in the prior 80 weeks are also stable without any abrupt changes (not shown). (B) Real time electrograms (top: ECG Lead I, middle: Atrial EGM, bottom: RV tip-RV ring) initially appear normal, however, with a provocative upper arm straining maneuver, artifact appears on the ECG tracing, the atrial channel is unaffected and noise appears on the near field EGM with ventricular oversensing suggesting a problem in the conductor or connection to the RV tip. Noise was not seen on the can to RV coil electrogram (not shown). Analysis of the extracted lead showed a fracture of the ring conductor.*

Table 15.3 *Impedance changes in evaluation of lead problems*

↑ Impedance	Impedance Unchanged	↓ Impedance
Conductor fracture	Conductor fracture	Insulation breach
Connection problem	Insulation breach-in pocket	
Calcium deposition at electrode-tissue interface (no lead problem in absence of sensing issues)	Insulation breach: inside out	

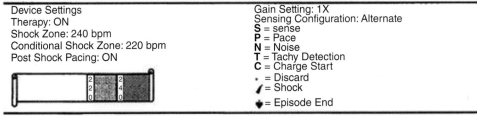

Device Settings
Therapy: ON
Shock Zone: 240 bpm
Conditional Shock Zone: 220 bpm
Post Shock Pacing: ON

Gain Setting: 1X
Sensing Configuration: Alternate
S = sense
P = Pace
N = Noise
T = Tachy Detection
C = Charge Start
. = Discard
/ = Shock
⬥ = Episode End

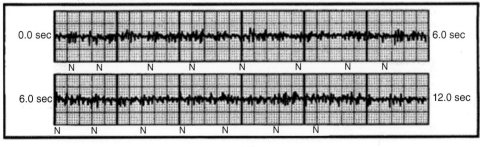

CAPTURED S-ECG: 01/05/2015 08:22:15 AM 25 mm/sec 2.5 mm/mV

0.0 sec   6.0 sec

N   N   N   N   N   N   N   N

6.0 sec   12.0 sec

N   N   N   N   N   N   N

(A)

Device Settings
Therapy: ON
Shock Zone: 240 bpm
Conditional Shock Zone: 220 bpm
Post Shock Pacing: ON

Gain Setting: 1X
Sensing Configuration: Primary
S = sense
P = Pace
N = Noise
T = Tachy Detection
C = Charge Start
. = Discard
/ = Shock
⬥ = Episode End

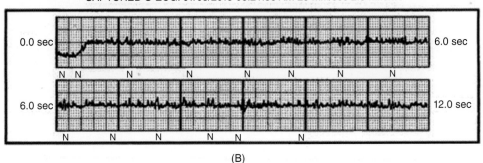

CAPTURED S-ECG: 01/05/2015 08:21:53 AM 25 mm/sec 2.5 mm/mV

0.0 sec   6.0 sec

N N   N   N   N   N   N   N

6.0 sec   12.0 sec

N   N   N   N   N   N

(B)

Figure 15.4 *Real time electrograms reveal "noise" signals on the alternate sensing vector (distal sense to proximal sense) (A) and primary sensing vector (proximal sense to can) (B) of a subcutaneous ICD (S-ICD, Boston Scientific Inc., Marlborough, MA) at 3 months follow up in a 17-year-old boy with hypertrophic cardiomyopathy and S-ICD for primary prevention of sudden death. The secondary vector (distal sense to can) is unaffected (C). At implant and at 1 month follow up, noise was not present on any of the three sense vectors. (D) Lateral view of the Chest X-ray at 3 months after implantation reveals that the subcutaneous electrode has retracted from its original position in the port probably secondary to a loose set screw. (E) Lateral view of the chest X-ray on day 1 after S-ICD implantation shows the subcutaneous electrode fully inserted in the port with the connector pin visible beyond the inner most connector ring. At implant, the secondary vector had been programmed in the sensing configuration, so oversensing and/or inappropriate shock did not occur.*

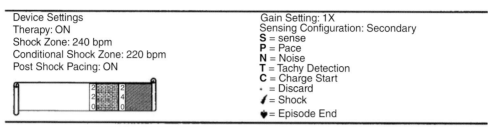

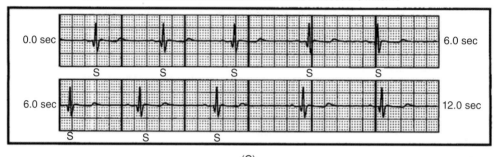

(C)

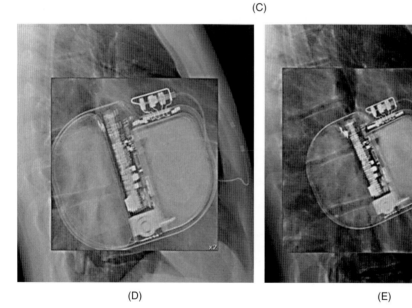

(D)   (E)

Figure 15.4 *(Continued)*

lengths. Evaluating the stored electrograms and associated marker annotations assists in identifying the source of the problem.

T-wave oversensing

T-wave oversensing is the most common over-sensing problem seen in ICDs and may cause inappropriate detection and therapy for VT or VF (Figure 15.5). Many pediatric patients who receive

an ICD have long QT syndrome or hypertrophic cardiomyopathy, two conditions that increase the risk of T-wave oversensing. Appropriate programming, vigilant remote monitoring, and exercise stress testing may serve to avoid this problem.[16] Programming appropriate ventricular sensing depends on the size of the R wave relative to the T wave. It may be necessary to investigate the various available bipolar sensing options when programming the sensing/detection

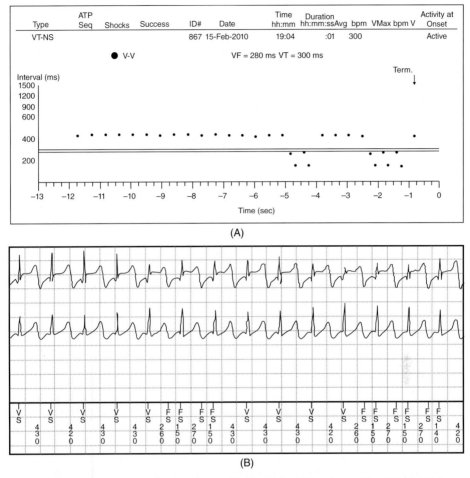

Figure 15.5 *Intermittent T-wave oversensing in a 12-year-old girl with long QT syndrome. The programmed R wave sensitivity was 0.3 mv and sensed R waves were 8 mv. A "railroad track pattern" on the plot of stored ventricular intervals is seen in (A). Cyclic oversensing often causes alternation of sensed ventricular cycle lengths that produces a characteristic railroad track pattern. (B) Following sensed normal sinus rhythm, the device intermittently senses events in the VF zone that correlate with T waves. From top to bottom, near field EGM, far field EGM, and markers. During T-wave oversensing, note that the R wave to T wave ratio has diminished in the near field EGM. In this case, decreasing the sensitivity to 0.45 mV corrected the problem but programming options may be limited if R waves are small. It is important that the near field EGMs are reviewed the ICD uses this signal for rate detection.*

channel. Along with tip to ring, additional options include tip to coil, and tip to can. If none of these maneuvers work, then ICD lead repositioning or replacement may be necessary.

P-wave oversensing

The sensing of atrial depolarization in the ventricular channel when there is 1:1 AV conduction results in double counting of the heart rate. However, oversensing of P waves during atrial fibrillation or atrial flutter can cause inappropriate detection and

therapy independent of the ventricular rate. P wave oversensing may occur when the distal coil of an integrated bipolar ICD lead is close to the tricuspid valve and the PR interval, interpreted as a sensed R-R, exceeds the ventricular blanking period. Children are particularly at risk due to their smaller intracardiac dimensions. This can be avoided by utilizing dedicated bipolar sensing, positioning the defibrillation lead in the RV apex, or when programmable, extending the ventricular blanking period.

R-wave double counting

R wave double counting occurs when the duration of the sensed ventricular electrogram exceeds the ventricular blanking period. The ventricular blanking period is typically 120–140 ms, though in some ICDs it is programmable. Patients are vulnerable to this event in the presence of QRS prolongation from fixed or rate related bundle branch block or from antiarrhythmic medications. Troubleshooting this problem may include adjusting medication or changing the sensing/detection channel.

Supraventricular tachycardia

Supraventricular tachycardia (SVT) often results in a rapid ventricular rate that exceeds the programmable rate detection zone. In adults, rapid conduction of atrial tachycardias misclassified by the ICD as ventricular tachycardia is the most common cause of inappropriate shocks.[17] While atrial fibrillation is uncommon in the pediatric population, sinus tachycardia from increased activity levels and elevated sinus rates exhibited in pediatric patients may result in inappropriate therapy. As patients with repaired congenital heart disease age, they are more likely to develop primary atrial arrhythmias, such as atrial flutter and atrial fibrillation.[18] Rapid ventricular response to these arrhythmias put them at risk for inappropriate shocks.

SVT-VT discriminators are a programmable feature of the detection algorithm that withholds therapy if the tachycardia is determined to be SVT. The features available are in part dependent on whether the patient has a dual chamber or single chamber device. Single chamber devices evaluate for interval stability, sudden onset, and analysis of ventricular electrogram morphology (Figure 15.6A–B). In single chamber ICDs,

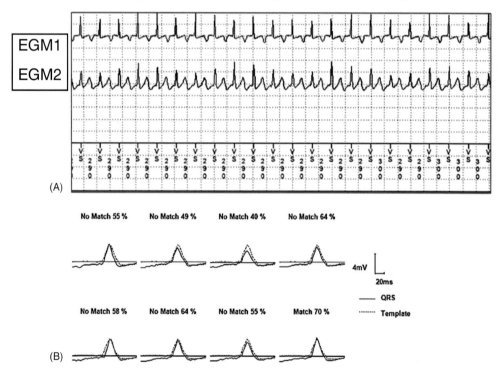

Figure 15.6 (A) Inappropriate detection of sinus tachycardia events as VT by Medtronic Wavelet ™ morphology alorithm due to electrogram attenuation issue. EGM1 is RV tip-RV ring (top), EGM2 is RV Coil-Can. Wavelet uses EGM2 as the source for template collection and comparison. The "match" threshold value was programmed to 70%. The programmed EGM2 R wave amplitude range was +/– 12 mV. (B) Wavelet™ requries at least three of the last eight QRS complexes to match the stored template, to withhold VT/VF detection but in this case only one QRS had a 70% match. Changing the R wave amplitude range to +/– 8 mV optimized Wavelet™ performance and resulted in correctly classifiying events as sinus tachycardia.

morphologic discriminators "stand alone," without any further discriminator, have been reported to correctly classify 75–90% of SVTs with a sensitivity for VT around 99%, that is superior to stability and onset working together (Figure 15.7A–D). They are to be used as single discriminators, with the others in "monitor mode" (passive) where available, so that they can be turned ON only when proven to add significant value to arrhythmia discrimination.[19] However, some discrimination failure modes may occur (Table 15.4). Dual chamber devices integrate single chamber discriminators with analysis of atrial rhythm. These features are automatic and designed to enhance sensitivity and specificity of detection, thus avoiding inappropriate therapy and delivering therapy when appropriate. The principles behind these algorithms can be applied by the clinician when evaluating an ICD patient who has received an ICD discharge or has events detected. In patients with a dual chamber device, if the detected atrial rate is greater than the ventricular rate, then the rhythm is almost certainly SVT. The exception is the development of VT in a patient with ongoing atrial flutter or atrial fibrillation. It is important that there is accurate sensing of atrial electrograms as atrial lead dislodgement, oversensing of far-field R waves, or atrial undersensing due to low amplitude electrograms, may result in misclassification of the arrhythmia. While the addition of an atrial lead may help distinguish SVT from VT, studies have demonstrated limited benefit and added expense when comparing dual-chamber to single-chamber ICDs with respect to inappropriate shocks.[20–22]

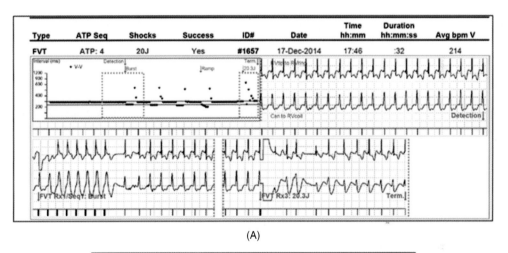

(A)

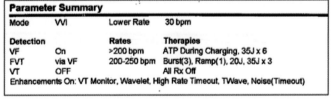

(B)

Figure 15.7 (A) Remote transmission showing ICD therapies (ATP followed by shock) for SVT (ventricular rate 214 bpm) in a 15-year-old boy with a single chamber ICD. (B) Ventricular tachycardia detection parameters and enhancements are shown. Note that SVT discrimination was programmed using the Medtronic Wavelet™ morphology algorithm. A high rate time out of 0.75 min was programmed (programmed length of time after which the device overrides SVT discrimination). (C) SVT was appropriately detected with the wavelet match. (D) Therapy was withheld for 51 s, after which the morphology algorithm timed out and tachycardia was subsequently detected in the fast VT zone. While this is an "inappropriate" ICD therapy for SVT, the ICD functioned exactly as it was programmed. From top to bottom, near field EGM, far field EGM, and markers.

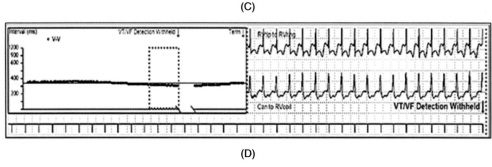

Wavelet Measurements Prior to Initial VT/VF Detection

Wavelet Result: SVT, but High Rate Timeout-VF Zone Only
Template Status: OK

-8. Match 82%
-7. Match 85%
-6. Match 79%
-5. Match 79%
-4. Match 79%
-3. Match 82%
-2. Match 82%
-1. Match 76%
0. Detection

(C)

(D)

Figure 15.7 *(Continued)*

Table 15.4 *Correcting ventricular electrogram morphology discriminator errors*

Potential Error	Possible Solution
• Inaccurate template	• Periodic template updates
• EGM truncation	• Adjust amplitude scale
• Alignment error	• Acquire template at tachycardia rates, alter minimum sensitivity, threshold start or threshold delay
• Myopotential oversensing	
• Rate related aberrancy	• Use alternate source of discriminator EGM
	• Reduce number of EGMs needed to exceed match threshold, reduce match score threshold (%), acquire template during aberrancy and consider deactivating automatic template updating

In pediatric and congenital heart disease patients, preventing sinus tachycardia from entering the programmed VT or VF zones has a significant impact on diminishing inappropriate ICD discharges. This can be achieved by limiting sinus tachycardia with beta blockade, setting a monitoring zone, and utilizing exercise stress testing to assess heart rate response.[16] Additionally, programming high detection rates and long detection duration results in a lower rate of inappropriate shocks without associated adverse events.[23] This has the added benefit of avoiding ICD therapy for episodes of nonsustained VT.

In summary, the three principal programming goals aimed to reduce inappropriate ICD shocks are to optimize SVT-VT discrimination, prevent oversensing, and prevent detection of nonsustained VT.[24] An additional strategy to decrease ICD shocks, whether appropriate or inappropriate, is to increase the use of antitachycardia pacing. This has been successfully expanded to rhythms categorized as rapid VT or VF zones, as the current ICDs provide antitachycardia pacing while the device is charging.[25] It is important to recognize the studies that demonstrated this benefit excluded patients considered unlikely to have the substrate for stable monomorphic VT. These conditions, particularly hypertrophic cardiomyopathy and long-QT syndrome, are common diagnoses in pediatric patients who receive an ICD.[4, 5]

Failure to deliver therapy

The failure of an ICD to deliver appropriate therapy in the event of VT or VF can have catastrophic
consequences. This may be due to ICD programming that result in failure to detect and/or treat VT
or VF, or unsuccessful therapy.

An avoidable and potentially tragic outcome
in a normally functioning device is the failure
to reprogram detection and therapy following a
surgical procedure or catheter ablation. ICDs are
routinely deactivated by programming therapy
to "off" or "monitor only" to avoid inappropriate
shocks if electrocautery or radiofrequency catheter
ablation is planned. It is critical to reprogram the
ICD to provide appropriate treatment following
the procedure. ICDs may be temporarily inhibited from providing therapy while a magnet is
applied over the pulse generator. Many of the
earlier generation ICDs could be deactivated by
30 s of magnet application. There are reports of
accidental deactivation by a magnetic field and
airport surveillance equipment resulting in patient
deaths.[26, 27] While temporary inhibition with a

magnet is still available, the feature of magnet
deactivation is not.

The basic algorithm for ICD therapy is the recognition of a ventricular rhythm that is categorized
as tachycardia by achieving a programmed rate.
It is possible to develop a slow VT that does not
meet the rate criterion (Figure 15.8A–C). Since the
heart rate criterion is a programmed feature, this is
dependent on how aggressively the physician sets
the device. The likelihood of developing a hemodynamically significant slow VT is greater in adults
with ischemic or non-ischemic cardiomyopathy
than in pediatric or congenital heart patients.[28]
It is important to consider the addition of antiarrhythmic medications which may decrease the rate
of clinical VT below the programmed detection
rate. Programming a monitoring zone will help
to identify this without increasing the delivery of
inappropriate ICD shocks.

Ventricular arrhythmias, particularly VF, may
be undersensed due to inadequately programmed
sensitivity, low amplitude electrograms, drug or
metabolic effects, or post-shock tissue changes.[29]

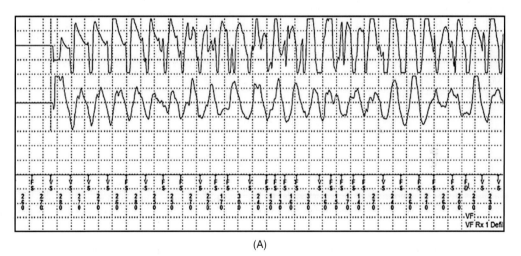

(A)

Figure 15.8 Failure of ICD therapy in a 16-year-old patient with hypertrophic cardiomyopathy. The ICD (EnTrust model
D154VRC, Medtronic., Inc.) was programmed with a single zone VF detection (rate greater than 222 bpm, initial number
of ventricular intervals detected 18/24, and 12/16 during redetection). From top to bottom, near field EGM, far field EGM,
and marker channels. (A) Correct detection of rapid VT as VF resulted in capacitor charging (VF Rx 1 Defib). (B) Note that
four out of five ventricular intervals (arrows) between capacitor charging and ending of charge cycle are greater than
310 ms (programmed VF interval + 60 ms). (C) The ICD shock was therefore aborted in accordance with manufacturer
specific device algorithm in which charge is delivered as a shock during the "confirmation" process only if the ventricular
cycle length after charging is less than the programmed VT interval + 60 ms. This algorithm was designed ostensibly to
prevent "committed shocks" for self-terminating arrhythmias. The patient was rescued with an automatic external
defibrillator shock and by-stander CPR.

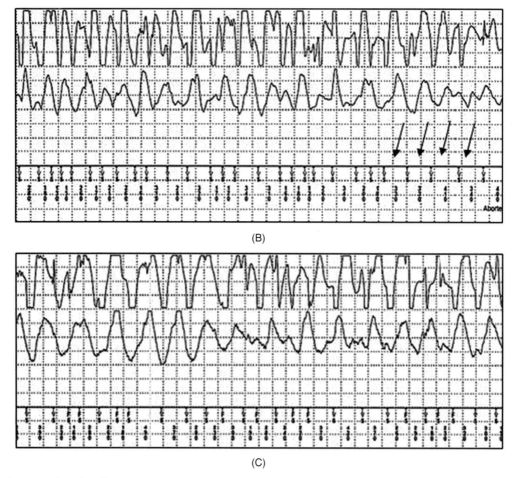

Figure 15.8 *(Continued)*

Clinically significant undersensing of VF is rare if the baseline R-wave amplitude is greater than 5 mV. However, in patients with degenerative myocardial disease such as arrhythmogenic right ventricular cardiomyopathy, the sensed R-wave amplitude may progressively diminish and compromise arrhythmia detection.[30]

Unsuccessful therapy

An ICD may appropriately detect VT or VF and deliver therapy, yet fail to terminate the ventricular arrhythmia. This may be due to patient related or ICD system related factors (Figure 15.9). Establishing defibrillation efficacy is performed at ICD implantation by inducing ventricular fibrillation and confirming that the implanted device is capable of successful defibrillation at various energy outputs.[31] Since defibrillation success is probabilistic, occasionally shocks fail to defibrillate, but failure of more than two maximum output shocks is rare if the safety margin is adequate. Patient related factors that raise defibrillation thresholds and may result in unsuccessful defibrillation include hyperkalemia, antiarrhythmic medications, ischemia, pericardial effusion, and progressive cardiac enlargement.

ICD system related causes of unsuccessful therapy include insufficient programmed shock strength, battery depletion, generator component failure, lead failure, device-lead connection failures, and lead dislodgment.[29] Interrogation of the device provides complete information regarding defibrillation settings, delivered shock strength,

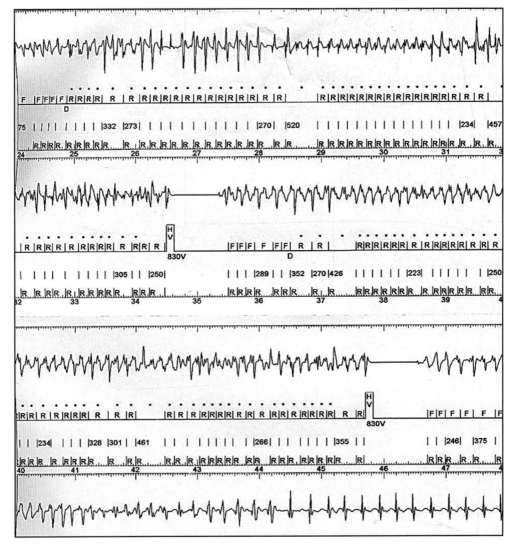

Figure 15.9 *Unsuccessful ICD therapy (2 shocks at 36 J) 3 months after implantation in a patient with rapid polymorphic VT correctly classified in the programmed VF zone (>222 bpm). After time marker 44, rhythm spontaneously converts to sinus. All ICD parameters were within normal limits suggesting that there was no lead of generator problem. Defibrillation threshold testing was successful at 10 J, suggesting that shock vectors were adequate. The most likely cause for inefficacious ICD therapy is a catecholamine triggered type ventricular tachycardia.*

battery strength, lead impedance trends, high voltage impedance, and the presence of noise due to a faulty connection. Lead failure rates are substantially higher in pediatric patients (5.6%/year) compared with adult patients (2%/year).[32] This may be due to mechanical stress exerted on the ICD leads as a result of somatic growth and increased activity in children. These factors may also contribute to lead dislodgment in pediatric patients, which can be typically diagnosed by chest X-ray. There are a number of pediatric and adult congenital patients who are not candidates for conventional transvenous leads because of small somatic size, limited venous capacitance, or structural heart disease with an intracardiac shunt or abnormal venous anatomy.[33] A variety of nontransvenous techniques have been reported including the use of a subcutaneous shock coil or the placement of an ICD lead within the pericardial space along the epicardial surface of the heart.[34] However, these various nontransvenous techniques have been reported to have a higher incidence of early failure rate compared with standard transvenous ICD systems.[35] Patients with these types of systems require careful surveillance to monitor for system failure.

Small caliber ICD lead failures

Small-diameter ICD leads, the Medtronic Sprint Fidelis, the St. Jude Riata, and Riata ST leads, were particularly attractive for pediatric patients because they were less likely to cause venous obstruction and tricuspid valve distortion. However, these leads were both recalled due to increased associated complications. The Fidelis lead had a high incidence of premature pace-sense conductor fracture, while the Riata leads were recalled due to premature insulation failure resulting in externalization of conductor cables.[36, 37] This problem was magnified in the pediatric population with a reported failure rate of these leads of 12.1%/year.[32] Complications associated with these leads include inappropriate shocks, failed shocks, cardiac perforation, inadequate sensing, and elevated pacing thresholds. Increased device surveillance, activation of the lead integrity alarm algorithms, and fluoroscopic evaluation are essential for identifying early lead failure.[3, 38]

ICD generator failures

ICD pulse generator failure, which fortunately is rare, may manifest as absence of telemetry, inappropriate shock, premature battery depletion, inability to interrogate or program, failure to charge or retain a charge, or failure to deliver therapy.[29, 40] Failed pulse generators should be explanted and returned to the manufacturer for analysis, and the incident should be reported to the FDA (Table 15.5). In the past two decades, a significant proportion of ICDs have been subject to FDA advisories. One pediatric study showed that 25% of ICD recipients had advisory/recalled devices at an average of 3.1 years of implant duration.[41]

Table 15.5 *ICD generator malfunction*

Components	Malfunction
Premature battery depletion	"No output" condition
Defective ICD crystal oscillator	Rapid pacing and induction of ventricular arrhythmia
Defective capacitor	Prolonged charge times
Weak header bonding	↑in shock coil impedance, associated with non-physiological noise
Fracture in ICD soldered connection	Loss of telemetry and device output
Hermetic seal disruption	Premature battery depletion, loss of telemetry and output
Jammed reed switch	Failure to deliver ICD therapy
Firmware abnormalities	Specific software malfunction

Conclusion

The implantable cardioverter-defibrillator has proven to be an extraordinary advancement in the treatment of patients at risk for life threatening ventricular arrhythmias. While technological improvements are continually introduced, these devices are not without problems. Improved outcomes and troubleshooting when necessary requires a thorough understanding of ICDs and ongoing patient surveillance, particularly in the pediatric and adult congenital population.

References

1 Goldberger Z, Lampert R. Implantable cardioverter-defibrillators: expanding indications and technologies. *JAMA* 2006; 295: 809–818.

2 Prystowsky EN, Nisam S. Prophylactic implantable cardioverter defibrillator trials: MUSTT, MADIT, and beyond. *Am J Cardiol* 2000; 86: 1214–1215.

3 Grimm W, Alter P, Maisch B. Arrhythmia risk stratification with regard to prophylactic implantable defibrillator therapy in patients with dilated cardiomyopathy. Results of MACAS, DEFINITE, and SCD-HeFT. *Herz* 2004; 29: 348–352.

4 Alexander ME, Cecchin F, Walsh EP, Triedman JK Bevilacqua LM, Berul CI. Implications of implantable cardioverter defibrillators in congenital heart disease and pediatrics. *J Cardiovasc Electrophysiol* 2004; 15: 72–76.

5 Etheridge SP, Sanatani S, Cohen MI, Albaro CA, Saarel EV, Bradley DJ. Long QT syndrome in children in the era of implantable defibrillators. *J Am Coll Cardiol* 2007; 50: 1335–1340.

6 Kozak LJ, Owings MF, Hall MJ. National hospital discharge survey: 2002 annual summary with detailed diagnosis and procedure data. *Viral Health Data* 2005; 13:1–199.

7 Shah MJ. Implantable cardioverter defibrillator-related complications in the pediatric population. *Pacing Clin Electrophysiol* 2009; 32: S71–S74.

8 Akar JG, Bao H, Jones P, Wang Y, Varosy P, Masoudi FA, et al. Use of remote monitoring is associated with lower risk of adverse outcomes among patients with implanted cardiac defibrillators. *Circ Arrhythm Electrophysiol* 2015; 114: epub.

9 Geiger MJ, O'Neill P, Sharma A, Skadsen A, Zimerman L, Greenfield RA, et al. Interactions between transvenous nonthoracotomy cardioverter defibrillator systems and permanent transvenous endocardial pacemakers. *Pacing Clin Electrophysiol* 1997; 20: 624–630.

10 Korte T, Koditz H, Niehaus M, Paul T, Tebbenhohanns J. High incidence of inappropriate ICD therapies in children and adolescents with implantable-cardioverter defibrillator. *Pacing Clin Electrophysiol* 2004; 27: 924–932.

11 Love BA, Barrett KD, Alexander ME, Bevilaqua LM, Epstein MR, Triedman JK, et al. Supraventricular arrhythmias in children and young adults with implantable cardioverter defibrillators. *J Cardiovasc Electrophysiol* 2001; 12: 1097–1101.

12 Lee SW, Moak JP, Lewis B. Inadvertent detection of 60-Hz alternating current by an implantable cardioverter defibrillator. *Pacing Clin Electrophysiol* 2002; 25: 518–551.

13 Sousa MD, Klein G, Korte T, Niehaus M. Electromagnetic interference in patients with implanted cardioverter-defibrillators and implantable loop recorders. *Indian Pacing Electrophysiol J* 2002; 2: 79–84.

14 Vlay SC. Fish pond electromagnetic interference resulting in an inappropriate resulting in an inappropriate implantable cardioverter defibrillator shock. *Pacing Clin Electrophysiol* 2002; 25: 1532.

15 Niehaus M, Neuzner J, Vogt J, Korte T, Tebbenjohanns J. Adjustment of maximum automatic sensitivity (automatic gain control) reduces inappropriate therapies in patients with implantable cardioverter defibrillators. *Pacing Clin Electrophysiol* 2002; 25: 151–155.

16 Cohen MI, Shaffer J, Pedersen S, Sims JJ, Papez A. Limited utility of exercise-stress testing to prevent T-wave oversensing in pediatric internal cardioverter

defibrillator recipients. *Pacing Clin Electrophysiol* 2011; 34: 436–442.

17 Thuens DA, Klootwijk AP, Goedhart DM, Jordaens L. Prevention of inappropriate therapy in implantable cardioverter-defibrillators: results of a prospective, randomized study of tachyarrhythmia detection algorithms. *J Am Coll Cardiol* 2004; 44: 2362–2367.

18 Trojinarska O, Grajek S, Kramer L, Gwizdala A. Risk factors of supraventricular arrhythmias in adults with congenital heart disease. *Cardiol J* 2009; 16: 218–226.

19 Boriani G, Occhetta E, Cesario S. Contribution of morphology discrimination algorithm for improving rhythm discrimination in slow and fast ventricular tachycardia zones in dual-chamber implantable cardioverter-defibrillators. *Europace.* 2008; 10: 918–925

20 Friedman PA, McClelland R, Bamlet W, Acosta J, Kessler D, Munger TM, et al. Dual-chamber versus single-chamber detection enhancements for implantable defibrillator rhythm diagnosis: The Detect supraventricular tachycardia study. *Circulation* 2006; 113: 2871–2879.

21 Thuens DA, Rivero-Ayerza M, Boersma E, Jordaens L. Prevention of inappropriate therapy in implantable defibrillators: a meta-analysis of clinical trials comparing single-chamber and dual-chamber arrhythmia discrimination algorithms. *Int J Cardiol* 2008; 125: 352–357.

22 Friedman PA, Bradley D, Koestler C, Slusser J, Hodge D, Bailey K, et al. A prospective randomized trial of single or dual-chamber implantable cardioverter-defibrillators to minimize inappropriate shock risk in primary sudden cardiac death prevention. *Europace* 2014; 16: 1460–1468.

23 Garnreiter JM, Pilcher TA, Etheridge SP, Saarel EV. Inappropriate ICD shocks in pediatrics and congenital heart disease patients: Risk factors and programming strategies. *Heart Rhythm* 2015; 12: 937–942.

24 Swerdlow CD, Freidman PA. Advanced ICD Troubleshooting: Part I. *Pacing Clin Electrophysiol* 2005; 28: 1322–1346.

25 Wathen MS, DeGroot PJ, Sweeney MO, Stark AJ, Otterness MF, Adkisson WO, et al; for the PainFree Rx II Investigators. Prospective randomized multicenter trial of empirical antitachycardia pacing versus shocks for spontaneous rapid ventricular tachycardia in patients with implantable cardioverter-defibrillators: Pacing fast ventricular tachycardia reduces shock therapies (PainFREE Rx II) trial results. *Circulation* 2004; 110: 2591–2596.

26 Junge M, Weckmuller J, Nagele H, Puschel K. "Natural death" of a patient with a deactivated implantable cardioverter defibrillator (ICD)? *Forens Sci Int* 2002; 125: 172–177.

27 Pires LA, Hull ML, Nino CL, May LM, Ganji JR. Sudden death in recipients of transvenous implantable cardioverter defibrillator systems: terminal events, predictors, and potential mechanisms. *J Cardiovasc Electrophysiol* 1999; 10: 1049–1056.

28 Bansch D, Castrucci M, Bocker D, Breithardt G, Block M. Ventricular tachycardia above the initially programmed tachycardia detection interval in patients with implantable cardioverter-defibrillators: Incidence, prediction, and significance. *J Am Coll Cardiol* 2000; 36: 557–565.

29 Swerdlow CD, Freidman PA. Advanced ICD Troubleshooting: Part II. *Pacing Clin Electrophysiol* 2006; 29: 70–96.

30 Mugnai G, Tomei R, Dugo C, Tomasi L, Morani G, Vassanelli C. Implantable cardioverter-defibrillators in patients with arrhythmogenic right ventricular cardiomyopathy: the course of electronic parameters, clinical features, and complications during long-term follow-up. *J Interv Card Electrophysiol* 2014; 41: 23–29.

31 Strickberger SA, Man KC, Souza J, Zivin A, Weiss R, Knight BP, et al. A prospective evaluation of two defibrillation safety margin techniques in patients with low defibrillation energy requirements. *J Cardiovasc Electrophysiol* 1998; 9: 41–46.

32 Janson CM, Patel AR, Bonny WJ, Smoots K, Shah MJ. Implantable cardioverter-defibrillator lead failure in children and young adults: a matter of lead diameter or lead design? *J Am Coll Cardiol* 2014; 63: 133–140.

33 Berul CI. Defibrillator indications and implantation in young children. *Heart Rhythm* 2008; 5: 1755–1757.

34 Stephenson EA, Batra AS, Knilans TK, Gow RM, Gradaus R, Balaji S, et al. A multicenter experience with novel implantable cardioverter defibrillator configurations in the pediatric and congenital heart disease population. *J Cardiovasc Electrophysiol* 2006; 17: 41–46.

35 Radbill AE, Triedman JK, Berul CI, Fynn-Thompson F, Atallah J, Alexander ME, et al. System survival of nontransvenous implantable cardioverter-defibrillators compared to transvenous implantable cardioverter-defibrillators in pediatric and congenital heart disease. *Heart Rhythm* 2010; 7: 193–198.

36 Hauser RG, Hayes DL. Increasing hazard of Sprint Fidelis implantable cardioverter-defibrillator lead failure. *Heart Rhythm* 2009; 6: 605–610.

37 Hauser RG, McGriff D, Retel LK. Riata implantable cardioverter-defibrillator lead failure analysis of explanted leads with a unique insulation defect. *Heart Rhythm* 2012; 9: 742–749.

38 Kallinen LM, Hauser RG, Tang C, Melby DP, Almquist AK, Katsiyiannis WT, Gornick CC. Lead integrity alert algorithm decreases inappropriate shocks in patients who have Sprint Fidelis pace-sense conductor fractures. *Heart Rhythm* 2010; 7: 1048–1055.

39 Dorman HG, van Opstal JM, Stevenhagen J, Scholten MF. Conductor externalization of the Riata internal cardioverter-defibrillator lead: tip of the iceberg? Report of three cases and review of literature. *Europace* 2012; 14: 1161–1164.

40 Lau KC, Shah MJ. Subcutaneous implantable cardioverter defibrillator device malfunction: first report of a "high current" condition triggering device failure. *J Interv Card Electrophysiol*. 2015 Jun; 43(1): 77.

41 Mahajan T, Dubin AM, Atkins DL, Bradley DJ, Shannon KM, Erickson CC, et al; Members of the Pediatric and Congenital Electrophysiology Society. Impact of manufacturer advisories and FDA recalls of implantable cardioverter defibrillator generators in pediatric and congenital heart disease patients. *J Cardiovasc Electrophysiol*. 2008 Dec; 19(12): 1270–1274.

16 CHAPTER 16

CRT device programming and optimization

Anoop Singh[1] and Seshadri Balaji[2]

[1]Director, Cardiac Electrophysiology, Children's Hospital of Wisconsin, Assistant Professor, Medical College of Wisconsin, Milkwaukee, WI, USA

[2]Director, Arrhythmias Pacing and Electrophysiology, Doernbecher Children's Hospital, Professor of Pediatrics (Cardiology), Oregon Health & Science University, Portland, OR, USA

Introduction

Cardiac resynchronization therapy (CRT) has been proven to be beneficial in adults with cardiomyopathy.[1, 2] In children, the utility of CRT is less certain, with evidence mainly coming from smaller studies in patients with cardiomyopathy secondary to congenital heart block, congenital heart disease, and dilated cardiomyopathy.[3–5] Once the patient has been selected and the CRT system implanted (discussed in previous chapters), the focus now shifts to programming the device and measuring the patient's response. This chapter details the initial programming of the CRT device in the peri-implant period; the subsequent optimization for poor responders; and the available techniques for monitoring response and guiding manipulation of resynchronization therapy.

At present, pediatric studies have focused mainly on patient selection and implantation techniques. Indeed, current literature searches reveal only a few case reports that detail optimization in children.[6–8] Thus, most evidence for CRT programming and optimization is derived from adult studies that are based primarily on patients with LBBB and ischemic or non-ischemic cardiomyopathy. Since pacing-induced cardiomyopathy[5] has been the commonest indication for CRT in pediatrics and ACHD, we must be circumspect in extrapolating adult data to pediatric and ACHD patients.

Programming the device

At the time of implant, atrial sensing and capture should be assessed by standard methods. Both right ventricular (RV) and left ventricular (LV) capture must be demonstrated independent of each other. This is best done by using VVI mode at a rate faster than the patient's intrinsic rate to assess ventricular threshold for the RV and then LV leads.

The electrocardiogram (ECG) can be useful to confirm pacing capture depending on the site of pacing. RVOT pacing demonstrates positive QRS complexes in the inferior leads; RV apical pacing shows a superior QRS axis with LBBB pattern; and LV pacing produces positive QRS complexes in the right precordial leads and a rightward axis (Figure 16.1). The exact QRS morphology with BV pacing varies depending on the sequential offset between RV and LV pacing, but BV pacing commonly produces a narrower QRS complex than RV or LV pacing alone. Malposition of the

Cardiac Pacing and Defibrillation in Pediatric and Congenital Heart Disease, First Edition.
Edited by Maully Shah, Larry Rhodes and Jonathan Kaltman.
© 2017 John Wiley & Sons Ltd. Published 2017 by John Wiley & Sons Ltd.
Companion Website: www.wiley.com/go/shah/cardiac_pacing

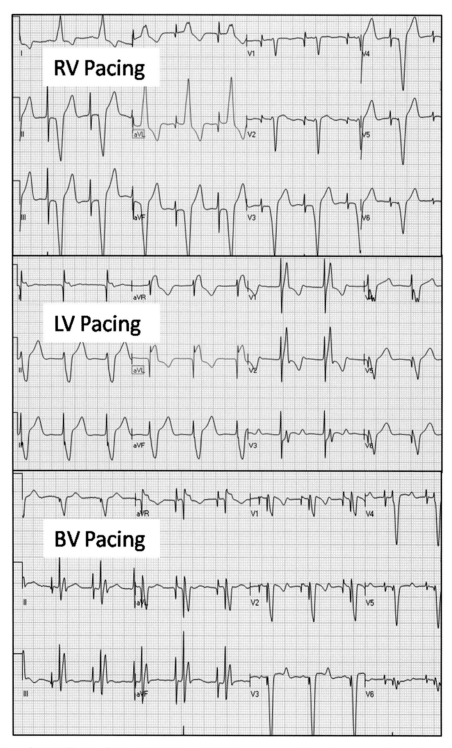

Figure 16.1 *Electrocardiogram during right ventricular (RV); left ventricular (LV) and biventricular (BV) pacing.*

heart within the thoracic cavity (e.g., mesocardia or dextrocardia) may alter the baseline ECG and invalidate these electrocardiographic patterns for confirming RV or LV capture. Moreover, in patients with single ventricles, ECG patterns with multi-site ventricular pacing will depend on the anatomy and positioning of the epicardial leads. The demonstration of three distinct, paced QRS morphologies is reasonable proof of ventricular capture from the individual RV and LV leads and their combined output resulting in BV capture.

AV delay

Dual chamber and multisite pacing systems are generally programmed in DDD mode, but VDD is acceptable in patients without sinus node dysfunction. Programming the AV delay should provide sufficient time for atrial contraction to augment ventricular filling while avoiding prolonged isovolumic contraction or loss of biventricular pacing (in the patient with intrinsic AV conduction). Previous studies evaluated invasive hemodynamic parameters such as LVEDP, LV + dP/dT, and blood pressure to guide AV delay programming.[9] While this data supports the concept of an ideal AV delay for each patient these methods are, by and large, impractical for clinicians. The SMART AV trial examined the issue of programming AV delay, comparing three different methods, and found no difference in LV end-systolic volumes between the three methods.[10] Our preferred technique is to use a sensed AV delay of 120 ms and a paced AV delay of 150 ms at implant for adolescents and adults. Subsequent AV delay adjustment can be performed with echocardiography utilizing pulsed Doppler techniques. The optimal AV delay should be long enough to avoid truncating the A-wave but short enough to avoid intrinsic conduction.

VV offset

Older CRT systems paced right and left ventricles simultaneously while current systems offer VV offsets that allow either RV or LV preactivation. Programming simultaneous ventricular pacing is reasonable at implant. However, if there is significant, pre-operative, interventricular dyssynchrony, this may need to be adjusted and sequential BV pacing may need to be programmed prior to hospital discharge. Subsequent modification of the AV

and VV delays using non-invasive techniques will be discussed later in the section on optimization.

Monitoring CRT response

Follow-up visits for devices evaluate the pacemaker pocket site and troubleshoot patient complaints that may be device related. We generally recommend a first follow up at 6 weeks post implant. All devices should have thresholds re-measured and biventricular pacing confirmed via ECG. Most responders to CRT demonstrate a narrower QRS complex compared to their pre-implant baseline. For new CRT systems, these visits also serve as the opportunity to quantify the response to resynchronization therapy. CRT response is assessed primarily by echocardiography, but patient symptoms must be reviewed. The patient's heart failure status is ideally corroborated by objective data such as an exercise stress test or a 6-minute walk test.

Ideally, all patients, regardless of functional status should have some testing to assess cardiac function. We prefer ejection fraction to fractional shortening, as the latter can give meaningless results in patients with septal to free wall dyssynchrony. EF, however, is hard to quantify by echocardiography, especially in patients with congenital heart disease. At least 2D fractional area change should be estimated/measured. Theoretically, 3D echocardiography provides a more accurate assessment of ventricular function than standard 2D techniques. In addition, 3D-derived RV volumes and ejection fractions are comparable to that obtained with MRI in patients with congenital heart disease.[11] For obvious reasons, MRI scanning is not practical as a way to follow ventricular function. CT scanning may be used, but, in most cases, the use of radiation is not worth the benefit. Nuclear medicine techniques (MUGA scan) can be a useful way to follow the global ventricular function in patients with poor echocardiographic windows.

CRT optimization

Any patient with a suboptimal response to CRT (based on clinical, functional or imaging parameters) should have adjustments to the CRT system (optimization) performed. Early adult studies in

CRT demonstrated a non-responder prevalence of up to 30% while the pediatric and adult congenital CRT studies show a non-responder prevalence of 12–19%.[3-5] Thus, there has been significant interest in improving the response to CRT, and consequently there has been much research effort investigating methods for optimization. This section reviews available options for optimization. As discussed previously, AV delay and VV offset are the two main optimization parameters. Although we will discuss them separately it should be noted that manipulation of VV timing could affect AV optimization.

AV optimization

The Ritter method for AV optimization was originally developed for dual chamber pacemakers. A pulse wave Doppler across the mitral valve is obtained at a long and short AV delay. QRS onset to A wave offset (QA) is measured at the long and short AV delays. The optimal AV delay = $AV_{long} - (QA_{short} - QA_{long})$.

The iterative technique for AV delay optimization was used in the CARE-HF trial.[1] A long AV delay is programmed during pulse Doppler across the mitral valve. The AV delay is shortened by 20 ms increments until A wave truncation occurs due to premature mitral valve closure. At this point the AV delay is increased by 10 ms increments until A wave truncation is no longer seen.

While the Ritter or iterative methods assess diastolic parameters, the aortic valve VTI technique evaluates systolic function. For each AV delay selected, VTI is calculated from the continuous wave Doppler across the aortic valve. The optimal AV delay results in the maximal VTI.

At present, fixed AV delays are recommended when programming devices. However, the optimal AV delay in the clinic setting may not equate to the optimal AV delay when patients are exerting themselves. Data suggests that the optimal AV delay at higher heart rates is shortened in patients with CRT systems.[12] Unfortunately, at present it is not clear how rate-adaptive AV delays should be programmed for patients with CRT systems.

VV optimization

Preactivation of the right or left ventricle can improve CRT response in some patients. Global assessment of function via EF or aortic VTI during VV manipulation may demonstrate obvious improvements. However, in non-responders we recommend an assessment of interventricular and intraventricular dyssynchrony.

M-mode: M-mode has been used to demonstrate dyssynchrony in selecting candidates for CRT and can give a rough assessment of intraventricular dyssynchrony. Septal to posterior wall motion delay can be calculated as the time in peak difference between the two segments (Figure 16.2). VV adjustments that result in shortened delay should improve synchrony.

Doppler: Interventricular dyssynchrony can be modified by comparing RV and LV ejection timing. Pulse Doppler of the RVOT and LVOT is performed and timing from QRS onset to ejection Doppler onset is measured (Figure 16.3). The VV offset is adjusted to minimize interventricular dyssynchrony.

Tissue Doppler: Unlike conventional Doppler that assesses high velocity signals from the blood pool, tissue Doppler measures the low velocity signals of myocardial movement. The timing to peak systolic contraction can be analyzed for multiple segments, providing a measure of ventricular synchrony. However, velocity assessment alone cannot distinguish hypokinetic segments

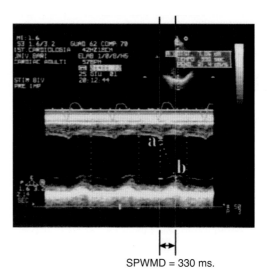

SPWMD = 330 ms.

Figure 16.2 *Use of M-mode echocardiography to assess intraventricular dyssynchrony. (Source: Pitzalis 2002. Reproduced with permission of Elsevier.)*

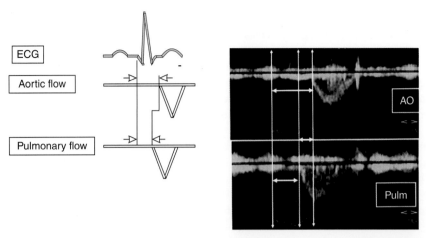

Figure 16.3 *Using Doppler echocardiography to assess interventricular dyssynchrony. (Source: Bax 2004. Reproduced with permission of Elsevier.)*

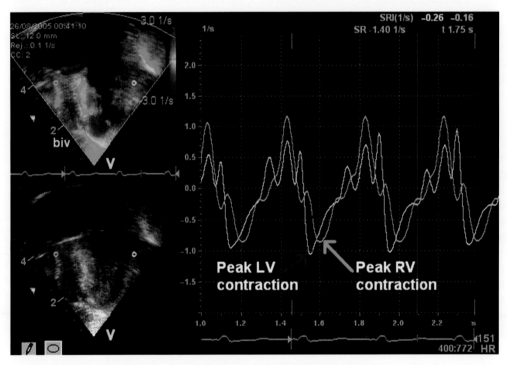

Figure 16.4 *Using strain and strain rate from tissue Doppler to evaluate dyssynchrony.*

from late activating myocardium. Strain and strain rate (Figure 16.4) can isolate these electrically dyssynchronous segments by evaluating contraction and expansion of discrete segments (strain) and the rate of deformational change (strain rate). Sogaard[13] used tissue Doppler assessment to create a 16 segment LV model for different VV delays. Longitudinal motion toward the apex was summed for the 16 segments. The VV offset that resulted in the largest, summed ventricular amplitude was chosen as the optimal VV setting. This VV optimization correlated with improved EF compared to simultaneous biventricular pacing.

Similarly, Tissue Synchronization Imaging uses tissue Doppler to measure timing to peak velocity of individual myocardial segments. A color-coded map is created that distinguishes early from late activating segments. Visual assessment of the color map guides VV manipulation with the aim of eliminating or minimizing electrically dyssynchronous areas.

Myocardial tissue has areas that reflect acoustic signals during ultrasound. These "speckles" can be tracked from frame to frame, producing an angle independent technique for calculating strain and strain rate. Speckle tracking of the right and/or left ventricle can assess radial, longitudinal, and circumferential strain. Radial strain signifies myocardial thickening in the short axis view, circumferential strain represents myocardial shortening in the short axis plane, and longitudinal strain characterizes myocardial shortening in the long axis plane. Segmental strain curves are plotted using software and the peaks are analyzed for timing. VV offset is adjusted to minimize the timing from earliest to latest contracting segments (Figure 16.5).

Three-dimensional echocardiography has been utilized as a technique for demonstrating dyssynchrony, guiding lead placement, and assessing acute response to CRT (Figure 16.6). A few studies have shown that 3D analysis of dyssynchrony can be done real-time and reasonably quickly. The main advantage of 3D is that it is a global rather than regional technique. However, there are some significant disadvantages including: acquisition time, patient cooperation for good windows, and the potential misinterpretation of data based on poor tracking in one segment that affects the entire geometry. Lastly, one main difference between 3D versus 2D is the lower frame rate that could lead to decreased accuracy of its findings, although, to date, studies have not shown any significant loss of fidelity from this. Future studies will likely investigate the potential for 3D echocardiography as a tool for optimization.

Electrocardiography is useful is selecting CRT candidates and remains an important tool in assessing the response. During follow-up visits, the VV offset is adjusted during ECG recordings. The optimal VV offset produces the narrowest QRS complex. This technique is a practical method for CRT optimization in the clinic setting and has shown promise when compared to TDI.[14]

At present there is no single method that has shown superiority and many optimization studies have used them as complementary techniques. Electrophysiology and echocardiography practitioners should focus on two or three of these techniques, based on the equipment and technology available at their center, and gain expertise as optimization is applied to their patients. Importantly, if a patient was identified as a candidate for CRT based on a particular technique then that methodology is the natural first choice for optimization.

Optimization in pediatrics and congenital heart disease

Optimization techniques have been applied with success in pediatric case reports.[6,7] For young children imaging windows may be superior to that seen with adults, but this advantage may be compromised in the uncooperative patient. Echocardiographic images need to be obtained at multiple AV and VV settings which can be time consuming and may affect the steady state of patient hemodynamics.

Systemic right and single ventricles pose a unique challenge for pediatric and adult congenital heart disease resynchronization. RV and single ventricle geometry differ from LV geometry, which is relevant for tracing borders in these patients. And while CRT can improve their EF, significant tricuspid (or AV valve) regurgitation can persist. Thus, CRT optimization in patients with systemic right or single ventricles should include assessment of tricuspid/AV valve regurgitation in addition to dyssynchrony.

Conclusion

The utility of CRT is undeniable but for some patients the benefit is minimal. For these patients, optimization techniques can improve the CRT response. Since no universal optimization technique exists it is important for the practitioner to familiarize him/herself with a few methods, apply them to the patients, and monitor their response.

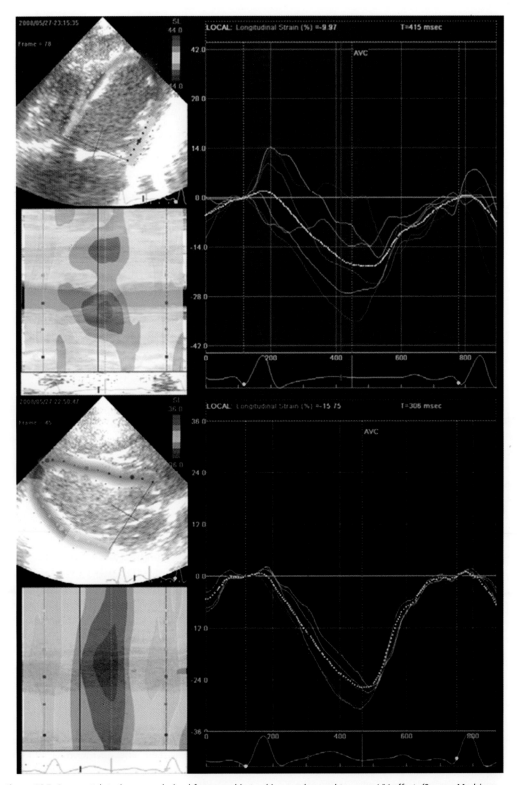

Figure 16.5 *Segmental strain curves derived from speckle tracking can be used to assess VV offset. (Source: Madriago 2010. Reproduced with permission of Elsevier.)*

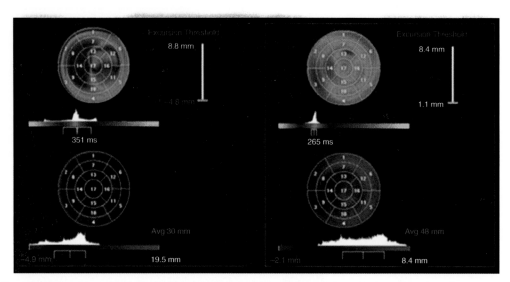

Figure 16.6 *Three-dimensional echocardiography can be used to assess dyssynchrony in three dimensions. (Source: Porciani 2008. Reproduced with permission of John Wiley & Sons, Inc.)*

References

1 Cleland JG, Daubert JC, Erdmann E, Freemantle N, Gras D, Kappenberger L, Tavazzi L. The effect of cardiac resynchronization on morbidity and mortality in heart failure. *N Engl J Med*. 2005; 352(15): 1539–1549.

2 Anand IS, Carson P, Galle E, Song R, Boehmer J, Ghali JK, et al. Cardiac resynchronization therapy reduces the risk of hospitalizations in patients with advanced heart failure: results from the Comparison of Medical Therapy, Pacing and Defibrillation in Heart Failure (COMPANION) trial. *Circulation*. 2009; 119(7): 969–977.

3 Cecchin F, Frangini PA, Brown DW, Fynn-Thompson F, Alexander ME, Triedman JK, et al. Cardiac resynchronization therapy (and multisite pacing) in pediatrics and congenital heart disease: five years experience in a single institution. *J Cardiovasc Electrophysiol*. 2009; 20(1): 58–65.

4 Dubin AM, Janousek J, Rhee E, Strieper MJ, Cecchin F, Law IH, et al. Resynchronization therapy in pediatric and congenital heart disease patients: an international multicenter study. *J Am Coll Cardiol*. 2005; 46(12): 2277–2283.

5 Janousek J, Gebauer RA, Abdul-Khaliq H, Turner M, Kornyei L, Grollmuss O, et al. Cardiac resynchronisation therapy in paediatric and congenital heart disease: differential effects in various anatomical and functional substrates. *Heart*. 2009; 95(14): 1165–1171.

6 Jeewa A, Potts MT, Sanatani S, Duncan WJ. Echocardiographic tools for pacemaker optimization of ventricular function in an infant following surgical repair for double outlet right ventricle. *Can J Cardiol*. 26(10): e353–355.

7 Madriago E, Sahn DJ, Balaji S. Optimization of myocardial strain imaging and speckle tracking for resynchronization after congenital heart surgery in children. *Europace* 12(9): 1341–1343.

8 Roofthooft MT, Blom NA, Rijlaarsdam ME, Bokenkamp R, Ottenkamp J, Schalij MJ, et al. Resynchronization therapy after congenital heart surgery to improve left ventricular function. *Pacing Clin Electrophysiol*. 2003; 26(10): 2042–2044.

9 Auricchio A, Stellbrink C, Block M, Sack S, Vogt J, Bakker P, et al. Effect of pacing chamber and atrioventricular delay on acute systolic function of paced patients with congestive heart failure. The Pacing Therapies for Congestive Heart Failure Study Group. The Guidant Congestive Heart Failure Research Group. *Circulation*. 1999; 99(23): 2993–3001.

10 Ellenbogen KA, Gold MR, Meyer TE, Fernndez Lozano I, Mittal S, Waggoner AD, et al. Primary results from the SmartDelay determined AV optimization: a comparison to other AV delay methods used in cardiac resynchronization therapy (SMART-AV) trial: a randomized trial comparing empirical, echocardiography-guided, and algorithmic atrioventricular delay programming in cardiac resynchronization therapy. *Circulation*. 122(25): 2660–2668.

11 Grewal J, Majdalany D, Syed I, Pellikka P, Warnes CA. Three-dimensional echocardiographic assessment of right ventricular volume and function in adult patients with congenital heart disease: comparison with magnetic resonance imaging. *J Am Soc Echocardiogr*. 23(2): 127–133.

12 Sun JP, Lee AP, Grimm RA, Hung MJ, Yang XS, Delurgio D, et al. Optimisation of atrioventricular delay during exercise improves cardiac output in patients stabilised with cardiac resynchronisation therapy. *Heart* 2012 Jan; 98(1): 54–59.

13 Sogaard P, Egeblad H, Kim WY, Jensen HK, Pedersen AK, Kristensen BO, Mortensen PT. Tissue Doppler imaging predicts improved systolic performance and reversed left ventricular remodeling during long-term cardiac resynchronization therapy. *J Am Coll Cardiol.* 2002; 40(4): 723–730.

14 Tamborero D, Vidal B, Tolosana JM, Sitges M, Berruezo A, Silva E, et al. Electrocardiographic versus echocardiographic optimization of the interventricular pacing delay in patients undergoing cardiac resynchronization therapy. *J Cardiovasc Electrophysiol.* 22(10): 1129–1134.

CHAPTER 17

Implantable syncope and arrhythmia monitors, and automated external defibrillators

John R. Phillips[1] and Pamela S. Ro[2]

[1]Chief, Pediatric Cardiology, Robert C. Byrd Health Sciences Center, Professor, Department of Pediatrics, WVU Children's Hospital, Morgantown, WV, USA

[2]Pediatric Electrophysiologist, North Carolina Children's Heart Center, North Carolina Children's Hospital, Associate Professor of Pediatrics, The University of North Carolina at Chapel Hill, Chapel Hill, NC, USA

Introduction

The practice of pediatric medicine is rarely an exact science. Unlike in the adult population, large scale, randomized, prospective studies are few in pediatrics. Through innovation and experience, pediatric cardiologists translate and mold adult practices to benefit the children they care for. In this way, implantable syncope and arrhythmia monitors, and automated external defibrillators have been added to the armamentarium of diagnostic and treatment options for children with arrhythmias. In this chapter, the utility of implantable syncope and arrhythmia monitors and automated external defibrillators will be discussed.

Implantable loop recorders

Indications for implantable loop recorders

Syncope and palpitations occur frequently in young patients and are a common reason for referral to pediatric cardiologists,[1–3] yet, syncope and palpitations are symptoms rather than diagnoses. Syncope is a transient, self-limited loss of consciousness and voluntary muscle tone. Palpitations refer to an appreciation of one's own heartbeat, due to an alteration in rate, rhythm, or strength of the contraction. Determining the etiology of these symptoms is often challenging and perplexing, particularly in the pediatric population where obtaining a history may be difficult. Although these symptoms are frequently benign, they are a source of anxiety for patients and their parents and may herald significant heart disease or potentially lethal problems. Studies have shown that patients with congenital heart disease have an increased incidence of malignant arrhythmias, including atrioventricular conduction disturbances, ventricular tachycardia, and rapid conduction of atrial arrhythmias.[4–7] Therefore, identifying underlying causes of syncope and palpitations is imperative to institute appropriate therapy.

Substrates for malignant arrhythmias may often be diagnosed by patient history, family history, and physical examination alone. Electrocardiography

Cardiac Pacing and Defibrillation in Pediatric and Congenital Heart Disease, First Edition.
Edited by Maully Shah, Larry Rhodes and Jonathan Kaltman.
© 2017 John Wiley & Sons Ltd. Published 2017 by John Wiley & Sons Ltd.
Companion Website: www.wiley.com/go/shah/cardiac_pacing

adds information by detecting diagnoses including Wolff–Parkinson–White syndrome, long QT syndrome, and Brugada syndrome. However, syncope and palpitations usually occur randomly or infrequently so that correlating the patient's rhythm with their symptoms proves difficult. Continuous rhythm assessment with ambulatory Holter monitors are useful in correlating symptoms with the heart rhythm only if the patient is symptomatic during the monitoring period.[8, 9] External loop recorders and transtelephonic monitors aid in recording a patient's rhythm during symptoms but their usefulness may be limited by the patient's ability to activate the device prior to cessation of symptoms, the physical size of the device, the patient's ability to sleep comfortably or participate in activities with the device, and sensitivity of the skin to long-term electrode placement. Studies show the diagnostic yield of external loop recorders ranging from 24–47% with the highest yield in patients with frequent events.[10-13] Evaluation of syncope with head upright tilt table testing can be useful. Tilt table testing attempts

to reproduce symptoms in a controlled setting while documenting the patient's rhythm and vital signs. However, symptoms can be induced in a large number of asymptomatic adolescents, thus decreasing the specificity of the test while failing to conclusively exclude a malignant etiology.[14]

The optimal diagnostic test for patients with recurrent syncope or palpitations must have the ability to monitor over long periods of time with automatic detection of abnormalities and manual capture of rhythm analysis during symptoms (Figure 17.1). The implantable loop recorder (ILR) has the capability of performing all of these actions. An ILR provides long-term monitoring of infrequent symptoms without external electrodes, and the device incorporates a continuous loop recording of the heart rhythm that can be stored automatically or when activated by the patient or a bystander.[15] Its use avoids compliance issues often seen with external monitoring devices. The ILR records a high fidelity bipolar ECG signal stored as a loop.[16] The use of an ILR was first reported in

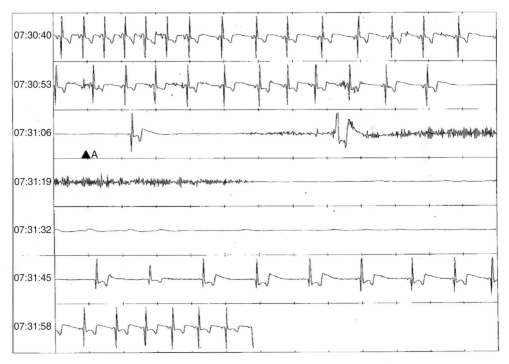

Figure 17.1 *ILR recording from a 4-year-old girl with multiple syncopal episodes. Previous work-up was negative or unable to be performed secondary to lack of patient cooperation.*

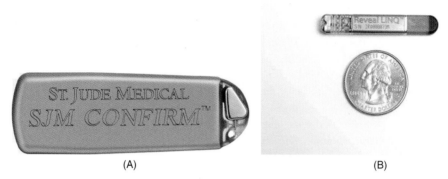

Figure 17.2 *(A) Example of an ILR model. (B) Example of a recent small ILR model.*

1997[10, 17, 18] with subsequent approval of the US Food and Drug Administration (FDA).[19]

Currently, there are two FDA approved ILRs. The device size ranges from 4.5–5.6 cm long, 0.7–1.9 cm wide, 0.4–0.8 cm thick, and weighs 2.5–12 g (Figure 17.2A and B). The battery life is approximately 3 years. Devices are implanted subcutaneously in the chest wall typically to the right or left of the sternum. Abdominal, submammary, and subaxillary implantation have been described in small children.[15, 20] The procedure may be done under local anesthetic depending on patient cooperation. Antibiotic prophylaxis generally is recommended. Prior to implantation, cutaneous mapping with the device is advised to optimize the sensed signal and decrease T-wave oversensing that may be falsely interpreted as a high rate episode. The duration of recording prior to and after an event is programmable with a total recording time of 48–50 min. As mentioned previously, ILR recordings can be auto-triggered or patient-activated.[21] Current versions of ILRs have programmable automatic detection of rapid and slow heart rate episodes as well as pauses.[22] The current algorithms sense R waves rather than signals originating from the atrium. Disadvantages of ILRs include sensing of muscle motion and other artifacts.

Implantable loop recorders first saw clinical use in the adult realm. The population was 16 adult patients who were highly symptomatic with recurrent unexplained syncope.[23] These patients had a mean of 8.4 ± 4.4 previous episodes of syncope. All patients had a negative work-up, including ambulatory Holter monitoring, tilt table testing, and electrophysiological studies. After undergoing device implantation, 15 of 16 patients (94%) had recurrent syncope during a mean of 13 ± 8.4 months of follow-up. For those 15 patients, a diagnosis was obtained in all with symptom-rhythm correlation in 9 patients (60%). Treatment was initiated in all with no recurrence of syncope at the time the study was terminated.

Adult trials utilizing ILRs

There have been two randomized trials utilizing ILRs in the adult population. Both studies compared the role of ILR with conventional investigation and management. The first, Randomized Assessment of Syncope Trial (RAST), involved 60 consecutive patients who were evaluated by a syncope service.[24] These patients had either recurrent unexplained syncope or a single episode of syncope with injury significant enough to warrant further investigation. Half the patients had an ILR implanted; the other half had prolonged external monitoring, tilt table testing, and electrophysiology study. If the original evaluation did not yield a diagnosis, the patients were offered the option of crossover to the alternative strategy. A diagnosis was established in 14 patients in the ILR arm versus 6 patients in the conventional arm (52% vs 20%, p = 0.012). There were 6 patients in the ILR arm and 21 patients in the conventional arm that crossed over. Overall, with combination of the primary arm and crossover, the ILR arm established a diagnosis in 55% of the patients compared with 19% in the conventional arm (p = 0.0014).

The second randomized study was the East-bourne Syncope Assessment Study (EasyAS).[25] There were 201 patients from a single institution who had recurrent syncope without a definitive diagnosis following initial clinical evaluation. The patients were randomly assigned to either ILR implantation n = 103 or conventional investigation n = 98. Forty-three patients (43%) in the ILR group proceeded to have further syncopal events compared to 32 patients (33%) in the conventional group. Thirty-three patients in the ILR group and four patients in the conventional group received an ECG diagnosis (33% vs 4%, HR 8.93, 95% CI 3.17 to 25.2, p < 0.0001). Follow-up data from the same group was reported at seventeen months.[26] Forty-three percent of the ILR group versus 6% of the conventional group eventually received an electrocardiographic diagnosis (HR 6.53, 95% CI 3.73 to 11.4, p < 0.0001). Of note, 37% of patients in the ILR group failed to capture their first syncopal event; however, after being trained on the device only 5% of those who had further syncope did not achieve a diagnosis by the end of the study.

The International Study of Syncope of Uncertain Origin (ISSUE) was a multicenter international observational study which assessed the etiology of syncope in four subgroups: recurrent syncope with a negative tilt test;[27] recurrent syncope with a positive tilt test; recurrent syncope with bundle branch block at baseline and negative electro-physiologic study;[28] and recurrent syncope with structural heart disease and negative electro-physiologic study.[29] The combined ISSUE studies determined that the greater the patient's baseline risk of a rhythm disturbance, the more likely that symptoms are indicative of an arrhythmia. The ISSUE studies led to the development of a classi-fication system to categorize rhythm disturbances detected by ILR.[16, 30] The rhythms are initially divided into categories of asystole, bradycardia, no or slight rhythm variations, and tachycardia, and then further classified thereafter. The syncope guidelines from the American Heart Associa-tion, the American College of Cardiology, and the European Society of Cardiology recommend the use of ILRs early in the diagnostic exami-nation, excluding patients at high risk who may

instead need anti-arrhythmic therapies, internal cardiac defibrillation, or other treatment.[31-33] The guideline recommendations reflect the acknowl-edgement that ILRs can document a significant arrhythmia at the time of pre-syncope, which has been noted as the gold standard criterion for the diagnosis of syncope.[34]

Pediatric studies utilizing ILRs

As is often true in pediatrics, there are very few studies evaluating the use of ILRs in children and adolescents and no randomized trials. One of the first pediatric studies retrospectively evaluated 21 patients from three pediatric centers.[15] The average age of the study population was 12.3 ± 5.3 years (range 0.8–22 years). The population was mixed, with five patients (24%) having structural heart dis-ease, two (10%) having a family history of sudden cardiac death, three (14%) having QT prolongation on electrocardiogram, and 11 with no cardio-vascular disease. Indications for ILR included recurrent syncope and near-syncope (15 patients), palpitations (2 patients), and acute life-threatening event (2 patients). Over a mean follow-up period of 8.4 ± 4.7 months, 14 patients (67%) continued to have symptoms and 7 patients (33%) had no symptoms following ILR placement. All 14 patients who continued to have symptoms were able to achieve symptom-rhythm correlation, including supraventricular tachycardia in 4 patients, ventric-ular tachycardia in 2 patients, torsades de pointes in 1 patient, asystole in 1 patient, junctional brady-cardia in 1 patient, and sinus rhythm in 5 patients. This study demonstrated that ILR placement is useful in determining the presence or absence of an arrhythmia during symptoms in young patients with and without structural heart disease when conventional diagnostic testing is inconclusive.

There are two groups of pediatric patients who may benefit from ILR placement: (1) patients with structural heart disease and primary electrical cardiac abnormalities who are at high risk for developing malignant ventricular arrhythmias, and (2) otherwise healthy patients whose clinical course is not consistent with neurocardiogenic syncope. Digital ILR is useful in children with unexplained syncope; however, the automatic detection algorithm can be imper-fect. Significant arrhythmias such as polymorphic ventricular tachycardia have been missed, and muscle tremors have been frequently misinterpreted as ventricular tachycardia or other high rate episodes. Also, secondary to continuous overwriting by the auto-detection, genuine arrhythmias may be over-recorded by artifact. In one report, the automatically activated recording was repetitively recorded over after a patient's death.[8] Interestingly though, most documented episodes from ILRs in pediatric patients are manually activated.[35]

Patients with congenital heart disease are a unique group of patients who have an increased incidence of malignant arrhythmias.[6, 7] These patients may have symptoms of syncope, presyncope, and palpitations. ILRs have been successfully utilized in this patient population regardless of underlying congenital heart defect or previous cardiac surgery.[36] Symptom-rhythm correlation can help determine which patients require pacemaker and/or defibrillator implantation (Figure 17.3). Further, ILRs can be particularly beneficial in patients with neurodevelopmental delay where symptom history is limited. Newer generations of ILRs have the improved ability to detect atrial fibrillation and other atrial arrhythmias, a growing concern in the adult realm. These newer detection algorithms may be particularly helpful in the growing population of adult congenital heart disease patients who are at risk for such arrhythmias.

Recent updates in ILRs

Improvements have been made to ILRs since their introduction. The newer generation of ILRs has been deemed safe for magnetic resonance imaging (MRI) use which in the past was an issue for patients with syncope requiring brain imaging.[32] One of the biggest complaints of ILRs, especially in children, has been the detection of inappropriate events. Newer sensing and detection schemes have been introduced, employing an automatically adjusted R-wave sensing threshold, enhanced noise rejection, and algorithms to detect asystole, bradyarrhythmia, and tachyarrhythmia.[37] Some groups have proposed to eliminate preoperative cutaneous mapping previously required prior to ILR implantation.[38] It has been proposed to implant the ILR in the left upper chest area midway between the supraclavicular notch and the left breast area. Only a minimal change in the

P-wave amplitude and peak-to-peak QRS amplitude was demonstrated. Previously, ILRs could not be downloaded transtelephonically, mandating the patient to return to clinic for interrogation.[39] Recently, remote transmission of ILR data has become available. Remote monitoring enhances the diagnostic effectiveness of the ILR by limiting the risk of memory saturation secondary to the high number of false detections and reducing the time to diagnosis.

External event recorders

Traditionally, transtelephoninc looping and non-looping monitors (TTM) have been utilized to capture events for symptom-rhythm correlation. Some disadvantages of TTMs are that they may have a maximum recording window of 30 days, lack of immediate display and patient compliance may be poor due to uncomfortable leads. Recently, the AliveCor Mobile ECG has been shown to be a viable alternative to a traditional transtelephonic monitor (TTM) for monitoring patients with arrhythmias (Figure 17.4A, B). It consists of software that can be downloaded to a smart phone and a phone cover with two large electrodes on the back which serve as electrodes analogous to a lead I. Touching the electrodes results in an instant ECG recording and display.

Automated external defibrillators

The importance of early defibrillation to treat sudden cardiac arrest is based on the principles that (1) ventricular fibrillation is the most common initial rhythm in witnessed sudden cardiac arrest; (2) electrical defibrillation is the most effective treatment of ventricular fibrillation; and (3) the probability of successful defibrillation diminishes rapidly over time.[40] In turn then, survival from sudden cardiac arrest is dependent on early defibrillation with the likelihood of surviving an event decreasing by 7–10% for every minute of delay in defibrillation.[40, 41]

History of automated external defibrillation

The first scientific description of defibrillation resulted from experiments on fibrillation. In 1900, Prevost and Batelli conducted research on ventricular fibrillation in dogs. In this study they

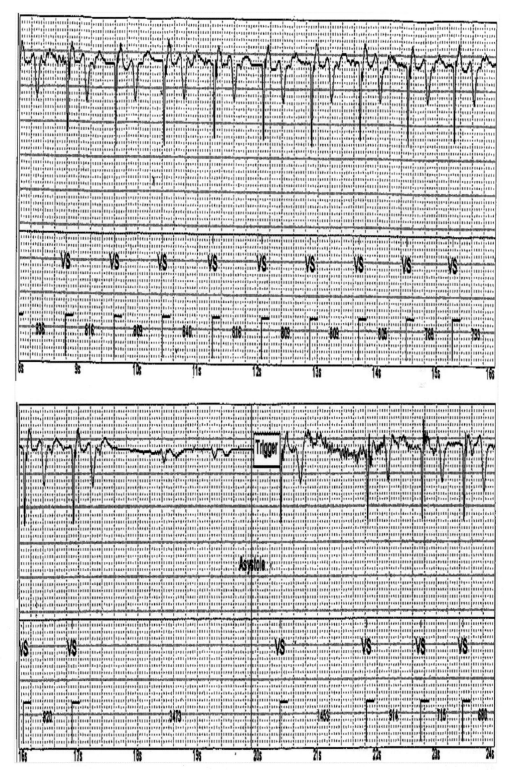

Figure 17.3 *ILR recording from an 11-year-old boy with history of tetralogy of Fallot status post repair with syncopal episodes. Baseline electrocardiogram demonstrates sinus rhythm with first-degree atrioventricular block and right bundle branch block with a PR interval of 480 ms. Patient had negative work-up including Holter monitor, exercise stress test, and external transtelephonic monitor.*

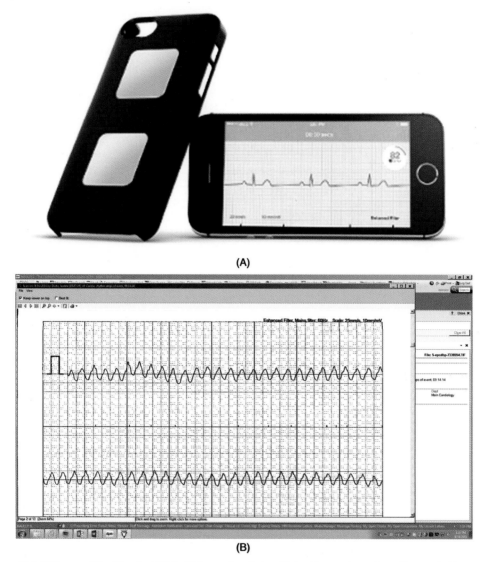

Figure 17.4 *(A) Image of the Alive Cor Mobile ECG recording device. (B) A wide complex tachycardia recorded by a patient with Wolff–Parkinson–White syndrome using the mobile ECG recording device. (Source: Dr. Maully Shah, Division of Cardiology, The Children's Hospital of Philadelphia, U.S.A. Reproduced with permission of Dr. Maully Shah.)*

described methods to fibrillate the heart using alternating (AC) and direct (DC) electrical currents. They noted that weaker currents were needed to fibrillate the ventricle compared to the stronger currents needed to defibrillate (or what they called "countershocking") ventricular fibrillation.

In 1947, Dr. Claude Beck put this information into clinical practice and performed the first successful human defibrillation using internal cardiac paddles on a 14-year-old boy who developed pulseless ventricular fibrillation during elective chest surgery.[42] The defibrillator used on this patient was made by James Rand, a friend of Beck, who made two defibrillators that year of 1947. The device had silver paddles (the size of large tablespoons) that could be directly applied to the heart (Figure 17.5).

In 1956, Paul Zoll used a more powerful unit to perform the first closed-chest defibrillation of a human.[43] In Belfast, ambulance-transported

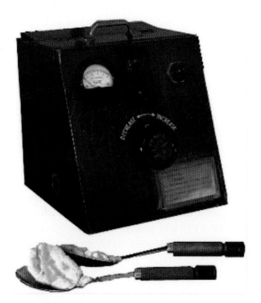

Figure 17.5 *Image of the first defibrillator used to successfully defibrillate a human.*

physicians first achieved pre-hospital defibrillation in 1966. Out-of-hospital defibrillation by emergency medical technicians (EMT), without the presence of physicians, was first performed in Oregon in 1969 and reported in 1972. The first prototype automated external defibrillators (AED) were developed in the early 1970s using an oral/epigastric electrode and placing a second electrode on the chest.[44] In 1982, the FDA approved EMT-defibrillation clinical trials. By the early 1990s, successful training and use of AEDs by police officers and first responders was reported. FDA approval of AED use by lay personnel and Good Samaritan legislation followed shortly after that. In May of 2003, New York State became the first state to mandate AEDs be placed in schools.

The mechanics of automated external defibrillators

As mentioned previously, the earliest models of AEDs required inserting an oral/epigastric electrode and placing a second electrode on the chest. Since then, these devices have advanced significantly with regard to ease of rescuer use, accuracy of rhythm analysis and efficacy of charge delivery.

Device mechanics: There are currently several manufacturers of AEDs in the United States with FDA approval for lay person use. The devices consist of essentially two components: the electrode pads and the device itself. Most current devices include voice prompts instructing the rescuer how to place the pads, whether a shock is advised and, in some models, when to perform CPR. It is important to note whether a device is semi-automated or fully automated. Semi-automated devices alert the rescuer that a shock is advised and then the rescuer must deliver the shock by pressing a button. Fully automated devices alert the rescuer that a shock is advised, asks rescuers to clear away from the victim and then automatically delivers a shock. This is an important distinction because the comfort of the rescuer influences the time to delivery of a therapy in a semi-automated device.

Placement location of the defibrillator pads is uniform for all devices with one pad being placed at the right sternal border and the other at the cardiac apex. The pads themselves are marked with a picture depicting where to place the pads on the chest. Several manufacturers offer attenuated pediatric pads for use in victims under the age of 8 years or weighing less than 25 kg (55 lb); however, therapy should not be delayed to determine the patient's exact age or weight. Once the pads are properly placed, the device will begin analyzing the victim's rhythm.

Rhythm analysis: AEDs are equipped with proprietary rhythm analysis algorithms. In general, analysis consists of filtering the electrocardiographic signal to reduce noise artifact, detecting and evaluating electrocardiographic characteristics including amplitude, frequency, and slope and calculating average heart rate. Some newer models include software for supraventricular tachycardia (SVT) discrimination adding to the sensitivity and specificity of rhythm analysis. From this information, a decision to advise the delivery of a shock, or not, is recommended by the device.

Clinical reports of individual manufacturers of AEDs demonstrate that rhythm analysis technology in adults has a sensitivity of near 100% (correct identification of shockable rhythms) and specificity near 98% (correct identification of non-shockable rhythms).[45] These findings have been corroborated using pediatric databases against AED rhythm detection algorithms that yielded sensitivities of greater than 99% and specificities greater than 96%.[46–48] Furthermore, they surpass the American Heart Association's adult algorithm recommendations.[49] In 2003, these findings led the International Liaison Committee on Resuscitation to expand AED use to include children 1–8 years of age who have no signs of circulation.[50]

Charge delivery: The majority of AEDs available on the market today deliver a biphasic defibrillation waveform. This means that the charge is delivered in one direction for half the shock and the electrically opposite direction for the second half. This form of defibrillation uses less energy with the same or superior effectiveness compared to a monophasic therapy.

Currently available AEDs are programmed to deliver 150–360 J of energy using standard adult pads depending on the impedance of the interface between the patient and the device. Pediatric pads

that attenuate energy output or adapters to reduce energy are available for use in victims less than 8 years of age or under 25 kg (55 lb). These pads deliver approximately 50 J of energy and have been shown to be effective and safe.[51]

Event recording: AEDs record and store rescue data for future analysis by the medical director or physician supervising its use. This data can be downloaded and document the victim's rhythm so as to aid in diagnosis and treatment of the victim. Figure 17.6 is the rhythm strip of a previously healthy 16-year-old high school student who collapsed during basketball practice. His school's AED was placed, recognized ventricular fibrillation, and successfully defibrillated him to a normal sinus rhythm. The young man survived the ordeal.

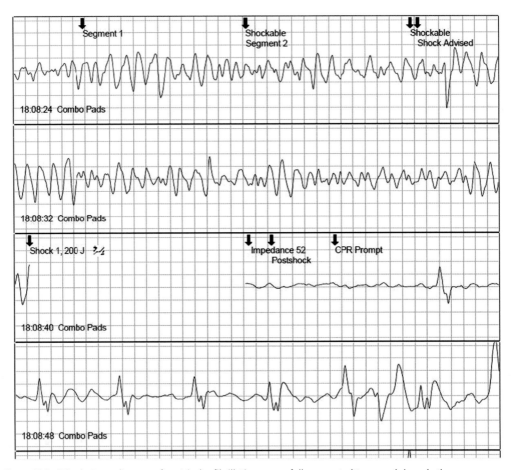

Figure 17.6 *AED electrocardiogram of ventricular fibrillation successfully converted to normal sinus rhythm.*

Public access defibrillation

Public access defibrillation has been shown to be an important part of successful recovery from out-of-hospital sudden cardiac arrest.[52–54] These findings led to wide spread placement of AEDs in settings highly populated with adults, such as airports, health centers, stadiums, and casinos. Consequently, at the urgency of parents and state legislators, AEDs began being placed in schools as well. By the age of 18 years, a person is estimated to have spent 35% of their days in school, about 18% of their waking hours. Thus, school-based AED programs have given us the most insight into the benefit of AEDs for children.

In 2004, 32% of United States schools reported having an AED.[55] Some individual states have an even higher prevalence: 54% in Washington state high schools in 2007[56] and 72.5% in North Carolina high schools in 2009.[57] A recent study conducted by Mercer et al. demonstrated an increased prevalence of AEDs in West Virginia public high schools from 33% in 2005 to 76% in 2010.[58]

Like their adult counter parts, school-based AED programs have been shown to be effective. In a large cross-sectional national survey of over 1700 high schools across the country, Drezner et al showed improved survival in high school student athletes and nonstudents who suffer sudden cardiac arrest.[59] These schools had Emergency Response Planning and AED access and 23 of 36 sudden cardiac arrest victims survived to hospital discharge. Survival was equal for both student athletes and older non-students. The annual incidence of sudden cardiac arrest in high school athletes was found to be 4.4/100,000 in this study.

In schools without an AED, school administrators cite cost as the main barrier to obtaining a device. Yet, data shows that most schools obtain devices through donations or grants, with a minority actually using school funds.[58, 60] This perceived barrier can be overcome, as there are many options for schools to acquire philanthropic funds to finance their school-based AED programs. The National Center for Early Defibrillation gives an in-depth outline on securing donations from local corporations and industries, civic organizations, private foundations, public charities, government grants, and traditional fund-raisers (www.early-defib.org). Perhaps most impressive is the ability of parents struck by the tragedy of a child with sudden death to implement change and policy. Parents have spearheaded change in state legislature, and parental and community programs provide material, information, and funds to aid interested groups in obtaining devices for their schools (i.e., Maura Rae Kuhl AED Foundation, KEN Heart Foundation, Project ADAM, Project SAVE).

With the growing prevalence of AEDs in schools throughout the country, it will fall on the shoulders of local pediatricians, family practitioners, and physician extenders to provide accurate medical knowledge and guidance to school administrators, personnel, students, and their families to ensure competent and effective school-based AED programs.

Personal use automated external defibrillators

In 2002, the FDA approved the first AED for home use with a prescription. Two years later, in 2004, the FDA allowed the sale of personal AEDs without a prescription. Today, there are a multitude of companies who provide information and sales of all the major AED devices and related supplies, making it easy for the lay person with the financial capability to purchase a personal AED.

In the clinical realm, placement of implantable cardioverter defibrillators (ICDs) in the pediatric population, particularly youngsters, remains a concern for practitioners secondary to complications and morbidity arising from inappropriate shocks and lead failure.[61] Personal use AEDs, therefore, may be considered in younger patients who are at high risk of complications from ICD placement. Further, as genetic identification of congenitally inherited diseases (i.e., long QT syndrome, hypertrophic cardiomyopathy, Brugada syndrome) increases, so do the number of asymptomatic family members with positive gene screening. This creates a conundrum for the practitioner with regard to treatment recommendations, exercise restrictions, and sudden death risk stratification. In these cases, personal AEDs, in addition to medical therapy and exercise restrictions, may be used to augment prevention of sudden death and treatment of malignant arrhythmias.

In rare instances, transvenous defibrillation with an ICD is unsuccessful, particularly in hypertrophic

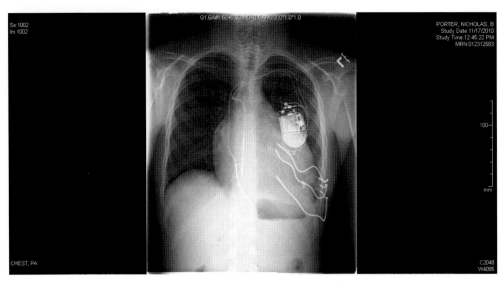

Figure 17.7 *Chest X-ray of a patient with hypertrophic cardiomyopathy and failure of an ICD to attain defibrillation thresholds.*

cardiomyopathy. Patients most at risk are those with massive left ventricular hypertrophy (wall thickness >45 mm) and/or concomitant amiodarone use.[62] Figure 17.7 shows the chest X-ray of a patient prescribed a personal AED after failure of his ICD to attain defibrillation thresholds. The patient is a 14-year-old boy with severe hypertrophic cardiomyopathy secondary to a mutation in the PRKAG2 gene who suffered chest pain and pre-syncope. His left ventricular lateral free wall measured 40 mm, the left ventricular posterior wall measured 37 mm, the ventricular septum measured 44 mm, and the apical wall measured 40 mm. He underwent placement of a transvenous ICD that failed to yield successful defibrillation thresholds. An additional azygous vein defibrillation coil was added but again did not provide successful defibrillation thresholds. Subsequently, a subcutaneous array was placed intraoperatively. Using a combination of energy vectors from the array and transvenous system, adequate defibrillation thresholds were not attained. The device was left in place and active but in the absence of sufficient defibrillation thresholds, a personal use AED was prescribed. This case demonstrates the utility of AEDs to augment conventional therapy methods.

Yet AEDs have their limitations with regard to continuous monitoring and prevention of malignant arrhythmias as well as cost when used in a home setting. The necessity of a bystander rescuer to activate the device, place the defibrillator pads and, in some instances, push a button to deliver a shock precludes AEDs from providing protection while the patient is asleep or alone. In this regard, the AED does not replace the efficacy of ICDs. It is worth noting that a wearable defibrillator is available that has been shown to be an effective bridge to implantable defibrillation therapy or cardiac transplant and provides patients around-the-clock rhythm analysis and treatment of malignant arrhythmias.[63, 64] Lastly, the ability of the patient or family to afford the purchase of a device may be an issue with the average cost of an AED falling between $1200 and $3000. The authors have had success prescribing AEDs with all or partial payment of devices by third-party payers.

Automated external defibrillator precautions

Whether an AED is prescribed for personal use or part of a public access defibrillation program, several precautions must be considered.

1 Victims should be unresponsive before an AED is applied. Emergency medical services should be activated immediately.

2 To prevent inappropriate therapies, CPR should be held while the unit is analyzing the victim's

rhythm. Most models have voice prompts that ask the rescuer to "Hold CPR"

3 An AED should not be used on a victim who is seizing and used with caution in a moving vehicle. Most units are designed to warn the rescuer of motion artifact or poor contact.

4 The victim should be placed in a dry location prior to use. The chest does not need to be shaved but should be dried prior to placing the pads. If possible, the pads should be placed at least (2.5 cm (1") from implanted devices and should not be placed over medicinal patches (i.e., nitroglycerin patches).

5 If a therapy is advised, provisions to protect the rescuer from inadvertent electrocution should be taken. The rescuer should discontinue CPR and not touch the victim when a shock is advised. Metal objects in contact with the victim should be avoided.

6 Radiofrequency interference from cellular phones, CB radios, and FM two-way radios may affect rhythm recognition. Wireless radiotelephones should not be used within 2 m of an AED.

7 Proper maintenance is important to assure that the unit's battery is properly charged and pads are attached, intact, and not expired. Individual manufacturer recommendations for scheduled maintenance should be followed. Most models perform scheduled self-tests to detect issues with the device and sound audible warnings to notify the owner of possible problems with the device.

Conclusion

Advances in medical technology include the advent of implantable syncope and arrhythmia devices and automated external defibrillators. In the realm of pediatric medicine, practitioners have developed innovative applications of these technologies to aid in the diagnosis and treatment of arrhythmias in the young and those with congenital heart disease.

References

1 Freed MD. Advances in the diagnosis and therapy of syncope and palpitations in children. *Curr Opin Pediatr* 1994; 6: 368–372.

2 Geggel RL. Conditions leading to pediatric cardiology consultation in a tertiary academic hospital. *Pediatrics* 2004; 114: e409–417.

3 Batra AS, Hohn AR. Consultation with the specialist: palpitations, syncope, and sudden cardiac death in children: who's at risk? *Pediatr Rev* 2003; 24: 269–275.

4 Lewis DA, Dhala A. Syncope in the pediatric patient: the cardiologist's perspective. *Pediatr Clin North Am* 1999; 46: 205–219.

5 Tanel RE, Walsh EP. Syncope in the pediatric patient. *Cardiol Clin* 1997; 15: 277–294.

6 Flinn CJ, Wolff GS, Dick M, et al. Cardiac rhythm after the Mustard operation for complete transposition of the great arteries. *N Engl J Med* 1984; 310: 1635–1638.

7 Walsh EP, Rockenmacher S, Keane JF, Hougen TJ, Lock JE, Castaneda AR. Late results in patients with tetralogy of Fallot repaired during infancy. *Circulation* 1988; 77: 1062–1067.

8 Kothari DS, Riddell F, Smith W, Voss J, Skinner JR. Digital implantable loop recorders in the investigation of syncope in children: benefits and limitations. *Heart Rhythm* 2006; 3: 1306–1312.

9 Ayabakan C, Ozer S, Celiker A, Ozme S. Analysis of 201 Holter records in pediatric patients. *Turk J Pediatr* 2000; 42: 286–293.

10 Hammill SC. Value and limitations of noninvasive assessment of syncope. *Cardiol Clin* 1997; 15: 195–218.

11 Linzer M. Incremental diagnostic yield of loop electrocardiographic recorder in unexplained syncope. *Am J Cardiol* 1990; 66: 214–219.

12 Kapoor WN. Evaluation and management of the patient with syncope. *JAMA* 1992; 268: 2553–2560.

13 Brown AP, Dawkins KD, Davies JG. Detection of arrhythmias: use of a patient-activated ambulatory electrocardiogram device with solid-state memory loop. *Br Heart J* 1987; 58: 251–253.

14 Lewis DA, Zlotocha J Henke L, Dhala A. Specificity of head-up tilt testing in adolescents: effect of various degrees of tilt challenge in normal control subjects. *J Am Coll Cardiol* 1997; 30: 1057–1060.

15 Rossano J, Bloemers B, Sreeram N, Balaji S, Shah MJ. Efficacy of implantable loop recorders in establishing symptom-rhythm correlation in young patients with syncope and palpitations. *Pediatrics* 2003; 112: e228–233.

16 Parry SW, Matthews IG. Implantable loop recorders in the investigation of unexplained syncope: a state of the art review. *Heart* 2010; 96: 1611–1616.

17 Krahn AD, Klein GJ, Yee R. Recurrent syncope: experience with an implantable loop recorder. *Cardiol Clin* 1997; 15: 313–326.

18 Waktare JE, Malik M. Holter, loop recorder, and event counter capabilities of implanted devices. *Pacing Clin Electrophysiol* 1997; 20: 2658–2669.

19 Sanatani S, Peirone A, Chiu C, Human DG, Gross GJ, Hamilton RM. Use of an implantable loop recorder in

the evaluation of children with congenital heart disease. *Am Heart J* 2002; 143: 366–372.

20 Bloemers BL, Sreeram N. Implantable loop recorders in pediatric practice. *J Electrocardiol* 2002; 35 (suppl): 131–135.

21 Potts JE, Rajagopalan K, Sanatani S. Minimally invasive approach to the child with palpitations. *Exp Rev Cardiovasc Ther* 2006; 4: 681–694.

22 Subbiah R, Gula LJ, Klein GJ, Skanes AC, Yee R, Krahn AD. Syncope: review of monitoring modalities. *Curr Cardio Rev* 2008; 4: 41–48.

23 Krahn AD, Klein GJ, Norris C, Yee R. The etiology of syncope in patients with negative tilt table and electrophysiological testing. *Circulation* 1995; 92: 1819–1824.

24 Krahn AD, Klein GJ, Yee R, Skanes AC. Randomized assessment of syncope trial: conventional diagnostic testing versus a prolonged monitoring strategy. *Circulation* 2001; 104: 46–51.

25 Farwell DJ, Sulke AN. A randomized prospective comparison of three protocols for head-up tilt testing and carotid sinus massage. *Int J Cardiol* 2005; 105: 241–249.

26 Farwell DJ, Freemantle N, Sulke N. The clinical impact of implantable loop recorders in patients with syncope. *Eur Heart J* 2006; 27: 351–356.

27 Moya A, Brignole M, Menozzi C, et al. Mechanism of syncope in patients with isolated syncope and in patients with tilt-positive syncope. *Circulation* 2001; 104: 1261–1267.

28 Brignole M, Menozzi C, Moya A, et al. Mechanism of syncope in patients with bundle branch block and negative electrophysiological test. *Circulation* 2001; 104: 2045–2050.

29 Menozzi C, Brignole M, Garcia-Civera R, et al. Mechanism of syncope in patients with heart disease and negative electrophysiologic test. *Circulation* 2002; 105: 2741–2275.

30 Brignole M, Moya A, Menozzi C, Garcia-Civera R, Sutton R. Proposed electrocardiographic classification of spontaneous syncope documented by an implantable loop recorder. *Europace* 2005; 7: 14–18.

31 The Task Force for the Diagnosis and Management of Syncope of the European Society of Cardiology (ESC). Guidelines for the diagnosis and management of syncope (version 2009). *Eur Heart J* 2009; 30: 2631–2671.

32 Auricchio A, Moccetti T. Electronic cardiac medicine: present and future opportunities. *Swiss Medical Weekly* 2010; 140: w13052.

33 Strickberger SA, Benson DW, Biaggioni I, et al. AHA/ACCF scientific statement on the evaluation of syncope: from the American Heart Association Councils on Clinical Cardiology, Cardiovascular Nursing, Cardiovascular Disease in the Young, and Stroke, and

the Quality of Care and Outcomes Research Interdisciplinary Working Group; and the American College of Cardiology Foundation: in collaboration with the Heart Rhythm Society: endorsed by the American Autonomic Society. *Circulation* 2006; 113: 316–327.

34 Brignole M, Vardas P, Hoffman E, et al. Indications for the use of diagnostic implantable and external ECG loop recorders. *Europace* 2009; 11: 671–687.

35 Al Dhahri KN, Pott JE, Chiu CC, Hamilton RM, Sanatani S. Are implantable loop recorders useful in detecting arrhythmias in children with unexplained syncope? *Pacing Clin Electrophysiol* 2009; 32: 1422–1427.

36 Kenny D, Chakrabarti S, Ranasinghe A, Chambers A, Martin R, Stuart G. Single-centre use of implantable loop recorders in patients with congenital heart disease. *Europace* 2009; 11: 303–307.

37 Brignole M, Bellardine Black CL, Bloch Thomsen PE, et al. Improved arrhythmia detection in implantable loop recorders. *J Cardiovasc Electrophysiol* 2008; 19: 928–934.

38 Grubb BP, Welch M, Kanjwal K, Karabin B, Kanjwal Y. An anatomic-based approach for the placement of implantable loop recorders. *Pacing Clin Electrophysiol* 2010; 33: 1149–1152.

39 Furukawa T, Maggi R, Bertolone C, et al. Effectiveness of remote monitoring in the management of syncope and palpitations. *Europace* 2011; 13: 431–437.

40 The American Heart Association in collaboration with the International Liaison Committee on Resuscitation Guidelines 2000 for Cardiopulmonary Resuscitation and Emergency Cardiovascular Care. Part 4: the automated external defibrillator: key link in the chain of survival. *Circulation* 2000; 102: I60–I76.

41 Larsen MP, Eisenberg MS, Cummins RO, Hallstrom AP. Predicting survival from out-of-hospital cardiac arrest: a graphic model. *Ann Emerg Med.* 1993; 22: 1652–1658.

42 Beck CS, Pritchard WH, Feil SA. Ventricular fibrillation of long duration abolished by electric shock. *JAMA* 1947; 135: 985–989.

43 Zoll PM, Linenthal AJ, Gibson W, et al. Termination of ventricular fibrillation in man by externally applied electric countershock. *N Engl J Med.* Apr 19 1956; 254(16): 727–732.

44 Diack AW, Welborn WS, Rullman RG, et al. An automatic cardiac resuscitator for emergency treatment of cardiac arrest. *Med Instrum.* Mar–Apr 1979; 13(2): 78–83.

45 Mattioni TA, Nademanee K, Brodsky M, et al. Initial clinical experience with a fully automatic in-hospital external cardioverter defibrillator. *Pacing Clin Electrophysiol.* 1999 Nov; 22(11): 1648–1655.

46 Cecchin F, Jorgenson DB, Berul CI, et al. Is arrhythmia detection by automatic external defibrillator accurate for children? Sensitivity and specificity of an automatic external defibrillator algorithm in 696 pediatric arrhythmias. *Circulation.* 2001; 103: 2483–2488.

47 Atkinson E, Mikysa B, Conway JA, et al. Specificity and sensitivity of automated external defibrillator rhythm analysis in infants and children. *Ann Emerg Med.* 2003; 42: 185–196.

48 Atkins DL, Scott WA, Blaufox AD, et al. Sensitivity and specificity of an automated external defibrillator algorithm designed for pediatric patients. *Resuscitation.* 2008 Feb; 76(2): 168–174.

49 Kerber RE, Becker LB, Bourland JD, et al. Automatic external defibrillators for public access defibrillation: recommendations for specifying and reporting arrhythmia analysis algorithm performance, incorporating new waveforms, and enhancing safety. *Circulation.* 1997; 95: 1677–1682.

50 Samson RA, Berg RA, Bingham R, et al. Use of automated external defibrillators for children: an update: an advisory statement from the pediatric advanced life support task force, International Liaison Committee on Resuscitation. *Circulation.* 2003 Jul 1; 107(25): 3250–3255.

51 Atkins DL, Jorgenson DB. Attenuated pediatric electrode pads for automated external defibrillator use in children. *Resuscitation.* 2005 Jul; 66(1): 31–37.

52 Caffrey SL, Willoughby PJ, Pepe PE, Becker LB. Public use of automated external defibrillators. *N Engl J Med.* 2002; 347: 1242–1247.

53 Page RL, Joglar JA, Kowal RC, Zagrodzky JD, Nelson LL, Ramaswamy K, et al. Use of automated external defibrillators by a U.S. airline. *N Engl J Med.* 2000; 343: 1210–1216.

54 Valenzuela TD, Roe DJ, Nichol G, Clark LL, Spaite DW, Hardman RG. Outcomes of rapid defibrillation by security officers after cardiac arrest in casinos. *N Engl J Med.* 2000; 343: 1206–1209.

55 Olympia R, Wan E, Avner J. The preparedness of schools to respond to emergencies in children: a national survey of school nurses. *Pediatrics.* 2005; 116: e738–e745.

56 Rothmier JD, Drezner J, Harmon JG. Automated external defibrillators in Washington State high schools. *Br J Sports Med.* 2007; 41: 301–305.

57 Monroe A, Rosenbaum DA, Davis S. Emergency planning for sudden cardiac events in North Carolina high schools. *N C Med J.* 2009 May–Jun; 70(3): 198–204.

58 Mercer C, Rhodes LA, Phillips JR. Automated external defibrillators in West Virginia schools. *WV Medical Journal.* 2012; 108(4): 18–24.

59 Drezner JA, Rao AL, Heistand J, et al. Effectiveness of emergency response planning for sudden cardiac arrest in United States high schools with automated external defibrillators. *Circulation.* 2009; 120: 518–525.

60 England H, Hoffman C, Hodgman T, Singh S, Homoud M, Weinstock J, et al. Effectiveness of automated external defibrillators in high schools in greater Boston. *Am J Cardiol.* 2005; 95: 1484–1486.

61 Berul CI, Van Hare GF, Kertesz NJ, et al. Results of a multicenter retrospective implantable cardioverter-defibrillator registry of pediatric and congenital heart disease patients. *J Am Coll Cardiol* 2008; 51: 1685–1691.

62 Almquist AK, Montgomery JV, Haas TS, et al. Cardioverter-defibrillator implantation in high-risk patients with hypertrophic cardiomyopathy. *Heart Rhythm.* 2005 Aug; 2(8): 814–819.

63 Rao M, Goldenberg I, Moss AJ, et al. Wearable defibrillator in congenital structural heart disease and inherited arrhythmias. *Am J Cardiol.* 2011 Dec; 108(11): 1632–1638.

64 Collins KK, Silva JN, Rhee EK, et al. Use of a wearable automated defibrillator in children compared to young adults. *Pacing Clin Electrophysiol.* 2010 Sep; 33(9): 1119–1124.

CHAPTER 18

Electromagnetic interference and implantable devices

Karen Smoots[1] and R. Lee Vogel[2]

[1]Electrophysiology Device Nurse, The Cardiac center, The Children's Hospital of Philadelphia, Philadelphia, PA, USA

[2]Staff Cardiologist, The Children's Hospital of Philadelphia, Professor of Clinical Pediatrics, Perelman School of Medicine, University of Pennsylvania, Philadelphia, PA, USA

Background

Electromagnetic radiation, both natural and manmade surrounds us and is part of our daily lives. Visible light, ultraviolet light, X-rays, and gamma rays are produced by the Sun and atomic particles whereas radio waves, television signals, microwave ovens, and radiofrequency ablation equipment are examples of manmade electromagnetic radiation. At the atomic level, electromagnetic radiation is produced when an energy source excites atoms causing the electrons to rise to a higher energy level. When the energy source is removed, the electrons fall back to the lower energy level releasing the energy as an electromagnetic wave. Manmade radio waves are produced when direct current is applied to a wire establishing a magnetic field which produces an electromagnetic wave. When the current is removed, another wave is produced. By sequentially turning the energy or current on and off, a continuous wave can be produced.

The three basic properties of electromagnetic waves are speed, frequency, and the ability to travel through a vacuum. All electromagnetic waves travel at the speed of light, 299,792 km/s. The number of waves that pass one point in one second is the frequency expressed in units of hertz (Hz). If a wave passes a point 1000 times in 1 s, the frequency is 1 KHz; 1,000,000 times in 1 s, the frequency is 1 MHz. The wavelength of a given electromagnetic wave can be calculated by dividing the speed of light by the frequency of the wave. The electromagnetic spectrum is a continuum with long wavelength, low frequency radio waves at one end and short wavelength, high frequency gamma waves at the other end. AM radio operates in the 535 KHz–1.8 MHz range, FM radio 88–106 MHz, microwaves 100 Hz–300 GHz, visible light $10^{14.7}$–10^{15} Hz, X-rays 10^{18} Hz, and gamma rays, 10^{20} Hz (Figure 18.1). Finally, sound waves need a medium to travel through such as air, water, or a solid. Electromagnetic radiation can travel through the vacuum of space and depending on characteristics of a specific wave, can travel through the human body and other solid objects.

Two features that have significantly improved the efficacy of modern permanent pacemakers and implantable cardioverter/defibrillators (ICD), known collectively as cardiovascular implantable electronic devices (CIEDs), are non-invasive

Cardiac Pacing and Defibrillation in Pediatric and Congenital Heart Disease, First Edition.
Edited by Maully Shah, Larry Rhodes and Jonathan Kaltman.
© 2017 John Wiley & Sons Ltd. Published 2017 by John Wiley & Sons Ltd.
Companion Website: www.wiley.com/go/shah/cardiac_pacing

Wavelength (meters)

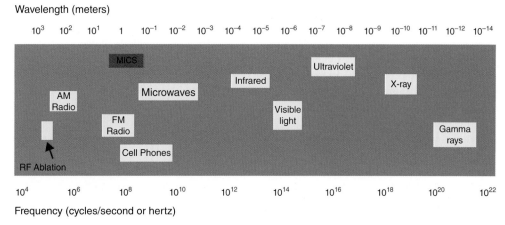

Figure 18.1 *Electromagnetic spectrum.*

programmability and non-invasive transmission of stored data. Having the ability to alter modes of pacing, output settings and treatment protocols and to review stored electrograms or conduct a non-invasive electrophysiology study through the ICD, has made it possible to customize the device to the patient. To achieve this functionality, CIED design engineers developed microelectronic systems that are activated by changes in the local magnetic field and respond to commands sent via electromagnetic waves. Additionally, the pacemaker or an ICD's stored data can be transmitted via electromagnetic waves back to a receiver that translates that data into a usable report. To accomplish this, the CIED must have a transmitter as well as an antenna.

As such, pacemakers and ICDs are vulnerable to electromagnetic interference (EMI) ubiquitous in our present environment. If one could assign a visible color to all the different electromagnetic waves that surround us, the collage of colors produced would create a painting worthy of display in any museum of modern art. EMI can interfere with normal pacemaker function affecting either pacing, sensing, or both. Reports of pacemaker interference by a cellular phone surfaced in the mid-1990s. Hayes et al. described the results of 5330 tests done on 980 pacemaker patients concluding that significant interference occurred in only 1.7% of the tests and only when the cellular phone was placed directly over the pacemaker pocket.[1] In an ICD, EMI may mimic a tachydysrhythmia initiating a programmed therapy that may lead to an inappropriate ICD discharge. In a typical hospital setting, EMI can be generated from bedside telemetry, radiofrequency ablation generators, lithotripsy equipment, magnetic resonance imaging equipment, cell phones, digital music players, radios, television, and security/surveillance equipment to name a few. To decrease the likelihood of EMI, manufacturers have incorporated into their devices titanium and stainless steel battery casings covered with an insulating coating, interference rejection circuits, feed through capacitors, noise reduction functions, Hall sensors, and other programmable sensing parameters.

The literature and pacemaker/ICD manufacturer's technical service archives contain numerous case reports and technical briefs of EMI produced by many different sources. It is highly recommended to those who care for patients with pacemakers or ICDs to maintain a close working relationship with the technical/clinical specialists representing the manufacturer of the device. They have intimate knowledge of their device and ready access to their product engineers. However, the ultimate responsibility of the care of a CIED patient lies with the clinician. For the patient who is experiencing a device malfunction secondary to suspected EMI, it is always important to obtain a thorough history. In most cases the source of EMI is obvious but in some, finding it may take a good deal of detective work.

For EMI to have an effect, three elements are necessary: a source of EMI, a device with an antenna capable of receiving the EMI (the pacemaker or

ICD) and a permissive environment for the EMI to have an effect. Physical obstacles like walls or buildings impede the progress of an electromagnetic wave. The effect of EMI varies indirectly with distance from the source to the pacemaker/ICD. Lawrentschuk noted that EMI generated more than one meter from medical equipment usually does not produce an adverse effect.[2] Similarly, the duration of time the EMI is produced is directly related to the development of an adverse effect on the pacemaker/ICD. In an operating room setting, very brief bursts of electrocautery are less likely to produce clinically significant EMI when compared to long, sustained applications.[3]

Just like surrounding electronic equipment can generate radiofrequency signals (electromagnetic waves) that affect CIEDs, CIEDs also produce radiofrequency signals when the device transmits stored data to the programmer or other receiving stations. Wireless communication between the device and the receiving station is becoming commonplace for the routine assessment and follow-up of implanted medical devices. To decrease the likelihood of the generated electromagnetic waves interfering with other electrical equipment and to assure that medical devices are allotted a specific location on the radio spectrum, the Federal Communications Commission, an independent agency of the United States government under the Congressional branch charged with overseeing all radio, television, wire, satellite, and cable communication within the United States and its territories, established the Medical Implant Communications Service in the 402–405 MHz band.[4] This wavelength band is shared with meteorological testing equipment and interference with medical devices is not expected.

When to suspect electromagnetic interference

Most pacemakers and ICDs function reliably. In the United States, the high standards set by the Food and Drug Administration and the manufacturers of these devices minimizes most of the potential problems. When troubleshooting a pacemaker or ICD, consider electromagnetic interference when there is evidence of:

1 Pacing inhibition

2 Triggered pacing and low rate pacing
3 An inappropriate ICD shock
4 Electric reset and mode change
5 Damage to the generator circuitry.[5]

Pacing inhibition in a pacemaker dependent patient is serious and an inappropriate ICD shock can be quite traumatic. Both can be caused by electromagnetic interference. In each case, the device incorrectly senses the extrinsic electrical activity as intrinsic cardiac activity. Pacemaker outputs may be inhibited due to oversensing the EMI. Depending on the frequency of the extrinsic signal, an ICD may incorrectly interpret it as ventricular tachycardia or fibrillation and initiate the programmed therapies. Figures 18.2 and 18.3 are the data download of a patient who received an ICD shock. Both the atrial and ventricular electrograms demonstrate non physiologic rate deflections that are misinterpreted as ventricular fibrillation. The capacitors ultimately charged at the end of the upper panel in Figure 18.3 and discharged at the beginning of lower panel on the same figure. In this case, the patient experienced a shock when entering his vacation trailer after swimming. Review of the ICD data download identified rapid sensed electrical activity that was interpreted as ventricular fibrillation and ultimately resulted in a shock. Detailed investigation of the case discovered that the shock occurred when the patient was wet and in bare feet after swimming. The fast ventricular rate counters started when he entered the trailer door. Nothing happened when he entered the trailer fully clothed in dry clothes earlier in the day. Further investigation found that his vacation trailer was connected to the campsite electrical outlet but the trailer was not properly grounded. Once proper grounding was established, the electrical current no longer flowed from the doorknob into the patient and he no longer experienced any inappropriate shocks.

Any single, strong electrical event can cause a pacemaker or ICD to experience an electrical reset or damage to the generator circuitry. The reset parameters are unique to the individual device and its significance depends on the individual patient. The common causes are external and internal defibrillation and electrocautery.[5] For this reason, each implanting institution should develop protocols for safely using electrocautery

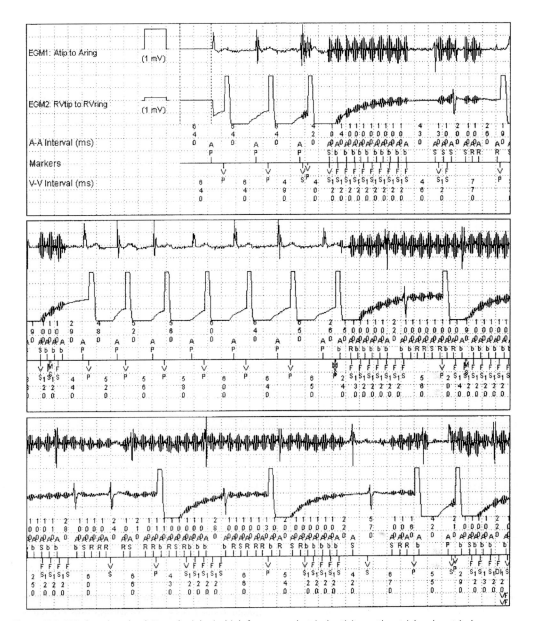

Figure 18.2 *ICD data download. Non-physiologic, high frequency electrical activity on the atrial and ventricular electrograms interpreted as ventricular fibrillation (FS).*

and performing elective and urgent DC cardioversion/defibrillation in patients with pacemakers or ICDs.[3]

Generally, before DC cardioversion/defibrillation, a complete patient and device history and device interrogation should be obtained particularly noting if the patient is pacemaker dependent and the reset parameters of the device.

Each pacemaker/ICD manufacturer makes recommendations for defibrillator pad placement with most recommending an anterior/posterior orientation. A surface electrocardiogram and pulse oximetry should be monitored. The delivered energy, preferably biphasic, should be the minimum necessary to achieve a successful cardioversion. Following cardioversion, the device

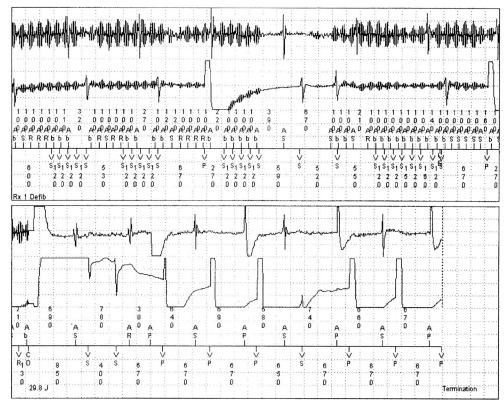

Figure 18.3 *ICD data download. In the upper panel, the capacitors are energized (CE). In the lower panel, the capacitors are discharged (CD).*

should be re-interrogated with threshold testing and re-programming if indicated.

Like DC cardioversion, manufacturers have specific recommendations for their devices that may be exposed to surgical electrocautery. Prior to surgery that may include electrocautery, a CIED patient should have a complete personal and device history with a device interrogation. A qualified medical team experienced in CIED management should make the recommendation whether a pacemaker dependent patient should have the device programmed into an asynchronous mode (VOO or DOO) or have the surgical team prepared to place a magnet over the device during electrocautery application. For ICD patients, suspending therapies before surgery or placing a magnet over the device during electrocautery may be appropriate. In all cases, re-interrogation of the device after the procedure is mandatory.

Avoidance of electrocautery is best but mostly impractical. Similarly, bipolar electrocautery is

preferred to unipolar electrocautery but surgeons rarely consider it a suitable alternative if significant cutting and dissection are necessary. To minimize the risk of unipolar electrocautery, the placement of the grounding pad should be about 15 cm from the device and lead and the current pathway between the grounding pad and the electrocautery tip should not crossover the device and lead. Finally, short bursts up to 5 s of electrocautery with a 10-s pause are better than long applications.[6]

In the DDD and VDD modes, electromagnetic interference may trigger ventricular activity causing inappropriate high rate ventricular pacing. If the frequency of the interference is high enough, mode switching may occur. Conversely, increased sensing in the atrial or ventricular channels during the respective refractory periods can lead to noise reversion. In this scenario, the refractory periods and blanking periods are constantly reset. This results in pacing at the low programmed rate. Moving away from the offending electromagnetic source and programming to a less sensitive setting using a bipolar sensing configuration if possible may resolve both of these problems.

Finally, external radiation therapy uses focused, high energy electromagnetic radiation with very short wavelengths to kill cancer cells. The wavelengths fall into the X-ray and gamma ray portion of the spectrum. Studies have shown that radiation therapy can degrade the silicon and silicon dioxide insulators within a pacemaker's microcircuitry resulting in malfunction or complete failure.[7] Unfortunately, the total dose of radiation that may cause a problem varies widely and the onset of device failure is unpredictable. Radiation therapy can be used but it is highly recommended that the entire radiation protocol developed by the radiation therapy team include significant input from the clinicians managing the patient's CIED. The daily dose should remain below 10 gray if possible and depending on the protocol, device interrogation may be necessary weekly with plans for long term serial device follow-up after the radiation therapy protocol concludes.[8] Citing the lack of extensive *in vitro* and *in vivo* data on the effect of radiation therapy on ICD function and integrity, Langer et al. presented the protocol used at his institution.[9] The protocol again emphasized the importance of complete co-operation of the radiation therapy and cardiovascular teams with input from the device manufacturer.

Sources of electromagnetic interference

It is beyond the scope of this chapter to list all the sources of electromagnetic interference. Further, not all forms of electromagnetic interference affect pacemaker or ICD's in a similar fashion. One of the best repositories of this information is the *Medtronic Electromagnetic Compatibility Table for Pacemakers and Defibrillators*.[10] Not only does it provide an exhaustive list of sources, it provides information on the potential effect of the electromagnetic interference and ways to eliminate or minimize the effect. Complementing this list is the *Consensus Statement on the Perioperative Management of Patients with Implantable Defibrillators, Pacemakers and Arrhythmia Monitors* from the Heart Rhythm Society and American

Society of Anesthesiologists.[3] This expert consensus thoroughly reviews the literature and provides a framework for developing protocols for safely managing patients with CIEDs. For any device, the implanting center should always solicit this information from the device manufacturer. While patient care is ultimately the responsibility of the clinical team, it cannot be emphasized enough the importance of maintaining a close relationship with the device manufacturer's technical service team. Each implanting center should maintain up to date data on the CIEDs they follow and have it readily available for patient safety and education.

The most useful list will contain sources that can occur at home, in the community/workplace and in a hospital setting. Tables 18.1–18.3 list potential

Table 18.1 *Potential sources of electromagnetic interference at home*

Cellular telephone
Digital music player
Electric toothbrush
Hand-held hair dryer
Corded electric razor
Large speakers
Invisible pet fences and dog shock collars
Electric golf carts
CB and Ham radio equipment
Metal detectors
Hand held video game controllers

Table 18.2 *Potential sources of electromagnetic interference in the community/workplace*

Electric welding equipment
Electric kilns
Battery and electric powered hand and bench power tools
Battery chargers
Car ignition systems
High voltage power lines
Hydroelectric plants
Tattoo machine
Electronic article surveillance/antitheft devices
House arrest monitors
Improperly grounded swimming pools
Recipient of an electronic stun gun discharge

Table 18.3 *Potential sources of electromagnetic interference in the hospital*

Magnetic resonance imaging
Electrocautery
RF ablation equipment
DC cardioversion
Radiation therapy
Electroconvulsive therapy
AC electrolysis equipment
TENS devices
Electromyography
Diathermy

sources of electromagnetic interference a device patient is likely to encounter. In most cases, the potential for a negative effect is small. Minimizing the effects of electromagnetic interference can usually be achieved by increasing the distance between the source and the device. The usual cited distance is 15 cm.[5, 10] For fixed sources, such as store antitheft systems, device patients are advised not to linger near the source and walk briskly through monitoring gates. Finally, like any list, it is incomplete and will become outdated as new electronic devices and gadgets are invented.

Cardiovascular implanted electronic devices and magnetic resonance imaging

At this time, there are no absolute uniform guidelines for MRI studies for patients with CIEDs. The American Heart Association 2007 guidelines state MRI studies should not be performed in pacemaker dependent and ICD patients unless there are "highly compelling circumstances."[11] Further, MRI studies in non-pacemaker dependent patients are discouraged unless there is a "strong clinical indication."[11] The same recommendation applies to those patients with epicardial lead systems or those patients with abandoned or fractured leads. In the USA, there is only one FDA approved MRI conditional pacemaker system and it is only approved if both the MR conditional lead and MR conditional generator are used together.[12] The MRI protocol must use a 1.5 Tesla magnet with limitations on the scanning protocol and strict

guidelines on the pre- and post-test assessment of the patient and the device.[13] There is no approved MR conditional ICD system currently in the USA.

As expected, the large static and pulsed magnetic fields generated by an MRI study can directly affect a non-MR conditional CIED.[14] Static fields can cause possible device movement with resultant pain and lead dislodgement. The status of the reed switch may be altered ~~and~~ resulting in unpredictable device behavior.[15] During the pulsed applications, device oversensing and undersensing with changes in normal CIED function may occur. Finally, the generated radiofrequency field may cause local heating resulting in thermal burns and inappropriate CIED function, including reset.

Despite these negative possibilities, Nazarian et al. developed and reported on an MRI protocol for CIED patients.[16] In this prospective study of 438 patients, 54% with pacemakers and 46% with ICDs, having 555 MRI studies, only three patients, one ICD, and two pacemakers, had power-on-reset events. The ICD patient felt a pulling sensation in the chest and the MRI was terminated. The other two patients were not pacemaker dependent and completed the MRI without difficulty. During long-term follow-up, all three patients had normal device function. This study was limited to adults and excluded patients with epicardial, fractured, or abandoned leads.

References

1 Hayes DL, Wang PJ, Reynolds DW, et al. Interference with cardiac pacemakers by cellular telephones. *New England Journal of Medicine* 1997; 336: 1473–1479.

2 Lawrentschuk N, Bolton DM. Mobile phone interference with medical equipment and its clinical relevance: a systematic review. *MJA* 2004; 181 (3): 145–149.

3 Crossley GH, Poole JE, Rozner MA et al. The Heart Rhythm Society (HRS)/American Society of Anesthesiologists (ASA) expert consensus statement on the perioperative management of patients with implantable defibrillators, pacemakers and arrhythmia monitors: facilities and patient management. *Heart Rhythm* 2011; 8(7): 1114–1154.

4 Establishment of a Medical Implant Communications Service in the 402–405 MHz band. Federal Communications Commission. Final rule. *Federal Register* Dec 1999; 64 (240): 69926–69934.

5 Kaszala K, Nazarian S, Halperin H. Electromagnetic interference and CIEDs. In: Ellenbogen KA, Kay

GN, Lau C, Wilkoff BL, eds. *Clinical Cardiac Pacing, Defibrillation and Resynchronization Therapy*, 4th Edn. Philadelphia: Elsevier Saunders, 2011: 1004–1027.

6 Ubee SS, Kasi VS, Bello D, Manikandan R. Implications of pacemakers and implantable cardioverter defibrillators in urological practice. *Journal of Urology* 2011; 186: 1198–1205.

7 Last A. Radiotherapy in patients with cardiac pacemakers. *British Journal of Radiology* 1998; 71: 4–10.

8 Wadasadawala T, Pandey A, Agarwal JP, et al. Radiation therapy with implanted cardiac pacemaker devices: a clinical and dosimetric analysis of patients and proposed precautions. *Clinical Oncology* 2011; 23: 79–85.

9 Langer M, Orlandi E, Carrara M, et al. Management of patients with implantable cardioverter defibrillator needing radiation therapy for cancer. *British Journal of Anaesthesia* 2012; 108(5): 881–882.

10 *Medtronic Electromagnetic Compatibility Table for Pacemakers and Defibrillators*. Medtronic, Inc. 4/16/2010

11 Levine GN, Gomes AS, Arai AE, et al. Safety of magnetic resonance imaging in patients with cardiovascular devices. *Circulation* 2007; 116: 2878–2891.

12 Shinebane JS, Colletti PM, Shellock FG. Magnetic resonance imaging in patients with cardiac pacemakers: era of "MR Conditional" designs. *Journal of Cardiovascular Magnetic Resonance* 2011; 13:63

13 Lobodzinski SS. Recent innovations in the development of magnetic resonance imaging conditional pacemakers and implantable cardioverter-defibrillators. *Cardiology Journal* 2012; 19(1): 98–104.

14 Dyrda K, Khairy P. Implantable rhythm devices and electromagnetic interference: myth or reality? *Expert Reviews Cardiovascular Therapy* 2008; 6(6): 823–832.

15 Beinart R, Nazarian S. Magnetic resonance imaging in patients with implanted devices. *Journal of Cardiovascular Electrophysiology* 2012; 23(9): 1040–1042.

16 Nazarian S, Hansford R, Roguin A, et al. A prospective evaluation of a protocol for magnetic resonance imaging of patients with implanted cardiac devices. *Annals of Internal Medicine* 2011; 155: 415–424.

CHAPTER 19

Quality of life, sports, and implantable devices in the young

Elizabeth Saarel

Ronald and Helen Ross Distinguished Chair, Pediatric Cardiology Cleveland Clinic, Professor of Pediatrics, Cleveland Clinic Lerner College of Medicine of Case Western Reserve University, Cleveland, OH, USA

Introduction

Chronic implantable cardiac devices including pacemakers and cardioverter defibrillators (ICDs) are accepted therapies for patients of all ages with cardiac arrhythmias. Indications for device placement have expanded and now include implantation as a mechanism for reduction in morbidity in addition to mortality. Despite a large body of literature supporting cardiac device use in pediatric and adult patients, the effect of device implantation on quality of life (QOL) was largely unexplored until the last decade. In a similar manner, the safety of sports participation for patients with pacemakers and ICDs remains fundamentally unstudied.

Description of the topic

Early research in cardiac pacing and internal defibrillation for both children and adults focused on advances in technology and improvement in hardware. The next era in cardiac pacing and internal defibrillation expanded research in cardiac monitoring and complex programming for implantable devices. Today, pacemaker and ICD options are sophisticated and useful for personalized treatment of unique pediatric and adult congenital heart

patients. The recent body of medical literature has reflected a growing concern for QOL and the safety of sports for patients with chronic implanted devices including pacemakers and ICDs.

Quality of Life

There have been few studies examining QOL in patients with pacemakers. All found improved QOL after pacemaker placement in adults regardless of pacing mode.[1] One investigation compared psychosocial outcomes in children with and without pacemakers and found no significant difference in standardized measures of self-esteem, anxiety, and self-competence.[2]

Numerous studies have compared QOL in adult patients with single or dual chamber pacemakers, and most found enhancement with dual chamber devices.[3] Of interest, one study compared QOL in those with pacemakers to those with ICDs and found no significant difference.[4] However, the methods by which QOL was measured vary in these studies and no single tool has been validated in cardiac device patients, so there has been recent interest in developing an accurate QOL outcome measure for use in future an investigation.[5–8]

Cardiac Pacing and Defibrillation in Pediatric and Congenital Heart Disease, First Edition.
Edited by Maully Shah, Larry Rhodes and Jonathan Kaltman.
© 2017 John Wiley & Sons Ltd. Published 2017 by John Wiley & Sons Ltd.
Companion Website: www.wiley.com/go/shah/cardiac_pacing

In contrast to dual chamber pacemakers, rate responsive pacing and dual rate sensors have a limited influence on QOL in adult studies.[9] Finally, there have been numerous prospective randomized trials proving enhanced QOL after cardiac resynchronization therapy in adult patients with severe left ventricular dysfunction and NYHA class III-IV symptoms, but none in the young heart failure population.

There is a growing body of medical literature examining QOL for patients with ICDs. Most studies in adult patients show a decrease in QOL for patients who receive ICDs compared to their pre-ICD state. In particular, patients who received multiple shocks, both appropriate and inappropriate, have worse quality of life than those who do not.[10-12] Post traumatic stress disorder has been well documented in a subset of adults with ICDs, usually those who have received multiple shocks.[13-15] Of relevance to the pediatric and adult congenital heart disease population, in most studies, young adult ICD patients (less than 50 years of age) were at increased risk for psychological distress.[16]

Studies examining QOL in pediatric patients with ICDs are few in number but are increasing in frequency. It is interesting and encouraging that initial results contrast adult ICD patients' experience. An early study by DeMaso et al. in 2004 documented relatively good QOL in pediatric patients with ICDs.[17] Despite lower physical functioning scores in those with ICDs, psychosocial functioning was comparable to a normal patient population and patients' QOL correlated with feelings of anxiety and depression and family functioning rather than severity of illness.[17, 18] Despite these reports there remains concern for worse psychosocial outcomes in pediatrics patients because of a higher rate of appropriate and inappropriate shocks. In addition, post-shock anxiety disorders have been well documented in the young.[19, 20] Investigators have recently initiated the development of a pediatric specific QOL measure to be validated in young patients with ICDs.[21]

Research evaluating psychosocial interventions in the adult ICD population shows promising results. Behavioral therapy, cardiac education, and cardiac rehabilitation are most effective in reducing anxiety in adult patients with ICDs.[22, 23] Although

the positive effects may be small regardless of methods used, levels of depression and anxiety and QOL improved significantly from baseline to after the intervention.[24]

Vigilance for the identification of psychosocial dysfunction and anxiety disorders in our young patients with implanted cardiac devices should be maintained. If pathology is suspected, appropriate referrals for evaluation and intervention by behavioral health providers are warranted. If future studies indicate a high rate of psychosocial dysfunction in this young population, routine screening should be considered.

Sports participation

Cardiac physical rehabilitation has been shown to be safe and effective for improving exercise tolerance in adult patients with ICDs, but published data about exercise in young patients or competitive sports participation in those with implanted cardiac devices remain sparse. Despite a dearth of research, published guidelines in the United States and Europe, based on expert opinion, recommend against competitive sports participation in activities more strenuous than bowling or golf (Class IA) for patients with pacemakers or ICDs (Figure 19.1).[25-29]

Subsequent to the publication of guidelines in 2005, a survey of Heart Rhythm Society members was performed to ascertain physicians' current practice regarding participation in sports for their patients with ICDs.[30] Seventy-one percent of electrophysiologists reported caring for patients who participated in sports or vigorous exercise including competitive athletics like basketball, running, and skiing.[30] Whereas 10% of electrophysiologists recommended against participation in all sports more physical than the 1A classification (commensurate with guidelines), 76% allowed participation in sports as long as patients avoid contact and 45% recommended avoidance of competitive sports.[30] Most physicians considered underlying heart disease when formulating sports restrictions for their patients with implanted cardiac devices.[30] Although ICD therapies during sports were common, few serious consequences were reported.[30] Of interest, the most common adverse events reported were lead damage due to

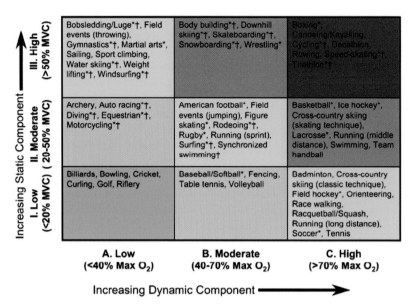

Figure 19.1 *The 36th Bethesda Conference Task Force 8: Classification of Sports (Adapted from Maron, BJ and DP Zipes, Introduction: eligibility recommendations for competitive athletes with cardiovascular abnormalities-general considerations. J Am Coll Cardiol, 2005.[25])*

repetitive motion activities such as weight lifting or golf.[30]

Another study surveyed 387 patients, ages 25–86 years, with ICDs.[31] Patients were queried regarding athletic activities and ICD shocks. Fifty-nine percent of patients participated in sports including biking, alpine hiking, swimming, skiing, jogging, gymnastics, soccer, tennis, and others.[31] The reported rate of ICD shocks during sports was 14%, higher than the rate of shocks during non-athletic activities, with biking, skiing, jogging, and hiking imparting the highest risk.[31]

In 2006, a prospective multicenter registry was launched to study the safety of sports participation for patients with ICDs.[32] This international investigation includes patients ages 10–60 years who received ICDs for primary or secondary prevention of sudden cardiac death. Diagnoses include inherited arrhythmia syndromes, inherited or acquired cardiomyopathies, congenital heart disease, and valvular heart disease. Three hundred and twenty-eight athletes were enrolled in the registry and over a median of 31 months, there were no occurrences of either death or resuscitated arrest or arrhythmia- or shock-related injury-during sports. There were 49 shocks in 37 participants (10% of

study population) during competition/practice, 39 shocks in 29 participants (8%) during other physical activity, and 33 shocks in 24 participants (6%) at rest leading the authors to conclude that many athletes with ICDs can engage in sports without physical injury or failure to terminate the arrhythmia despite the occurrence of both inappropriate and appropriate shocks.[33]

Unpublished data from a prospective registry in our pediatric and adult congenital heart center includes 15 young patients with ICDs who regularly participate in competitive or vigorous sports (great than IA for dynamic and/or static component). Our data show no mortality and no increase in morbidity after 2 years.[34] Patients' choice of athletics include running, jogging, alpine hiking, swimming, skiing, snowboarding, rock climbing, basketball, football, baseball, gymnastics, and other sports. One teen with congenital heart disease experienced two appropriate ICD shocks for treatment of ventricular tachyarrhythmias during basketball and then decided to withdraw from competitive athletics. No other patients have had an increased incidence of ICD therapies during athletics, either inappropriate or appropriate. We have seen no increased rate of damage to the ICD system during organized sports. Of note, most of our patients with ICDs are on beta blocker therapy to prevent inappropriate ICD shocks due to sinus or supraventricular tachycardias, and most underwent formal exercise testing to screen for arrhythmia prior to sports participation.

A recent study by Aziz et al, reviewed 212 pediatric genotype positive long QT syndrome patients who engaged in sports including 6 patients with ICDs. While the numbers are small, no patients had an appropriate ICD discharge while playing organized sports or experienced sports related injury to the ICD system.[35]

When questions arise about sports participation it is our practice to counsel patients and families about the risks, including potential for increased rate of ventricular tachyarrhythmias and damage to the pacemaker or ICD system. Counseling is patient specific; the underlying cardiac disease, type of device, indication for implant, position of leads and pulse generators, underlying heart rhythm, patient age, and type of athletic activity are considered when estimating risk.

The potential benefits of sports participation for young patients include decreased risk for obesity, metabolic syndrome, coronary and peripheral artery disease, stroke and diabetes.[36] The centers for Disease Control and Prevention recommend at least 30 minutes of moderate to vigorous physical activity on most days in order to decrease risk for cardiovascular disease.[37] Indeed, the relative risk of cardiovascular disease associated with physical inactivity ranges from 1.5 to 2.4, an increase comparable to that observed for high blood cholesterol, high blood pressure, or cigarette smoking.[37]

There are additional benefits of exercise including a positive effect on general mental health, decreasing risk for depression and overall improvement in wellbeing, all of which affect quality of life.[38] Exercise and resistance training also improve bone density. Sports participation has been shown to increase healthy behaviors in adolescents in the United States including decreased rates of recreational drug use and teen pregnancy.[39] Ultimately, the importance of sports participation to each patient's quality of life must be estimated by the individual and their family.

In summary, the risk of sports participation for our patients with implanted cardiac devices may include an increased tachyarrhythmia burden, injury after loss of consciousness from cardiac device function or malfunction, and permanent damage to the implanted device system during sports. Sports that evoke a high potential for serious injury to one's self or others if a patient were to experience syncope, including those using motor vehicles, should be discouraged. In the future, our estimates of risk should be guided by research rather than opinion.[40] The risks of sports participation must be weighed against the benefits, including potential for improved quality of life, for all young patients with implanted cardiac devices.

References

1 Lopez-Jimenez, F, Goldman L, Orav EJ, et al. Health values before and after pacemaker implantation. *Am Heart J*, 2002; 144(4): 687–692.

2 Alpern D, Uzark K, Dick M, 2nd. Psychosocial responses of children to cardiac pacemakers. *J Pediatr*, 1989; 114(3): 494–501.

3 Newman D, Relationships between pacing mode and quality of life: evidence from randomized clinical trials. *Card Electrophysiol Rev*, 2003; 7(4): 401–405.

4 Duru F, Buchi S, Klaghofer R, et al. How different from pacemaker patients are recipients of implantable cardioverter-defibrillators with respect to psychosocial adaptation, affective disorders, and quality of life? *Heart*, 2001; 85(4): 375–379.

5 Beery TA, Baas LS, Matthews H, et al. Development of the implanted devices adjustment scale. *Dimens Crit Care Nurs*, 2005; 24(5): 242–248.

6 Stofmeel MA, Post MW, Kelder JC, Grobbee DE, van Hemel NM. Quality-of-life of pacemaker patients: a reappraisal of current instruments. *Pacing Clin Electrophysiol*, 2000; 23(6): 946–952.

7 Stofmeel MA, Post MW, Kelder JC, Grobbee DE, van Hemel NM. Psychometric properties of Aquarel. a disease-specific quality of life questionnaire for pacemaker patients. *J Clin Epidemiol*, 2001; 54(2): 157–165.

8 Stofmeel MA, van Stel HF, van Hemel NM, Grobbee DE. The relevance of health related quality of life in paced patients. *Int J Cardiol*, 2005; 102(3): 377–382.

9 van Hemel NM, Holwerda KJ, Slegers PC, et al. The contribution of rate adaptive pacing with single or dual sensors to health-related quality of life. *Europace*, 2007; 9(4): 233–238.

10 Sears SF, Hazelton AG, St Amant J, et al. Quality of life in pediatric patients with implantable cardioverter defibrillators. *Am J Cardiol*, 2011; 107(7): 1023–1027.

11 Irvine J, Dorian P, Baker B, et al. Quality of life in the Canadian Implantable Defibrillator Study (CIDS). *Am Heart J*, 2002; 144(2): 282–289.

12 Passman R, Subacius H, Ruo B, et al. Implantable cardioverter defibrillators and quality of life: results from the defibrillators in nonischemic cardiomyopathy treatment evaluation study. *Arch Intern Med*, 2007; 167(20): 2226–2232.

13 Sears SE, Jr., Conti JB. Understanding implantable cardioverter defibrillator shocks and storms: medical and psychosocial considerations for research and clinical care. *Clin Cardiol*, 2003; 26(3): 107–111.

14 von Känel R, Baumert J, Kolb C, Cho EY, Ladwig KH. Chronic posttraumatic stress and its predictors in patients living with an implantable cardioverter defibrillator. *J Affect Disord*, 2011; 131(1–3): 344–352.

15 Sears SF, Hauf JD, Kirian K, et al. Posttraumatic stress and the implantable cardioverter-defibrillator patient: what the electrophysiologist needs to know. *Circ Arrhythm Electrophysiol*, 2011; 4(2): 242–250.

16 Sears SF, Jr., Conti JB. Quality of life and psychological functioning of ICD patients. *Heart*, 2002; 87(5): 488–493.

17 DeMaso DR, Lauretti A, Spieth L, et al. Psychosocial factors and quality of life in children and adolescents with implantable cardioverter-defibrillators. *Am J Cardiol*, 2004; 93(5): 582–587.

18 Zeigler VL, Nelms T. Almost normal: experiences of adolescents with implantable cardioverter defibrillators. *J Spec Pediatr Nurs*, 2009; 14(2): 142–151.

19 Sears SF, St Amant JB, Zeigler V. Psychosocial considerations for children and young adolescents with implantable cardioverter defibrillators: an update. *Pacing Clin Electrophysiol*, 2009; 32(Suppl 2): S80–S82.

20 Stefanelli CB, Bradley DJ, Leroy S, et al. Implantable cardioverter defibrillator therapy for life-threatening arrhythmias in young patients. *J Interv Card Electrophysiol*, 2002; 6(3): 235–244.

21 Zeigler VL, Decker-Walters B. Determining psychosocial research priorities for adolescents with implantable cardioverter defibrillators using Delphi methodology. *J Cardiovasc Nurs*, 2010; 25(5): 398–404.

22 Pedersen SS, van den Broek KC, Sears SF, Jr., Psychological intervention following implantation of an implantable defibrillator: a review and future recommendations. *Pacing Clin Electrophysiol*, 2007; 30(12): 1546–1554.

23 Pedersen SS, Spek V, Theuns DA, et al. Rationale and design of WEBCARE: a randomized, controlled, web-based behavioral intervention trial in cardioverter-defibrillator patients to reduce anxiety and device concerns and enhance quality of life. *Trials*, 2009; 10: 120.

24 Sears SF, Sowell LD, Kuhl EA, et al. The ICD shock and stress management program: a randomized trial of psychosocial treatment to optimize quality of life in ICD patients. *Pacing Clin Electrophysiol*, 2007; 30(7): 858–864.

25 Zipes DP, Camm AJ, Borggrefe M, et al. ACC/AHA/ESC 2006 guidelines for management of patients with ventricular arrhythmias and the prevention of sudden cardiac death: a report of the American College of Cardiology/American Heart Association Task Force and the European Society of Cardiology Committee for Practice Guidelines (Writing Committee to Develop Guidelines for Management of Patients With Ventricular Arrhythmias and the Prevention of Sudden Cardiac Death). *J Am Coll Cardiol*, 2006; 48(5): p. e247–346.

26 Maron BJ, Zipes DP. Introduction: eligibility recommendations for competitive athletes with cardiovascular abnormalities-general considerations. *J Am Coll Cardiol*, 2005; 45(8): 1318–1321.

27 Pelliccia A, Fagard R, Bjørnstad HH, et al. Recommendations for competitive sports participation in athletes with cardiovascular disease: a consensus document from the Study Group of Sports Cardiology of the Working Group of Cardiac Rehabilitation and Exercise Physiology and the Working Group of Myocardial and Pericardial Diseases of the European Society of Cardiology. *Eur Heart J*, 2005; 26(14): 1422–1445.

28 Pelliccia, A. Implantable cardioverter defibrillator and competitive sport participation. *Eur Heart J*, 2009; 30(24): 2967–298.

29 Mitchell JH, Haskell W, Snell P, et al. Task Force 8: classification of sports. *J Am Coll Cardiol*, 2005; 45(8): 1364–1367.

30 Lampert R, Cannom D, Olshansky B. Safety of sports participation in patients with implantable cardioverter defibrillators: a survey of heart rhythm society members. *J Cardiovasc Electrophysiol*, 2006; 17(1): 11–15.

31 Kobza R, Duru F, and Erne P. Leisure-time activities of patients with ICDs: findings of a survey with respect to sports activity, high altitude stays, and driving patterns. *Pacing Clin Electrophysiol*, 2008; 31(7): 845–849.

32 Lampert R. *ICD Sports Registry*, Yale University. 2010.

33 Lampert R, Olshansky B, Heidbuchel H, Lawless C, Saarel E, Ackerman M, et al. Safety of sports for athletes with implantable cardioverter-defibrillators: results of a prospective, multinational registry. *Circulation*. 2013 May 21; 127(20): 2021–2030

34 Saarel EV. *Pediatric and Adult Congenital Heart Disease ICD Sports Registry*. 2011.

35 Aziz PF, Sweeten, T, Vogel RL, Bonney WJ, Henderson J, Patel AR, Shah MJ. Sports participation in genotype positive children with long QT syndrome. *JACCCEP*. 2015; 1(1): 62–70.

36 Lloyd-Jones D, Adams RJ, Brown TM, et al. Heart disease and stroke statistics – 2010 update: a report from the American Heart Association. *Circulation*, 2010; 121(7): p. e46–e215.

37 Pate RR, Pratt M, Blair SN, et al. Physical activity and public health. A recommendation from the Centers for Disease Control and Prevention and the American College of Sports Medicine. *JAMA*, 1995; 273(5): 402–407.

38 Landers, D. The Influence of Exercise on Mental Health. *The President's Council on Physical Fitness and Sports*, 1997; 2(12).

39 Pate RR, Trost SG, Levin S, et al. Sports participation and health-related behaviors among US youth. *Arch Pediatr Adolesc Med*, 2000; 154(9): 904–911.

40 Zipes DP, Link MS, Ackerman MJ, Kovacs RJ, Myerburg RJ, Estes NA 3rd. American Heart Association Electrocardiography and Arrhythmias Committee of Council on Clinical Cardiology, Council on Cardiovascular Disease in Young, Council on Cardiovascular and Stroke Nursing, Council on Functional Genomics and Translational Biology, and American College of Cardiology. Eligibility and Disqualification Recommendations for Competitive Athletes With Cardiovascular Abnormalities: Task Force 9: Arrhythmias and Conduction Defects: A Scientific Statement From the American Heart Association and American College of Cardiology. *Circulation*. 2015 Dec 1; 132(22): e315–e325.

CHAPTER 20

Device innovations and the future of device therapy for arrhythmia and heart failure management

Michael P. Carboni[1] and Ronald J. Kanter[2]

[1] Pediatric Electrophysiologist, Duke Children's Hospital and Health Center, Assistant Professor of Pediatrics, Duke University School of Medicine, Durham, NC, USA

[2] Director, Pediatric Electrophysiology, Nicklaus Children's Hospital, Miami, FL, USA

Introduction and the legacy of cardiac rhythm management devices

Improvements in cardiac rhythm management device (CRMD) therapy for children remain on a steep slope. It is useful to think about the major issues surrounding future developments in five categories:

1 Hardware – those components which are physically and electrically interactive with the patient, including but not limited to the battery, EMI filtered feedthroughs from the connector block to the circuitry, the enclosure ("casing"), capacitors, engineered components (silicone semiconductors for microelectronics, plastic connector block, and all assemblies), and leads (conductors, insulators, and physiological sensors);

2 Software design and implementation for more physiologically accurate pacing in children and those having congenital heart disease and for therapeutic strategies for heart failure;

3 Out-patient device monitoring;

4 Recognition and treatment of behavioral and emotional impact of device therapy; and

5 Global accessibility of devices for underserved children.

A comprehensive consideration of the emerging progress in all aspects of CRMD therapy for children is obviously impractical. This chapter will therefore highlight several issues for which information is available.

To briefly reiterate this textbook's opening chapter, myocardial pacing has been in existence for more than 50 years.[1,2] The first clinical application of cardiac pacing was performed during the 1950s and used external power sources. The first self-contained implantable pacemaker, developed by Wilson Greatbatch and William Chardack, used a rechargeable nickel-cadmium battery and was first implanted in a human in Buffalo, NY, in 1960. This inefficient energy source was replaced in the 1960s by the zinc-mercury battery, and the life span of these devices was more than two years, quite an improvement by the standards of the day.

Cardiac Pacing and Defibrillation in Pediatric and Congenital Heart Disease, First Edition.
Edited by Maully Shah, Larry Rhodes and Jonathan Kaltman.
© 2017 John Wiley & Sons Ltd. Published 2017 by John Wiley & Sons Ltd.
Companion Website: www.wiley.com/go/shah/cardiac_pacing

However, electrolyte generation in this battery resulted in release of hydrogen gas, requiring that the device be vented. This resulted in fluid leak, shorting of electronic components, and premature device failure, often without a premonitory voltage decay. The 1970s brought a change in battery and pacing lead technology which extended the service life of pacemakers almost tenfold. Programmability of devices was also introduced during this period. Starting about 1973, nuclear batteries, using metallic plutonium (^{238}Pu), and, later, ceramic plutonium oxide were implanted for a period of time. The slow decay of the isotope emits alpha particles, which interact with the device casing, generating heat. The semiconductor, bismuth telluride, is used for thermoelectric energy conversion. Despite an estimated half-life of 87 years, production of these physically large devices was halted for regulatory and public health reasons. Tracking of the devices as patients traveled between states and countries and proper disposal at device explantation were chief among these. As discussed next, the year 1972 heralded the application of the lithium iodine battery in cardiac pacemakers and which are still in use today. In the subsequent decades, miniaturization of electronics and changes in materials technology have resulted in smaller, more efficient devices (especially pertinent to children); dramatic increase in data storage capacity and telemetry; and more complex programmability. The 1990s was the decade of the implantable cardioverter-defibrillator, and the 2000s, the decade of cardiac resynchronization therapy. Advances in nanotechnology and cellular therapy now offer even greater possibilities for the future of cardiac rhythm management.

Toward a better energy source

Cardiac pacemaker battery design presents a collection of unique challenges related to shelf life, service life, internal resistance, specific energy (watt-hours/kg), specific power (watts/kg), safety, weight, physical dimensions, reliability, biocompatibility, and accurate end-of-life battery predictions. Electrochemical fuel cells have heretofore been the only source of cardiac pacemaker energy (thermoelectric batteries using radioactive plutonium being the only exception). Changes in battery technology have played a major role in the evolution of today's devices. The advent of the lithium battery significantly extended the life of pacemakers and allowed for production of smaller devices. The solid electrolyte lithium iodine battery (actually, lithium iodone-polyvinylpyridine, PVP) has long been the power source of cardiac pacemakers to this point, and the standard by which other power sources are compared. The coating of the anode, lithium, by layers of PVP underwent iterative improvements in the 1970s (Greatbatch, Inc.; Clarence, NY) and in the 1980s (Medtronic, Inc.; Minneapolis, MN) to greatly enhanced the battery's discharge characteristics. The self-discharge rate of lithium iodine batteries is very low resulting in a long shelf life. In addition, they have a stable voltage through their service life with a gradual and predictable reduction over time. This allows a reliable method for predicting replacement time. There is no production of heat, gas, or acid with battery use, making it an acceptable source of power for sealed implantable devices. Other lithium compounds are used as batteries in implantable cardioverter-defibrillators. Specifically, lithium silver vanadium oxide (SVO) is used in St. Jude Medical and some Biotronik devices, and lithium manganese dioxide is used by Boston Scientific and some Biotronik devices.

Two competing needs have been a constant challenge for device engineers: physical miniaturization and longer service life. Smaller devices leave less space for the power source; therefore, batteries with a smaller footprint are needed. Smaller batteries typically generate less power and have a reduced service life. In addition, new innovations in device connectivity and other device features (i.e., hemodynamic monitoring, autoprogrammability, myocardial contraction modulation, wireless monitoring) require the rapid availability of higher energy outputs and place increasing demands on the current lithium iodine batteries.

A newer type of solid electrolyte battery using lithium carbon monofluoride (CFx) offers higher power density at a smaller size and appears suitable for meeting the demands of future pacing devices.[3] It can deliver energy in the milliamp range without appreciable voltage drop. This battery technology has been successfully used in drug pumps. Other lithium-based systems also appear promising,

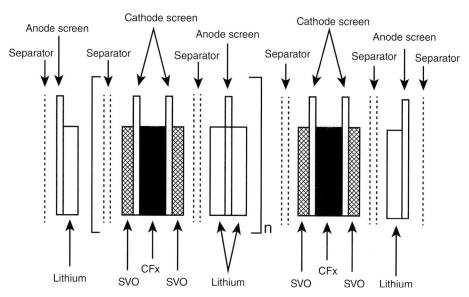

Figure 20.1 *Schema of the cathodal-anodal elements of the "Q technology." The hybrid cathode of silver vanadium oxide (SVO) and carbon monofluoride (CFx) combines the capacity for rapid delivery of high energy as well as maximizing the energy density necessary for all other functionalities, including bradycardia pacing. This battery is used in many of the newly designed implantable cardioverter-defibrillators. (Source: Curtis F. Holmes, Greatbatch Medical; Alden, NY. Reproduced with permission of Curtis F. Holmes.)*

but with some limitations. Unlike all previously described compounds, lithium-polycarbon fluoride and lithium manganese dioxide use liquid electrolyte. These batteries offer even higher power densities, in the tens of milliamps. However, the liquid component requires special attention to sealing in order to prevent leakage. In particular, gamma butyrolactone is a volatile component of the lithium polycarbon fluoride battery. New and practical techniques are being developed for detection of leak of this substance. Another liquid electrolyte, lithium thionyl chloride, has even higher power density, but with heightened concern for preventing leakage, because thionyl chloride is toxic and corrosive.

Due to increased use of memory necessary to store intrinsic cardiac electrical activity, need for faster and longer-term telemetry, newer sensors, and newer high power therapies, modern implantable cardiac devices have higher peak power requirements than previously and greater than can be achieved by lithium iodine batteries. Recently developed at Greatbatch Medical (Clarence, NY) is the "Q technology." QHR ("Q High Rate") batteries utilize cathodal chemistry

that blends CFx and SVO (Figure 20.1). Silver vanadium oxide allows rapid delivery of the large pulse required for defibrillation and a more gradual and reliable discharge rate over the lifespan of the battery; carbon monofluoride maximizes energy density necessary for all other functionalities, including bradycardia pacing. This battery provides higher current and faster charge times, while also ensuring optimum predictability of battery performance. These hybrid batteries have energy density equivalent to the lithium iodine battery but 40 times the power. Intended to provide greater longevity, these batteries are being used in the next generation of ICDs. They are also likely to figure prominently in the development of ICDs that are compatible with magnetic resonance imaging.

In the past, rechargeable batteries for home and commercial electronic equipment were primarily nickel cadmium (NiCad). NiCad batteries require complete discharge and recharge to maintain full capacity, have a relatively high self-discharge rate, and are physically large devices. Since Sony Corporation introduced the lithium-ion technology in 1992, there has been interest in the development of rechargeable batteries for use in cardiac pace-makers. Rechargeable lithium-ion batteries are already in use in some neurologic stimulators and in some left ventricular assist devices, but not yet in CRMDs. These batteries would have several desirable features: They have high energy density (twice that of NiCad); they can partially charge or discharge without affecting battery capacity; they are high voltage (4 V); their self-discharge rate is low (1%/month); their charge/discharge cycle rate is in the thousands before significant capacity reduction; and they may maintain function for over 10 years. Lithium-ion batteries may be used in addition to a primary battery, for example, to serve as the high power component of an ICD (charging the capacitor), or it may be the primary energy source in a small device (so long as the patient or family is capable of performing recharge responsibilities). Lithium-ion batteries contain no metallic lithium. Instead, lithium ions shuttle between positive cathodal (e.g., cobalt oxide) and negative anodal (e.g., graphitic carbon) poles. The spent battery is recharged by transcutaneous electromagnetic induction, using a wound wire in the device (secondary coil) and an external primary coil. Required recharge time is in the order of hours. Declining voltage during gradual discharge would have to be monitored telemetrically by the patient, and the time between required recharges shortens as a function of number of prior recharge sessions.

Due to limitations in battery technology, the search for alternative energy sources has been ongoing.[4] The idea of harvesting the power of the body's natural processes to run cardiac pacing devices makes sense. One obvious source of energy is motion, either from cardiac or body movement. Kinetic motion has been used to run wrist watches and charge or power other electric devices. Piezo-electric crystals are used to turn mechanical energy into electrical energy from deformation of the crystal. Additionally, nanogenerators with more than a million zinc oxide nanowires in proximity to a platinum electrode can convert vibrations into electrical energy.[5, 6] Theoretically, mechanical energy can also be harvested in this way from energy produced by blood flow or cardiac contraction.

Another available source of energy is heat. Thermocouples convert heat energy into electrical energy that can then be used to charge a battery. Innovations in materials technology have led to the development of thermoelectric materials produced on a nanoscale as a thin film. Thousands of these thermoelectric generators can be built into an implantable chip and, via semiconductor technology, be used to trickle charge batteries of an ICD or directly power a pacemaker. For such a biothermal device to perform optimally, a 2°C temperature difference is needed across it. Considering that at least a 5°C difference exists in the skin, implantation of these devices could be conveniently implanted in relative proximity to the device, itself. These power systems have the potential to run for 30 years. The sealed battery used for cardiac pacemakers consumes about 10 mcW, and these technologies produce at least 20 mcW. Devices using mechanical or thermal energy are not yet far enough along in development for human application.

Another alternative energy source under investigation are biofuel cells. Interest in this technology has been generated by the need for very large energy sources – up to 200 mcW – that are estimated to be necessary to power the proposed implantable artificial kidney and roboticized artificial urinary sphincter. These systems are capable of directly transforming chemical to electrical energy from biochemical reactions. Such systems require enzymes and redox mediators assembled into relatively large electrodes and which function at a physiologic pH in the extracellular space. One such system uses glucose and dioxygen from the body's extracellular fluid to generate power.[7] This system has been implanted in a rat and generated enough power to meet the energy requirements of a pacemaker. Longevity of the systems has yet to be determined, but theoretically should remain operational for years.

Preserving vascular access in our young patients

Miniaturization and simplification of pacing devices is best represented by Medtronic's prototype mini-pacemaker, a vitamin capsule-sized device which is leadless and implanted into the

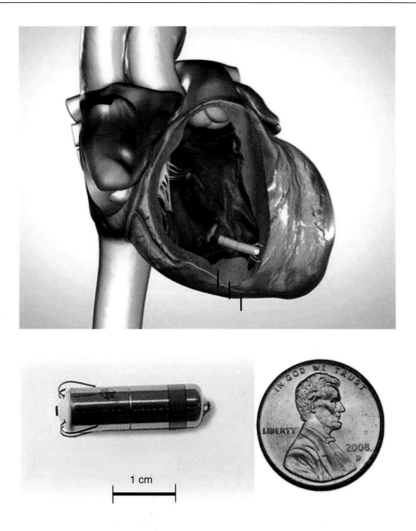

Figure 20.2 *Diagrams of the prototype leadless pacemaker with relative dimensions. Just entering human trials, this device has been in development by Medtronic, Inc. (Minneapolis, MN). (Source: Reproduced with permission from Medtronic, Inc.)*

right ventricle via catheter delivery (Figure 20.2).[8] The device is expected to have a 7-year battery, telemetry capability, and programmability. This device was simplified and has a reduced cost for use in developing countries, which often have limited resources and expertise. Because of the size and ease of implantation, this device may have a variety of applications. Unfortunately, transvenous delivery will require a very large sheath, so pediatric application will likely require alternate means of delivery. Additionally, the field of miniaturization will play a large role in the development of pacemakers for fetal heart block which could be placed *in utero* preventing hydrops and fetal demise.

Feasibility studies have been underway to explore pacing using ultrasound from a transcutaneous (ultimately, subcutaneous) generator to an unattached (ultimately, implanted) receiver in the chamber(s) of choice. In human studies, a customized receiver and sonoelectric converter was mounted into the 4 mm hemispherical platinum/iridium tip electrode of a standard, 6 Fr, bipolar temporary electrophysiology catheter (EBR Systems, Inc., Sunnyvale, CA). The ultrasound generator and external transmitter produced a low frequency (313–385 kHz) timed ultrasound field, delivered via a customary wand using coupling gel at the chest surface. Ultrasound transmission amplitude was limited by an output corresponding to a mechanical index (MI = peak negative pressure ÷ ultrasound frequency) of 1.9 (maximum FDA recommended MI for all non-ophthalmological ultrasound human applications to ensure biosafety). Data collection instrumentation was interfaced with the transmitter and receiver. In Lee's initial experience with 24 adults[9] undergoing standard electrophysiologic testing, 80 sites (including right atrium, right ventricle, endocardial left ventricle, and great cardiac vein) were paced by both ultrasound-mediated energy and by standard programmed electrical stimulator at 400 to 600 ms cycle length and at a pulse width of 0.5 ms. Consistent capture was observed in 77 of 80 sites using ultrasound-mediated pacing, and, when compared, the pacing threshold was comparable between techniques (1.01 + 0.64 V for ultrasound versus 0.97 + 0.67 V for standard). The advantages of this technology are that ultrasound energy is not influenced by electromagnetic interference, and there is no attenuation of ultrasound energy by distance and little attenuation by bone at these low ultrasound frequencies. However, major challenges are evident by the observation of great beat-to-beat receiver electrode output, likely related to cardiac and pulmonary motion, and by ultrasound reflection by the lungs. In addition, as with all systems having a component which is attached to myocardium, the long-term interactions between the receiver electrode and the heart will be potentially efficacy-limiting. Finally, the efficiency of energy conversion was very poor in this study; receiver electrode output energy versus transmitted energy was only 0.063%. The value of such a system in children who have a lifetime of pacing ahead of them is obvious, but the obstacles are daunting.

The old yet ingenious concept of induction pacing would permit leadless energy transmission from a subcutaneous transmitter (primary coil) to a receiver (secondary coil) attached to the myocardial conductor. The subcutaneous coil creates a rotating magnetic field, of which some portion of the generated energy is directly converted into voltage by the receiver. In theory, this is a far more efficient means by which to transfer energy compared with, say, an electrolytic battery used to charge a capacitor, which, in turn, is discharged for pulse generation. Conceptually, the shape of the pulse (i.e., the familiar pulse width and amplitude) is determined by the characteristics of the receiver coil plus the generated magnetic field. Wieneke and co-workers demonstrated the feasibility of such a system in a porcine model.[10] In their prototype, the transmitter consisted of a 6 cm diameter ring-shaped coil (40 turns of a copper strand) inserted subcutaneously over the heart. The strength of the magnetic field (H) is determined by the current (i), the number of turns (N), the radius of the coil (R), and the distance from the center of the coil (z) as: $i \times N \times R^2 / 2 \times (R^2 + z^2)^{2/3}$. The induced voltage (U) is related not to H, but rather to the temporal change in the magnetic flux (dB) and the area (A) as: $n \times A \times dB / dt$ (Faraday's induction law). Wieneke et al. generated the desired dB using an H-bridge circuit (including a small pulse generator). The receiver consisted of a cylindrical coil (2500 turns) of 15 mm length and 2.5 mm diameter, a high impedance hemispherical head, and either a passive or (electrically inactive) screw tip. The transmitter could generate a magnetic field strength of 0.5 mT, resulting in unipolar pulses of 0.4 ms pulse width, amplitude of 0.6–1.0 V, and energy consumption of up to 1 mJ at a distance of 3 cm. The induction field in this model should not be impacted by contemporary occupational and residential magnetic field exposure, due to the low-frequency (10–50 Hz) of alternating fields in our environment. However, this issue would always have to be considered with future technological advances in energy creation and manipulation for science and industry and the resulting exposure to such environmental energy fields.

Patients at risk for life-threatening ventricular arrhythmias, for whom anti-tachycardia pacing will not be necessary or successful, and who do not have chronotropic incompetence may benefit from a pure cardioverter-defibrillator. Such a system obviates all of the complications attendant to transvenous and intracardiac hardware. The system must reliably sense the ventricular electrograms and only ventricular electrograms, reliably discriminate ventricular from supraventricular tachycardia, and successfully depolarize the entire ventricular mass at a sufficiently low energy. The entirely subcutaneous implantable cardioverter-defibrillator (S-ICD) has been in development for over 10 years and has just become available for clinical application in the United States. Following testing of temporarily implanted devices in small series of adults from 2001–2004 and again in 2004–2005, Bardy et al. identified the optimum hardware configuration in the thorax.[11] Subsequent permanent implantation of 61 devices in New Zealand and Europe in 2008–2009 was performed. All 155 episodes of VF were appropriately detected at implantation, and two consecutive episodes were successfully defibrillated in 58 of 59 patients. At follow-up (10 months), there were no inappropriate discharges and successful therapies occurred in all three patients requiring it. The device (S-ICD™ System, Boston Scientific, Inc., Natick, MA) consists of an ICD positioned in the subcutaneous left lateral chest wall and a 3 mm tripolar lead, positioned vertically in the left parasternal subcutaneous tissue (1–2 cm left of midline). The distal electrode is superior and the shock coil is 8 cm in length, flanked by the distal and proximal electrodes (Figure 20.3). It is capable of conditional discrimination of supraventricular

tachycardia (SVT), and the minimum VT rates are from 170 to 240 bpm. In the current iteration, it delivers only an 80 J shock, and it is recommended that it be tested at 65 J. It can demand pace post-shock at 50 bpm for up to 30 s at a bipolar output of 200 mA. Subsequent comparison of the S-ICD™ with standard transvenous systems with respect to specificity of SVT discrimination (the START study) actually demonstrated superiority of the S-ICD™ system.[12] There are ongoing trials to evaluate factors impacting clinical outcome and cost effectiveness of the S-ICD (EFFORTLESS S-ICD Registry).[13] Despite early enthusiasm for this technology, recent experience with younger patients (10–48 years) has shown a relatively high incidence of early reoperation (3/16), inappropriate shocks (4/16), and delayed VF detection.[14] The S-ICD™ could have value in children and teenagers having certain high risk channelopathies and in all patients having congenital heart disease and requiring only primary or secondary prevention of sudden death. Substantial obstacles remain for this population, however, including need for downsizing the ICD for children, consideration of atypical shock vectors in some patients having congenital heart disease, and need for more robust programmability of VT rate detection.

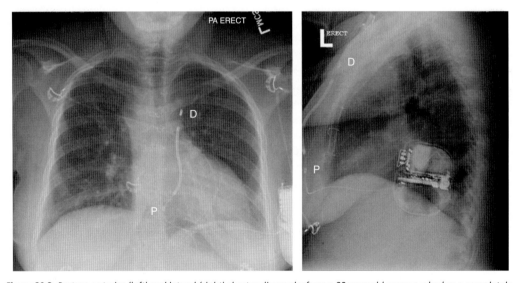

Figure 20.3 *Postero-anterior (left) and lateral (right) chest radiographs from a 22-year-old woman who has a completely subcutaneous implantable cardioverter-defibrillator. She has single ventricle physiology and had undergone lateral tunnel-style Fontan procedure at 3 years of age. She recently experienced resuscitated sudden arrhythmic death. D = distal electrode; P = proximal electrode.*

Even the most modern bradycardia pacing systems are fraught with some combination of lead complications, need for reoperation, hemodynamically imperfect ventricular activation, and lack of response to neurohumoral demands. These problems are amplified in children and in some patients having congenital heart disease. Therefore, the ultimate therapy for chronotropic incompetence is the biologic pacemaker.[15, 16] The goal is to recreate stable and reliable pacing function of biologic tissue without the need for batteries or leads. This tissue would exhibit physiologic responsiveness as seen in native conduction tissue. The two general approaches that have been considered are: (1) the use of explanted differentiated cells that have automaticity properties (such as sinoatrial node cells), or (2) development of stem cell- or mesenchymal cell-derived cardiac-type cells, which are genetically engineered to express the cardiac channels of interest. The former construct is restricted to that particular cell type and its channel endowment, and it also must consider tissue source and availability and host immune responses. The latter requires the modern tools of bioinformatics and molecular biology but could ultimately allow generation of tissue having biophysical properties customized to the patient's needs. Therefore, gene therapy and stem cell models have been the primary technology to replicate the function of the sinus node.[17] Such a model could also be applied to the ventricle or AV junction in the case of heart block. Once engineered, theoretically, a properly functioning and critical volume of tissue need only establish appropriate gap junctions to neighboring cells to be operative. By far, the HCN channel (generating the I_f or "funny current") has generated the most interest. This channel accounts for at least a portion of sinoatrial node automaticity; it has mixed Na/K permeability in response to hyperpolarization; and it has a cyclic nucleotide binding domain making it responsive to sympathetic and parasympathetic stimulation. There are four isoforms, each having characteristic current magnitudes, voltage activation, and activation kinetics. HCN2 and HCN2/HCN1 chimera have received the most attention in in vivo, in vitro, and in computer model studies. Some concerns exist with regards to the use of viral vectors and transmission of illness or carcinogenic mutations, neoplasm development from implanted stem cells, and proarrhythmia from automaticity of the tissue. Early in vivo studies have also shown a disappointingly slow discharge rate from the engineered automatic tissue.[15] Although the biologic pacemaker should function for a lifetime, the actual duration of stable pacemaker activity is unknown. Experts believe that clinical application of biological pacemakers has a 10-year horizon.

Leads and conductors

The emphasis of research and development in the field of CRMD leads and conductors over the last 20 years has been placed on high voltage conductors for ICDs and on transvenous leads for the cardiac veins supplying the subaortic ventricle for ventricular resynchronization therapy. There remains an ongoing need for improved lead technology for the growing population of patients having single ventricle physiology and chronotropic incompetence. If anything, the current surgical trend of reducing and even eliminating a portion of atrial mass on the systemic venous side of the circulation during Fontan operation further mitigates transvenous approaches for treatment of sinoatrial node dysfunction. Incorporation of the entire ventricular mass into the pulmonary venous side of the circulation prevents transvenous placement of ventricular leads for AV block, as well. Placement of the currently best performing epicardial lead (the steroid-eluting, bifurcated, passive fixation Medtronic 4968 leads) is suboptimal in this patient group due to prior repeat thoracotomy or sternotomy and the presence of excessive epicardial fibrosis. The ideal conductors for these patients would be a bipolar lead capable of active fixation, having high pacing impedance, and having a stable and low pacing threshold. Ideally, this lead could be introduced percutaneously via a transthoracic introducer sheath. Asirvatham et al. described an experimental intramyocardial bipolar lead, in which an electrically active external helix and central pin comprise the electrodes[18] (Figure 20.4). Although this lead was designed to optimize local sensing and pacing and is actually a transvenous construction, this sort of innovation will get us closer to the "holy grail" for single ventricle patients and children requiring epicardial pacing.

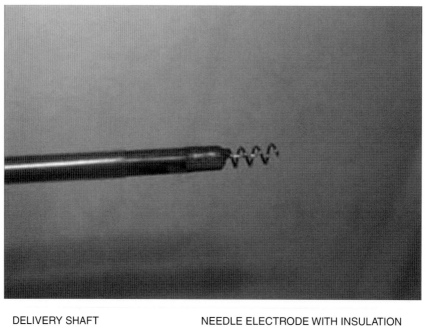

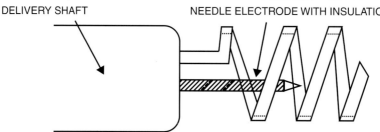

DELIVERY SHAFT　　　　　NEEDLE ELECTRODE WITH INSULATION

Figure 20.4 *A photograph (top) and diagram (bottom) of an experimental entirely intramyocardial bipolar lead, in which an electrically active external helix and central pin comprise the electrodes. Designed to optimize pacing and sensing characteristics, the pin is coated with a polyimide insulation and has micropores, to prevent electrical shorting. (Source: Asirvatham 2007. Reproduced with permission of Elsevier.)*

Advances in lead design are at the forefront of developing CRMDs compatible with diagnostic magnetic resonance imaging (MRI). Magnetic resonance imaging and angiography are now ubiquitous diagnostic instruments in all fields of pediatric medicine. Application to persons have congenital heart disease is supplanting echocardiography in many instances; for example, to monitor the effects of chronic pulmonary regurgitation following repair of tetralogy of Fallot. The potential deleterious effects of MRI on CRMDs include those from the static magnetic field (reed-switch closure, generator displacement), the radiofrequency field (alterations of pacing rate, inappropriate tachyarrhythmia detection, electrical reset, tissue heating at lead/tissue interface, heating of casing or device components), and the time-varying magnetic gradient field (inappropriate pacing from induction voltage, reed-switch closure, and heating of casing or device components). Tissue heating at the lead/tissue interface is related to lead design and lead length. Although restrictive algorithms have been published that advocate careful application of MRI in selective situations,[19] it has heretofore been generally recommended that MRI be avoided in patients having in situ CRMDs or retained leads. Recent advances in lead design are addressing this tenet. For example, it has been shown that radiofrequency energy heating can be reduced by: (1) reducing the area of lead tips; (2) increasing the lead conductor resistance; and (3) increasing outer lead insulation

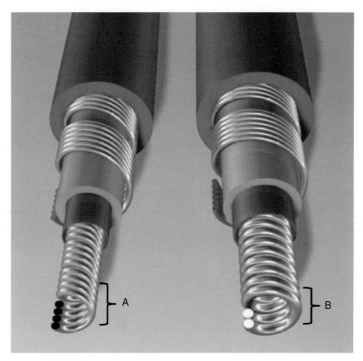

Figure 20.5 *Artistic rendering of the construction of a standard bipolar pacing lead (model 5076, Medtronic, Inc.; Minneapolis, MN) (left) and an MRI-compatible bipolar pacing lead (CapSure Fix^{TM} MRI lead, model 5086, Medtronic, Inc.) (right). The standard lead has four tendrils per turn: (A) within the inner coil, compared with two (B) in the MRI-compatible lead. (Source: Reproduced with permission from Medtronic, Inc.)*

conductivity.[20] A recent multi-institution trial has shown no adverse impact on patient safety or pacemaker system function after controlled exposure to 1.5 T MRI of a newly designed pacing system by Medtronic, Inc.[21] This system, the Revo SureScan™ Pacing System and CapSure Fix MRI™ lead, was designed specifically for MRI compatibility. Specific modifications include: (1) lead characteristics that reduce radiofrequency lead tip heating; (2) internal circuit changes to reduce cardiac stimulation; (3) decreased ferromagnetic material in construction; (4) internal circuit protection to prevent disruption of internal power supply; and (5) reed switch replacement by a Hall sensor, whose behavior in static magnetic field is predictable. Specific changes in lead design reduce transmission of induced energy as heat. This was accomplished by reducing the number of tendrils per turn from four to two. To compensate, the diameter of the inner coil (compared with the manufacturer's previous design) was increased from 0.026" to 0.036" in order to maintain good

torque (Figure 20.5). The leads are 5.3 Fr with both active and passive fixation choices. They are only available in specific MR-conditional lengths. Future advances will hopefully allow patients having ICDs to also be candidates for magnetic resonance imaging. Clearly, those having retained leads and lead fragments represent a very difficult group due to the potential for such hardware acting as electromagnetic antennae.

The interface between bradycardia pacing, antitachycardia therapies, and congestive heart failure (including all cardiomyopathy-related low cardiac output syndromes) heretofore has involved two areas: (1) progressively more sophisticated sensors (lead components) that can detect diminishing ventricular function/cardiac output and/or increasing cardiac output requirements; and (2) anatomical optimization of pacing sites to improve cardiac function (interatrial, atrioventricular, and inter-/intraventricular). Lead-based sensors of presumed oxygen extraction and ventricular myocardial responses to changes in autonomic tone are considered elsewhere in this textbook. In the presence of a normally functioning sinus node, one could imagine that similar real-time interpretation of cardiovascular autonomic tone could be derived from standard heart rate variability parameters of sympathetic and parasympathetic innervation.[22] If one imagines eventual cardiac device therapy as a closed loop system, currently the "afferent limb," as just described, is far advanced compared with therapy options, the "efferent limb." The only therapies currently available are chronotropic responses and optimized mechanical coordination of the cardiac chambers. Directed vagus nerve ganglion stimulation has been used to modify the ventricular response to atrial fibrillation in humans,[23] and such pacing has been shown to reduce the ventricular tachycardia burden[24] and improve long-term survival[25] in an animal model. Future directions must include a broader scope of device-based therapies, including local delivery systems for pharmaceuticals.

Out-patient monitoring

The irretrievable suddenness of asystole or ventricular fibrillation places demands on CRMD reliability unrivaled by other medical technologies. The schedule of the out-patient, on site evaluations of implanted devices is individually determined based upon multiple factors, including occurrence of symptoms, underlying hemodynamic status, rhythm stability, somatic growth, conductor function trends, battery status, and emotional response to CRMD therapy. Although there is no substitute for an in-person out-patient clinical assessment of a child having a device, and most clinicians recommend that such visits be scheduled annually, at minimum, more frequent visits are inconvenient and costly to families. These competing issues mandated development of ambulatory methods of heart rhythm monitoring. Transtelephonic monitoring (TTM) of the cardiac rhythm was first reported in patients having CRMDs in 1971,[26] and the Centers for Medicare and Medicaid Services in the United States established guidelines for frequency of TTM in 1984. The hardware required to perform TTM, including various types of metal contacts applied to the wrists of adults for rhythm transmission, were easily adapted to children and even infants. This technology enabled accurate identification of pacemaker failure (with positive predictive value of 93%)[27] and critical battery depletion[28] but was far less effective in identifying other device complications, when compared to in-office follow-up.[29]

Remote monitoring of programmed, telemetered, and real-time data via a radiofrequency transmitter within ICDs was first reported in 2004.[30] This feature was added more recently to pacemakers, and its efficacy in identifying actionable device or rhythm abnormalities compared with TTM in adults (66% versus 2%) was demonstrated in the PREFER (Pacemaker Remote Follow-up Evaluation and Review) trial.[31] Currently, each major CRMD company offers this feature for ICDs and some bradycardia devices: Biotronik's CardioMessenger, Boston Scientific's LATTITUDE, Medtronic's Care-Link, and St. Judes' Merlin@home. All information which the provider can download in person during an office visit is similarly transmittable by this process. Device data may be downloaded by a patient's family using a land-based telephone or, automatically, by a wireless receiver/transmitter placed within proximity of the patient, usually in their bedroom. Information is processed by the company and sent by Internet to the provider, with the option of alerting the provider urgently for pre-specified abnormalities.

This powerful analytical tool will likely be used to help direct optimal clinical and business practice. For example, the Medtronic Discovery ™ Link initiative hopes to use remote monitoring technology as a population-based strategy to address diverse issues involving bradycardia pacing, anti-tachycardia therapy, and cardiac resynchronization therapy. Application of contemporary and emerging remote monitoring technologies may be applied to children and patients having congenital heart disease similarly. As examples, trends in patient transmission rates may help inform methods to improve overall health care and cardiac care for children in at risk circumstances. More complete ascertainment of ventricular tachyarrhythmias may help refine anti-tachycardia therapies in young patients having ICDs. Determining the long-term burden of ventricular pacing in children who had under-gone pacemaker implantation for post-operative AV block and who later seemingly regained con-duction may help identify those who later do not require device replacement. The potential for actual reprogramming of devices remotely also exists. Safeguards against rogue reprogramming and myriad other safety issues will need to be addressed before this becomes a reality.

Cardiac rhythm management devices in low and middle income countries

It is now recognized that non-communicable dis-eases account for more deaths worldwide than do infectious diseases. It was reported by the World Health Organization in 2010 that cardiovascular disease was the primary category of mortality from non-communicable etiologies, accounting for 17 million global deaths per year, including 30% of all deaths in low and middle income countries. More than two-thirds of deaths attributable to cardiovascular causes worldwide occur in middle and low income countries. The recent changes in the demographic distribution of cardiovascular diseases are accelerating due to the combination of industrialization, globalization, and urban-ization. These factors are thought to result in increased tobacco use, unhealthy dietary patterns, hyperlipidemia, decreased physical activity, and hypertension. In response to myriad international directives dating back 20 years, the Institute of Medicine (of the National Academies of Science) convened the Committee on Preventing the Global Epidemic of Cardiovascular Disease: Meeting the Challenges in Developing Countries. Chaired by Valentin Fuster, the findings and recommendations from this committee were published in the exhaus-tive treatise, *Promoting Cardiovascular Health in the Developing World: A Critical Challenge to Achieve Global Health.*[32] The processes necessary to reduce this global epidemic must start with placing emphasis on chronic illness (often a lower priority in developing countries) and aligning the associated population needs with other develop-ment priorities. The committee's 12 categorical recommendations appear in Table 20.1.

Table 20.1 *Recommendations for governments in low and middle income countries, global health funders, and development agencies to achieve synchrony in order to give cardiovascular disease and related chronic diseases greater priority. (From: Fuster V, Kelly BB, Eds. Promoting Cardiovascular Health in the Developing World: A Critical Challenge to Achieve Global Health. 2010 National Academies Press. Washington, DC)*

1 Recognize chronic diseases as a development assistance priority
2 Improve local data
3 Implement policies to promote cardiovascular health
4 Include chronic diseases in health systems strength-ening
5 Improve national coordination for chronic diseases
6 Research to assess what works in different settings
7 Disseminate knowledge and innovation among sim-ilar countries
8 Collaborate to improve diets
9 Collaborate to improve access to CVD diagnostics, medicines, and technologies
10 Advocate for chronic diseases as a funding priority
11 Define resource needs
12 Report on global progress

A juxtaposition of CRMD availability to children in developing countries with the recommendations in the Table may not, at first glance, be intu-itive. Indeed, known sources of human pathology resulting in CRMD requirement in the young does not generally comprise a public health pri-ority. However, the principles articulated in all of these recommendations are equally applica-ble to the pediatric patients considered herein. As non-governmental organizations (NGOs; mostly philanthropic) are beginning to coop-erate with governmental agencies, international organizations, and each other, several of the recom-mendations by Fuster and his colleagues are already being realized. An example is the NGO, Heartbeat International Foundation, Inc (HBI). Originally, Heartbeat International Worldwide, it originated in 1984 as a repository for pacemakers and, later, ICDs in developing countries. Now with 32 device "banks" in 15 countries, it has resulted in over 11,000 device implants – many in children – in 25 countries. Since 2007, when each of these banks became independent organizations, HBI's emphasis has shifted more toward development of continuing education programs for healthcare professionals and education and prevention programs for the general population throughout its geographic footprint. More to the point of this discussion, HBI is developing strategic alliances, and together, helping to elevate awareness of chronic cardiac disease, improve local reporting of disease activity, disseminate knowledge and innovation among similar countries, collaborate to improve access to cardiovascular diagnostics and technology, advocate for chronic disease as a funding priority, define resource needs, and report global progress; all actions enumerated in Table 20.1. The newly formed organization, the Global Cardiovascular Alliance, in association with HBI and other nonprofit organizations, corporations, and other strategic alliances is a sterling example of how grassroots organizations will, going forward, influence global healthcare.

References

1 Beck H, Boden WE, Patibandla S, Kireyev D, Gupta V, Campagna F, Cain ME, Marine JE. 50th Anniversary of the first successful permanent pacemaker implantation in the United States: Historical review and future directions. *Am J Cardiol* 2010; 106: 810–818.

2 Furman S. The early history of cardiac pacing. *Pacing Clin Electrophysiol* 2003; 26: 2023–2032.

3 Mallela VS, Ilankumaran V, Rao NS. Trends in cardiac pacemaker batteries. *Indian Pacing Electrophysiol J* 2004; 4: 201–212.

4 Bhatia D, Bairagi S, Goel S, Jangra M. Pacemakers charging using body energy. *J Pharm Bioallied Sci.* 2010; 2: 51–54.

5 Karami MA, Inman DJ. Powering pacemakers from heartbeat vibrations using linear and nonlinear energy harvesters. *Applied Phys Lett* 2012; 100: 042901.

6 Qi Y, McAlpine MC. Nanotechnology-enabled flexible and biocompatible energy harvesting. *Energy Environ Sci* 2010; 3: 1275–1285.

7 Cinquin P, Gondran C, Giroud F, Mazabrard S, Pellissier A, et al. A glucose biofuel cell implanted in rats. *PLoS ONE* 2010;5: e10476.

8 Medtronic. Website. Available at: www.medtronic.com/innovation-au/smarter-miniaturization.html (accessed July 26, 2016): 2012.

9 Lee KL, Lau CP, Tse HF, Echt DS, Heaven D, Smith W, Wood M. First human demonstration of cardiac stimulation with cardiac ultrasound energy delivery: implications for wireless pacing with implantable devices. *J Am Coll Cardiol* 2007; 50: 877–883.

10 Wieneke H, Konorza T, Erbel R, Kisker E. Leadless pacing of the heart using induction technology: a feasibility study. *Pacing Clin Electrophysiol* 2009; 32: 177–183.

11 Bardy GH, Smith WM, Hood MA, Crozier IG, Melton IC, Jordaens L, et al. An entirely subcutaneous implantable cardioverter-defibrillator. *N Engl J Med* 2010; 363: 36–44.

12 Gold MR, Theuns DA, Knight BP, Sturdivant JL, Sanghera R, Ellenbogen KA, et al. Head-to-head arrhythmia discrimination performance of subcutaneous and transvenous ICD arrhythmia detection algorithms: the START Study. *J Cardiovasc Electrophysiol* 2012 Apr; 23(4): 359–366.

13 Pedersen SS, Lambiase P, Boersma LV, Murgatroyd F, Johansen JB, Reeve H, et al. Evaluation oF FactORs ImpacTing CLinical Outcome and Cost EffectiveneSS of the S-ICD: design and rationale of the EFFORTLESS S-ICD Registry. *Pacing Clin Electrophysiol* 2012; 35: 574–579.

14 Jarman JW, Lascelles K, Wong T, Markides V, Clague JR, Till J. Clinical experience of entirely subcutaneous implantable cardioverter-defibrillators in children and adults: cause for caution. *Eur Heart J* 2012 Jun; 33(11): 1351–1359.

15 Robinson RB. Engineering a biological pacemaker: in vivo, in vitro and in silico models. *Drug Discovery Today: Disease Models*, 2009; 6(3): 93–98.

16 Rosen MR, Brink PR, Cohen IS, Robinson RB, Biological pacemakers based on If. *Med Biol Eng Comput.* 2007 Feb; 45(2): 157–166.

17 Miake Jm Marbán E, Nuss, HB. Gene therapy: biological pacemaker created by gene transfer. *Nature* 2002; 419: 132–133.

18 Asirvatham SJ, Bruce CJ, Danielsen A, Johnson SB, Okumura Y, Kathmann E, et al. Intramyocardial pacing and sensing for the enhancement of cardiac stimulation and sensing specificity. *Pacing Clin Electrophysiol* 2007; 30: 748–754.

19 Nazarian S, Roguin A, Zviman MM, Lardo AC, Dickfeld TL, Calkins H, et al. Clinical utility and safety of a protocol for noncardiac and cardiac magnetic resonance imaging of patients with permanent pacemakers and implantable-cardioverter defibrillators at 1.5 tesla. *Circulation* 2006; 114; 1277–1284.

20 Nordbeck P, Fidler F, Friedrich MT, Weiss I, Warmuth M, Gensler D, et al. Reducing RF-related heating of cardiac pacemaker leads in MRI: Implementation and experimental verification of practical design changes. *Magn Reson Med* 2012; 68(6): 1963–1672.

21 Wilkoff BL, Bello D, Taborsky M, Vymazal J, Kanal E, Heuer H, et al. Magnetic resonance imaging in patients with a pacemaker system designed for the magnetic resonance environment. *Heart Rhythm* 2011; 8: 65–73.

22 Landolina M, Gasparini M, Lunati M, Santini M, Rordorf R, Vincenti A, et al. Heart rate variability monitored by the implanted device predicts response to CRT and long-term clinical outcome in patients with advanced heart failure. *Eur J Heart Fail* 2008; 10: 1073–1079.

23 Rossi P, Bianchi S, Valsecchi S, Porcelli D, Sgreccia F, Lucifero A, et al. Endocardial vagal atrioventricular node stimulation in humans: reproducibility on 18-month follow-up. *Europace* 2010; 12: 1719–1724.

24 Zheng C, Li M, Inagaki M, Kawada T, Sunagawa K, Sugimachi M. Vagal stimulation markedly suppresses arrhythmias in conscious rats with chronic heart failure after myocardial infarction. *Conf Proc IEEE Eng Med Biol Soc* 2005; 7: 7072–7075.

25 Li M, Zheng C, Sato T, Kawada T, Sugimachi M, Sunagawa K. Vagal nerve stimulation markedly improves long-term survival after chronic heart failure in rats. *Circulation* 2004; 109: 120–124.

26 Furman S, Parker B, Escher DJ. Transtelephone pacemaker clinic. *J Thorac Cardiovasc Surg* 1971; 61: 827–834.

27 Gessman LJ, Vielbig RE, Waspe LE, Moss L, Damm D, Sundeen FY. Accuracy and clinical utility of transtelephonic pacemaker follow-up. *Pacing Clin Electrophysiol* 1995; 18: 1032–1036.

28 Platt S, Furman S, Gross JN, Andrews C, Benedek M. Transtelephone monitoring for pacemaker follow-up 1981–1994. *Pacing Clin Electrophysiol* 1996; 19: 2089–2098.

29 Sweesy MW, Erickson SL, Crago JA, Castor KN, Batey RL, Forney RC. Analysis of the effectiveness of in-office and transtelephonic follow-up in terms of pacemaker system complications. *Pacing Clin Electrophysiol* 1994; 17: 2001–2003.

30 Schoenfeld MH, Compton SJ, Mead H, Weiss DN, Sherfesee L, Englund J, Mongeon LR. Remote monitoring of implantable cardioverter defibrillators: a prospective analysis. *Pacing Clin Electrophysiol* 2004; 27: 757–763.

31 Crossley GH, Chen J, Choucair W, Cohen TJ, Gohn DC, W. Johnson B, et al, PREFER Study Investigators. Clinical benefits of remote versus transtelephonic monitoring of implanted pacemakers. *J Am Coll Cardiol* 2009; 54: 2012–2019.

32 Fuster V, Kelly BB, eds. *Promoting Cardiovascular Health in the Developing World: A Critical Challenge to Achieve Global Health*. Washington DC: National Academies Press, 2010.

Glossary

Ampere (amp: A) – The amount of electrical current flowing past a point in a conductor when 1 V of potential is applied across 1 Ω of resistance. In pacing, these currents are so small that they are expressed in terms of milliamperes (one thousandth of an ampere, abbreviated to mA) and microamperes (one millionth of an ampere, abbreviated to μA).

Amplitude – The maximum absolute value attained by an electrical waveform, or any quantity that varies periodically. Pacemaker amplitudes express the value of the potential difference (in V) or the current flow (in A). Pacemaker output pulses have typically averaged 5 V and 10 mA.

Asynchronous – A pacemaker that stimulates at a fixed, preset rate independent of the electrical and/or mechanical activity of the heart. Examples: AOO and VOO.

Atrial Synchronous (VAT) – A duel chamber pacemaker which senses atrial activity and paces only in the ventricle. The rate of ventricular stimulation is directly synchronized to sensed atrial activity.

Atrial Tracking – A pacing mode (e.g., VDD, DDD) in which the ventricles are paced in synchrony with sensed atrial events.

A-V Sequential (DVI) – A duel chamber pacemaker that paces at a programmed rate in the atrium and senses and paces in the ventricle.

A-V Universal (DDD) – A duel chamber pacemaker which can pace and sense in both atria and the ventricles.

Blanking Period – The interval of time during which the pacemaker cannot sense any events. For example, the first part of the refractory period in demand pacemakers is a blanking period.

Capacitors – A device used to store electrical charge. It is made of two conductors separated by an insulator.

Capture – Depolarization of the atria and/or ventricles by an electrical stimulus delivered by an artificial pacemaker. One-to-one capture occurs when each electrical stimulus causes a corresponding depolarization. (See **Stimulation Threshold**.)

Cardiac Index (CI) – Measurement of a patient's cardiac output (CO) per square meter of body surface area (BSA). CI = CO (l/min) ÷ BSA (m^2).

Conductors – Materials that have relatively large number of free electrons and therefore pass an electric current well.

Coulomb (C) – A unit of charge that is positively or negatively charged: one negative Coulomb (−1 C) represents the charge of approximately 6.4 × 1018 electrons.

Cross Talk – The phenomenon that can occur in dual-chamber pacemakers in which a stimulus from the atrial lead is sensed by the ventricular lead, or vice versa, e.g., inhibition or resetting of the refractory period.

Demand (or Inhibited) – Any pacemaker that, after sensing a spontaneous depolarization, withholds its pacing stimulus. Examples: AAI and VVI.

Cardiac Pacing and Defibrillation in Pediatric and Congenital Heart Disease, First Edition.
Edited by Maully Shah, Larry Rhodes and Jonathan Kaltman.
© 2017 John Wiley & Sons Ltd. Published 2017 by John Wiley & Sons Ltd.
Companion Website: www.wiley.com/go/shah/cardiac_pacing

End of life (EOL) – The point at which the pacemaker signals that it should be replaced because its battery is nearing depletion.

Evoked Response – Area underneath an R wave is deoendentdependent upon the rate of myocardial depolarization. A decrease in cumulative R wave area calls for an increase in pacing rate.

Farad – It is a unit of capacitance. It is equal to a capacitor having a potential difference of 1 V between its plates when it is charged with 1 C.

Hysteresis – A pacing parameter that usually allows a longer escape interval after a sensed event, giving the heart a greater opportunity to beat on its own. For example, a pacemaker that is set to pace at a rate of 70 bpm. will allow the intrinsic heart rate to drop to 60 bpm. before delivering a pacing stimulus. If the hysteresis period elapses and no natural depolarization occurs, the pulse generator will revert to its faster rate (i.e., 70 bpm.) and begin pacing at this rate. In some antitachycardia pacing devices, the hysteresis period will be shorter rather than longer.

Impedance – The total opposition that a circuit presents to an alternating electrical current. Impedance and resistance are often inappropriately used as equivalent terms in pacing.

Insulators – Materials that have relatively small number of free electrons and therefore pass an electric current poorly.

Joule (J) – A unit of work or energy. In a pacing system, the energy released (J) = voltage × current × time.

Microampere (μA) – The unit of measure for very small electrical currents (one millionth of an ampere). Depending on its circuit design, most pacemakers typically draw 10–30 μm microamps continuously from a battery.

Microjoule (μJ) – The unit of measure for very small amounts of electrical energy (one millionth of a joule). The output of an implanted pacemaker ranges 1–50 μJ.

Ohm (Ω) – The unit of resistance: 1 Ω is the resistance that results in a current of 1 A when a potential of one volt1 A is placed across the resistance.

Ohm's law – V = IR. Voltage (V) is equal to the product of current (I) and resistance (R).

Output – The electrical stimulus generated by a pulse generator and intended to trigger a depolarization in the chamber of the heart being paced.

Overdrive Pacing – Pacing the heart at a rate faster the patient's intrinsic rhythm: to suppress a tachycardia, to gain electrical control of the heart, or to suppress PVCs.

Oversensing – Inhibition of a pacemaker by events other than those which that the pacemaker was designed to sense, e.g., myopotentials, electromagnetic interference, T-waves, crosstalk, etc.

Pacemaker Mediated Tachycardia (PMT) – A rapid paced rhythm that can occur with atrial tracking pacemakers. It begins with and is sustained by ventricular events with are conducted retrograde (backwards) to the atria. The pacemaker senses this retrograde atrial depolarization and then delivers a stimulus to the ventricle, causing a ventricular depolarization, which again is conducted retrograde to the atria. This cycle repeats itself to produce a tachycardia.

Polarization – Refers to layers of oppositely charged ions that surround the electrode during the pulse stimulus. It is inversely related to the surface area of the electrode.

Rate Responsive (Also Rate Adaptive, Rate Variable) – Term used to describe implantable pacemakers that change pacing rate in response to detected changes in the body to meet the body's metabolic need for greater blood flow. Examples are AAIR and VVIR. Additional examples of rate responsive pacemakers include: AOOR, VOOR, DDDR, VDIR, and DOOR.

Refractory Period (Pacemaker) – The time during which the pacemaker's sensing mechanism becomes nonresponsive (in full or in part) to cardiac activity, e.g., to a retrograde P wave in a DDD pacemaker.

Resistance (R) – The opposition to the flow of electric current.

Safety Pacing (Ventricular) – In some A-V sequential (DVI) and A-V universal (DDD) pacemakers, following atrial pacing, the pacemaker is designed to trigger a ventricular pacing output if ventricular sensing occurs during the first portion (e.g., 110 ms) of the programmed A-V interval. This feature insures a ventricular depolarization if the event sensed was electrical interference.

Slew Rate – The amount of change in voltage that occurs in a given segment of an intracardiac waveform divided by the period of time over which the change occurs. Graphically, it is the slope of the waveform and is expressed in millivolts per millisecond or volts per second.

Standard Load – The resistance conventionally placed across the terminals of a pulse generator when testing pacemaker operation (usually 500 Ω).

Stimulation Threshold – The minimum electrical stimulus needed to consistently elicit a cardiac depolarization. It can be expresses in terms of amplitude (V, mA), pulse width (ms), or energy (µJ).

Underdrive Pacing – Pacing at a rate below the tachycardia rate, for the purpose of interrupting the heart's tachy circuit with randomly times stimuli so as to gain control of the heart and restore its natural rhythm.

Undersensing – Failure of the pacemaker to sense the P wave or R wave; may cause the pacemaker to emit inappropriately timed impulses.

Upper Rate – In atrial tracking dual-chamber pacemakers (VDD and DDD), a programed limit to the rate at which the ventricles are paced in response to atrial activity. Thus, 1:1 tracking will prevail until the upper rate limit is exceeded; at this point the pacemaker will slow its rate of ventricular pacing to avoid tachycardia, by the Wenckebach operation, 2:1 block, etc.

V-A Interval – (DVI, DDD) With dual-chamber pacemakers, the period of time elapsing from a ventricular event (sensed or paced) to the next scheduled atrial pace. Also used to describe the physiologic retrograde conduction time.

Volts (V) – The unit of measure of electrical potential or electromotive force.

Watt (W) – The unit of power and rate at which work is done. 1 W = 1 J/s or voltage × current.

Wenckebach (Upper Rate Behavior) – In a DDD pacemaker, an operational function with limits the average ventricular pacing rate when intrinsic atrial rates rise above the prodrammed-programmed upper rate. The pacemaker does this by gradually prolonging the pacemaker's AV interval until one of the atrial events falls into the atrial refractory period and is not sensed. Since no A-V interval is started, there will be no ventricular output synchronized to this atrial event.

Index

Page references in *italics* refer to Figures; those in **bold** refer to Figures

35N LT® conductor   17
AAI pacing (atrial inhibited pacing)
    45, 72, 74, 75, 202, 214, 216
AAIR pacing   45, 72, 74, 214, 216,
    251
abandoned leads   145, 183, 190, 248,
    302
ablation   42, 64, 219
    AV nodal   99, 235
    catheter   39, 63, 64, 69, 152, 267
    photoablation   194
    radiofrequency   296, 297
aborted sudden death   65, 69, 75,
    233, 234
abrasions   18
accelerometers   74, 121, 122, 123,
    214
Accufix lead   188
action potentials   92, 95, 207
active fixation leads   16, *17*
Adapta pacemaker   55
adults
    ICD therapy, indications   **65**
    trials utilizing implantable loop
        recorders   284–5
    ventricular synchrony in heart
        failure   100–3, *100–1*
Advanced Hysteresis   54
afterpotentials   20
air embolism   176, 177–8
alerts   30, 32, 188, 250, 252, 289
algorithms
    ICD   30
    antitachycardia pacing   216–17
    atrial preference pacing
        (Medtronic)   214
    automatic mode switch   242

dynamic atrial overdrive (St. Jude)
    214
RV Lead Noise Discrimination
    30
Alive Cor Mobile ECG recording
    device   286, *288*
allergies   183
amiodarone   42, 128, 205, 240, 292
amyloidosis   39
anodal stimulation   15
antiarrhythmic drugs, effect on DFTs
    22, **22**
    hemodynamic compromise and
        63
antibiotics   136, 145, 183, 184
anti-SSA/Ro antibodies   40
antitachycardia pacing (ATP)   26–8,
    42, 255
    burst   26
    burst+   27
    ramp   27
    scan   27
antitachycardia pacing algorithms
    216–17
aortic stenosis   63
arrhythmias during implantation
    178–9
arrhythmogenic right ventricular
    cardiomyopathy   *29*
arrhythmogenic right ventricular
    dysplasia/cardiomyopathy
    (ARVD/C)   70–1
arteriovenous fistula   178
aspirin   45, 182
asynchronous mode   237
atrial antitachycardia pacing (ATP)
    55–6

atrial arrhthymias
    pacing to prevent   152
    pacing to terminate   152
atrial asynchronous pacing (AOO)
    202, 237
atrial blanking period   242
atrial electrograms   14, 75, 199, 201,
    242, 243, 265
atrial fibrillation   51, 53, 55, 72, 75,
    99, 152, 178, 216, 237, 263–5,
    286
atrial flutter   237, 263, 264, 265
atrial inhibited pacing (AAI) pacing
    see AAI pacing
atrial isomerism   40
atrial kick   95
atrial oversensing   243
atrial preference pacing (Medtronic)
    algorithm   214
atrial tachycardia   216
atrioventricular block   151
atrioventricular delay   275
atrioventricula node dysfunction
    67
atrioventricular optimization
    276
atrioventricular search hysteresis
    (AVSH)   74
atrioventricular septal defect   40
atrioventricular synchrony   151
Autocapture   53, 217
Autocapture system   251
automated external defibrillators
    (AED)   286–91
    history of   286–9
    mechanics of   289–90
    personal use of   291–2

Cardiac Pacing and Defibrillation in Pediatric and Congenital Heart Disease, First Edition.
Edited by Maully Shah, Larry Rhodes and Jonathan Kaltman.
© 2017 John Wiley & Sons Ltd. Published 2017 by John Wiley & Sons Ltd.
Companion Website: www.wiley.com/go/shah/cardiac_pacing

automated external defibrillators
	(AED) (*continued*)
	precautions 292–3
	public access defibrillation 291
Automatic Capture system   53
AV Search Hysteresis (AVSH)   54,
	74, 216
AV sequential (DVI pacing)   243
axillary approach   50
axillary vein   140, *141*

Bachmann's bundle   143
batteries
	depletion 186–7
	history of 5
	longevity 20
Becker's muscular dystrophy
	39–40
beta-blockers   39, 43, 66–7, 68, 74,
	219, 233–4, 266, 307
BIOTRONIK CardioMessenger
	320
BIOTRONIK ICD key programmable
	features **228–30**
bipolar pacing system   15–16, *16*
Boston Scientific AV Search
	Hysteresis 216
	Search AV+ (SAV+) 54
Boston Scientific Energen™   76
Boston Scientific ICD key
	programmable features
	222–4
brachiocephalic vein occlusion   *186*
bradyarrhythmias   178–9
bradycardia   40
bradycardia pacing   42
brain natriuretic peptide (BNP)   102
Brugada syndrome   67, 68–70, *69*,
	124, 254, 283, 291
bundle branch block   92, 264
	abnormal activation sequence
		during 97–8
	left 97, 98, 100, 101, 102–3, 157,
		178
	post-surgical 74
	right 103, 106, 178
burst (ATP)   26
burst pacing   26
burst+ (ATP)   27

cable conductor   17
caffeine   68
calsequestrin 2 gene (CASQ2)   68
capture threshold   217
CaptureManagement system   53
cardiac output   121
cardiac resynchronization therapy
	(CRT) device programming
	273–5, *274*

AV delay   275
	monitoring CRT response 275
	VV offset 275
cardiac resynchronization therapy
	(CRT) optimization 275–8
	AV optimization 276
	VV optimization 276–8, *277*
		3D echocardiography 278, *280*
		Doppler 276
		electrocardiography 278
		M-mode 276
		speckle tracking 278, *279*
		Tissue Doppler 276–8
cardiac resynchronization therapy
	157–9
	device implantation 161–2
	effectiveness 158–9
	recommendations for 157
	transvenous vs epicardial approach
		161–2
	see also cardiac resynchronization
		therapy (CRT), restoring
		synchrony
cardiac resynchronization therapy
	(CRT), restoring synchrony
	adult heart failure 100–2
	pediatric and CHD 103–11
		failing LV 102–5
		failing single ventricle 109–10,
			109
		failing V 106–9
		short and midterm outcomes
			110–11
cardiac rhythm management device
	(CRMD) therapy
	energy source 311–13
	improvements in 310–11
	leads and conductors 317–20
	in low and middle income
		countries 321–2
	out-patient monitoring 320–1
	preserving vascular access
		313–17
cardioversion   28
CARE-HF trial   276
catecholaminergic polymorphic
	ventricular tachycardia
	(CPVT) 67–8, 124, 254
cathodal stimulation   15
centroseptal subdivision of LBB   93
Chagas disease   39
chronaxie   12
cold flow   18
complications, device-related
	174–95, **175**
compression set   18, *18*
conduction system disease   67
conductor coil   17, *17*
conductors   17

congenital heart block   9
	escape rhythms in 40–1
	rate-adaptive pacing system in
		121
congenital heart disease (CHD)
	63–5, **64**, **65**, 149–62
	cardiac resynchronization therapy
		157–9
	congenitally corrected
		transposition of the great
		arteries (CCTGA) 40
	device implantation 153–5
		device, leads and device location
			153
		location of device 154–5
		pacemaker/ICD generator
			selection 155
		patient anatomy 154
		patient size 153–4
		standard approach 155
		transvenous versus epicardial
			leads 153
	dextrocardia 153
	dyssynchrony, assessment of
		159–61
		evaluation of AV synchrony
			159, *160*
		evaluation of inter-ventricular
			dyssynchrony 160–1
		intra-ventricular synchrony,
			evaluation of 159–60
		single ventricular lead for CRT
			161
	Ebstein anomaly 63
	indications for pacemaker
		placement in 149–50
	L transposition of great arteries
		63
	Mustard operation 41, 63
	pacemakers 149–50
	pacemaker/ICD implantation
		155–7
		bioprosthetic tricuspid valves
			and transvenous pacemaker
			156
		high threshold with epicardial
			device placement 155–6
		implantable cardioverter
			defibrillator in challenging
			vascular access 157
		in D-transposition of great
			arteries post Mustard or
			Senning procedure 63,
			156–7, *157*
		L transposition of great arteries
			63
		left sided superior vena cava and
			156, *156*

recommendations for implantable cardioverter defibrillator in 152–3
recommendations for pacemaker placement in 150–2
atrioventricular block 151
hypertrophic cardiomyopathy 151–2
pacing to prevent atrial arrhthymias 152
pacing to terminate atrial arrhythmias 152
pause dependent ventricular arrhythmias 151
post cardiac transplant 152
sinus node dysfunction 150
syncope 150–1
congestive heart failure 5, 100, 218, 230, 320
biventricular pacing in 101
countershocking 288
crush injury 18

DDD pacing 47, 55, 215, 216, 231, 234, 237, 243, 275, 300
DDDR pacing 51, 54, 72, 74, 215
DDI pacing 55, 217
DDI pacing with rate hysteresis 55
DDIR pacing 217
defibrillation 28–30
defibrillation threshold (DFT) 22, 30, 124–5
determination in paediatrics and CHD 126
effect of anti-arrhythmic agents on **22**
factors affecting 128
follow-up in non-transvenous ICD configurations 129
lowest energy tested (LET) strategy 125–6, *125*
retesting 129
treatment options 128–9, **128**
DETECT trial 75
diabetes 64, 307
dofetilide 128
Doppler imaging 276
dynamic atrial overdrive algorithm (St. Jude) 214
dyssynchrony, assessment of 159–61
evaluation of AV synchrony 159, *160*
evaluation of inter-ventricular dyssynchrony 160–1
intra-ventricular synchrony, evaluation of 159–60
single ventricular lead for CRT 161

Eastbourne Syncope Assessment Study (EasyAS) 285
elective replacement indicator (ERI) 20
electrical activation during sinus rhythm 92–4, *93*, *94*
electrocardiographic imaging (ECGI) 111
electrocardiography 278
electromagnetic interference (EMI) 256–7, 296–302
cardiovascular implanted electronic devices and MRI 302
sources of electromagnetic interference 301–2
troubleshooting 298–301
EMPIRIC trial 224
end of life (EOL) 20
end of service (EOS) 20
endless loop tachycardia (ELT) 242–3, *243*
endocardial pacing 202
indications 202
limitations 202
technical considerations 202
endocarditis 184
EnRhythm pacemaker 55
environmental stress cracking 18
epicardial leads 44, 45, 175–6
epicardial pacing 202–9
indications 202–5
limitations 208–9
technical considerations 205–8
epinephrine 68
Evolution® Shortie 194
excitation-contraction (E-C) coupling 94, *95*
exercise, basic physiology 120–1
exit block 13
expectation effect 43
external event recorders 286

fast VT (FVT) 28
fibrosis on intravascular leads *191*
flecainide 68
Fontan operation 41, 45, 72
Frank-Starling relationship 95
functional 2:1 AV block 67

Glenn shunt 167
Great batch Medical Myopore® Sutureless, Screw-In bipolar epicardial lead 82
Guidant devices 83
Guidant Endotak® lead failure 78
guidelines for implantation of cardiac pacemakers and antiarrhythmia devices 7

heart block
acquired 39–40, 215
AV block in 151
AV synchrony in 159
bradycardia in 98
congenital 9, 40–1, 121, 165, 273
medications causing 39
post-operative 4, 205, 208
single vs dual chamber pacing 51, 197
VDD lead in 49
VVIR in 52–3
hemodynamics of pacing, site-specific 98–100
LV apical pacing 99–100
RV apical pacing 98
RV septum pacing (His pacing) 98–9
RVOT pacing 99
hemothorax 176–7
His–Purkinje disease 51
history of cardiac pacing and defibrillation 1–19
hypercholesterolemia 64
hypertension 64
hypertrophic cardiomyopathy (HCM) 65–6, 151–2

ICD code 71
ICD generator construction and components 26, **27**, *28*
ICD generator selection 71–83
dual-chamber or single-chamber device 72–5
atrial arrhythmias 75–6
bradycardia pacing 72–4
cardiac resynchronization therapy (CRT) 74
unique conditions 74–5
maximum shock output 76
size and longevity 76, **77**
ICD lead selection 76–82, **79–80**
dual versus single coil ICD lead 81
lead survival 78
novel leads to consider for alternative configurations 81–2
true bipolar versusintegrated bipolar lead 78–80
ICD leads
active fixation design *23*
coaxial construction 24, *26*
coil electrode 24, *24*, *25*
construction and components 22–5
DF-1 connector *23*, *23*, *24*
DF-4 connector system *23*, *23*
dual coil passive fixation lead *24*

ICD leads (*continued*)
  dual-coil leads   25
  flat shocking coil electrode   24, *25*
  GORE-TEX sleeves   24, *24*
  integrated pace/sense bipolar
    configuration   23
  multi-lumen design   24, *26*
  no fixation mechanism   *23*
  passive fixation design   *23*
  single coil electrode   23, *24*, 26
  single lumen design   24, *25*
  true bipolar pace/sense
    configuration   23
ICD programming   217–31
  arrhythmia treatment   221–30
  arrhythmia detection   218–21
  arrhythmia re-detection   230
  heart failure detection   230–1
  pacemaker function   231
ICD testing   124–9
  DFT determination   126
  equipment and personnel
    readiness   127–8
  factors affecting DFT   128
  fibrillation and defibrillation
    124–5
  follow-up in non-transvenous ICD
    configurations   129
  lowest energy tested (LET) strategy
    125–6
  retesting   129
  treatment options iin high DFT
    128–9, **128**
  upper limit of vulnerability (ULV)
    126–7
ICD therapy, indications
  in adults   **65**
  in arrhythmogenic right
    ventricular
    dysplasia/cardiomyopathy
    (ARVD/C)   70–1
  in Brugada syndrome (BrS)
    68–70, *69*
  in catecholaminergic polymorphic
    ventricular tachycardia
    (CPVT)   67–8
  in congenital heart disease (CHD)
    63–5, **64, 65**
  in hypertrophic cardiomyopathy
    (HCM)   65–6
  in long QT syndrome (LQTS)
    66–7
ICD troubleshooting and follow-up
  254–70
  failure to deliver therapy   267–8,
    267–8
  ICD generator failure   270, **270**
  ICD therapy   255–6

nonphysiologic oversensing
  256–9, *257–62*
physiological oversensing
  259–62
  extracardiac signals   259
  intracardiac signals   259–62
  P-wave oversensing   263
  R-wave double counting   264
  small caliber ICD lead failures
    270
  supraventricular tachycardia
    264–6, *264, 265–6*
  T-wave oversensing   262–3, *263*
  unsuccessful therapy   268–70,
    269
impedance   15
implantable cardioverter defibrillator
  (ICD)
  basic concepts   21–2
  history of   8–9
implantable cardioverter-defibrillator
  (ICD) *see under* ICD
implantable loop recorder (ILR)
  282–6, *283, 284, 287*
  adult trials utilizing   284–5
  indications for   282–4
  pediatric studies utilizing   285–6
  recent updates   286
indifferent electrode   15
International Study of Syncope of
  Uncertain Origin (ISSUE)
  285
intra-atrial reentrant tachycardia
  (IART)   41–3, 55, 216
intrinsic deflection   14
Intrinsic RV Study   74
IS-1 in line lead connectors   19, *19*

Jervell Lange-Nielsen syndrome   67

Kawasaki disease   39
Kearns-Sayre syndrome   40

lead   82
lead extraction   190–5
lead INDEX   48
lead maturation   13
lead perforation   178–82
  acute perforation   178–80
  chronic perforation   180, *180*
  lead placement into systemic
    circulation   180
  lead dislodgement   180–2
lead selection   43–9
  active versus passive fixation   46,
    46
  epicardial versus transvenous
    pacing   43–6, *44*
  lead size   47–8

lumenless leads   48–9
steroid eluting leads   46
unipolar versus bipolar
  configurations   46–7, **47**
VDD lead (single-pass lead)   49
leadless pacemakers   21, *22*
lead-related failures   187–90
  failure to capture   187–8
  insulation break   189–90
  lead failure   188
  lead fracture   188–9
leads
  construction and components
    15–19, *15*
  four-pole connector system   19,
    19
  history of   5
  insulation   17–19, **18**
left atrial isomerism   40, 41
left bundle branch block (LBBB)   97,
  98, 100, 101, 102–3, 157, 178
left cervical sympathetic denervation
  (LCSD)   66
LIA™ (Lead Integrity Alert)   30
lithium-idiode cells   5, 20
locking stylets   191, *193*
long QT syndrome (LQT)   41, 43,
  66–7. 124 254, 283
lowest energy tested (LET) strategy
  125–6
Lyme disease   39

magnetic resonance Imaging (MRI)
  conditional pacemakers   21,
    247–9, **248**
Managed Ventricular Pacing (MVP)
  54, 72, 74, 216
mechanical activation during sinus
  rhythm   94–7, *95, 96*
Medtronic 4968® epicardial bipolar
  pace/sense lead   81
Medtronic Adapta model   55
Medtronic AT500 pacemaker   55
Medtronic bipolar coaxial   6495 206
Medtronic EnRhythm model   55
Medtronic EveraTM   76
Medtronic Fidelis ICD lead   188
Medtronic ICD key programmable
  features   **218–20**
Medtronic Kappa platform
  (accelerometer)   121
Medtronic pacemakers   55
Medtronic Protecta® devices   76
Medtronic Rate Drop Response   55
Medtronic Search AV+   216
Medtronic SelectSecure™ lead   17,
  17
  3830 lead   141

Medtronic Sprint Fidelis® ICD lead 24, 78, 154, 188, 270
Medtronic Sprint Quattro Secure® lead failure   78
metal ion oxidation   18
miniaturization   6
M-mode   276
MP35N® conductor   17
MP35N® silver cored conductor   17
MUGA scan   275
Multicenter Insync Randomized Clinical Evaluation (MIRACLE) trial   110
multiprogrammability   6
Multisite Stimulation in Cardiomyopathy (MUSTIC) trial   101
myocarditis, viral   39
Myopore® Sutureless, Screw-In bipolar epicardial lead   82
myotonic muscular dystrophy   39

noninvasive programmed stimulation (NIPS)   56
non-looping monitors (TTM)   286
nonphysiologic oversensing   256–9, 257–62
North American Society of Pacing and Electrophysiology (NASPE)   7–8
Norwood palliation   109

optimization in pediatrics and CHD   278
oversensing   238–9, 255, **256**, 256–62

pacemaker codes   6–7
pacemaker crosstalk   245–6, 247, 248
pacemaker follow-up   249–50
  ancillary testing   252
  database   252
  frequency of pacemaker monitoring   **249**
  pacemaker device evaluation   250–2, 251
  patient evaluation   250
  threshold margin test   249
pacemaker generator construction and components   19–21, 20
pacemaker mediated tachycardia (PMT)   242–4
pacemaker programming   211–17
  antitachycardia pacing for atrialarrhythmias   216–17
  automatic adjustments to lead parameters   227

AV node dysfunction   215
  reducing unnecessary ventricular pacing   225–6
  sinus node dysfunction   214–15
pacemaker pulse generator, selection of   49–56
  advanced device features   53–6
  atrial antitachycardia pacing (ATP)   55–6
  automatic pacing output adjustment   53
  basic device features   52–3
  general device consideration   49–50, **50**
  mode switching   53
  MRI compatibility   51–2
  preferential intrinsic ventricular conduction   54
  rate responsive pacing   52–3
  rate-adaptive AV delay adjustment   53–4
  single versus dual chamber pacing   51
  size considerations   50–1
  sleep mode and hysteresis rates   54
  sudden bradycardia response   54–5
pacemaker sensing   13–14
pacemaker troubleshooting   233–52
  automatic mode switch algorithms   242
  loss of capture issues   240
  MRI   247–9, **248**
  maladaptive pacemaker function in young/repaired CHD   239–40
  noise reversion   246–7, 248
  pacemaker crosstalk   245–6, 247, 248
  pacemaker mediated tachycardia (PMT)   242–4
  programming
    complex congenital heart disease   235–7
    in hypertrophic cardiomyopathy   235
    in long QT syndrome (LQTS)   233–4
    neurocardiogenic syncope   235
    pallid breathholding   235
  sensing   237–9
  upper rate behaviors   240–2
pacemakers, history of   1–5
Pacesetter Microny generators   53
pacing modes, history of   5–6
pacing system analyzer (PSA)   178
PainFREE RX and RXII trials   227–30

passive fixation   16, 17
pause dependent ventricular arrhythmias   151
permanent epicardial pacing   165–72
  complications   171, 172
  high risk patient with complete congenital AV block   168–9, 168
  lead longevity and implantation   167–8
  lead placement and cardiomyopathy   167
  leads and implantation approaches   170–1, 170
  after multiple cardiac surgeries   169–70, 169
  patient anatomy and physiology   166–7
  patient size   165–6
  primary indications   **166**
permanent pacing implantation, indications for   37–43, **38**, **42**
  acquired heart block   39–40
  congenital heart block   40–1
  intraatrial reentrant tachycardia (IART)   41–3, 55
  long QT syndrome   43
  sinus node dysfunction   41
  vasovagal syncope   43
peroneal muscular atrophy   40
physiological oversensing   259–62
  extracardiac signals   259
  intracardiac signals   259–62
pneumothorax   140, 176
polarization   16, 16
polyurethane leads   190
post cardiac transplant   152
post-surgical bundle-branch block   74
post-ventricular atrial refractory period (PVARP)   241, 243
PREPARE study   218–19
protein losing enteropathy (PLE)   41
public access defibrillation   291
pulse amplitude   12
pulse duration   12
pulse generator pocket   182–4
  chronic pocket pain   183
  dehiscence   184
  device erosion   183, 183
  ecchymosis   182
  infection   183–4
  pocket hematoma formation   182–3
Punctua™ family of devices   76
Purkinje-myocardial junctions   93
P-wave oversensing   263

quality of life   304–5

Random-access memory
        (RAM)/Read only memory
        (ROM) chips   21
RandomizedAssessment of Syncope
        Trial (RAST)   284
Rate Drop Response (Medtronic)
        54, 55
rate responsive pacing system, ideal
        121
recommended replacement time
        (RRT)   20
Regency generators   53
remote monitoring   30–1
renal failure   64
repetitive nonreentrant
        ventriculoatrial synchronous
        rhythm   243
rheobase   12
rheumatic fever   39
Right Ventricular (RV) Lead Noise
        Discrimination algorithm
        30
Ritter method for AV optimization
        276
RockyMountain spotted fever   39
Ross-Konno procedure   39
RV Lead Noise   30
R-wave double counting   264
ryanodine receptor 2 gene (RyR2)
        68

sarcoidosis   39
sarcoplasmic reticular Ca²⁺
        adenosine triphosphatase
        (SERCA)   94
scan (ATP)   27
Seldinger technique   5, 138
SelectSecure lead   48–9
Senning operation   41, 156–7, 236,
        237
sensing threshold   14
sensor driven pacing   119–23, **120**
sensors   121–2
   accelerometer   233
   chest impedance of 'minute
        ventilation'   122
   myocardial conductance   22
   practical consideration   122
sheaths   191–3
   mechanical   191–2, *193*
   powered   192–3, *194*
sickle cell disease   64
silicone leads   190, *190*
single ventricle physiology   63
Single-Chamber External Pulse
        Generators   202, *203*

sinus node dysfunction (SND)   41,
        67, 150
sinus tachycardia   75
slew rate   15
SMART AV trial   275
sotalol   42, 128
speckle tracking   278, *279*
   strain analysis, 2D   111
sports participation   305–8
St. Jude Durata lead   25
St. Jude Ellipse™ ICD   76
St. Jude Fortify® family of ICDs   76
St. Jude key programmable features
        225–7
St. Jude lead   19
St. Jude Medical Microny generator
        51
St. Jude Medical ships anodal devices
        76
St. Jude Medical, Capsure®   4698
        172
St. Jude Riata lead   24, 25, 270
   failure rate   78
St. Jude Riata leads   25, 270
St. Jude Riata ST lead   24, 25
St. Jude Riata ST Optim™ lead
        18–19, 25
St. Jude Riata® ICD Lead   78
Staphylococcus aureus   184
Staphylococcus epidermidis   184
START study   317
steroid eluting leads   13, *13*, 14
stimulating electrode   15
stimulation threshold   12–15
   factors affecting   13, **14**
strength-duration curve   12
structurally normal heart,
        transvenous pacemaker,
        permanent   135–46
   device location and pocket
        creation   144–5
   equipment for device pocket
        creation   136
   generator change   145–6
   lead placement in structurally
        normal heart   140–4, *141*,
        142
   procedural requirements and
        patient selection   135–8
   single vs dual chamber pacing
        137
   transvenous access and site
        selection   138–40
subclavian crush syndrome   140
subcutaneous ICD   84
sudden bradycardia response   54
supraventricular tachycardia   75,
        264–6, *264*, *265–6*
SureScan system   52

syncope   150–1
systolic dyssynchrony index (SDI)
        159

tachyarrhythmias   178
'tachycardia-bradycardia syndrome'
        42
TARGET study   102
Teletronics Accufix pacemaker lead
        188
temporary cardiac pacing (TCP)
        197–209
   complications   **213**
   indications   **198**
tetralogy of Fallot (TOF)   39, 63,
        64
three-dimensional echocardiography
        111, 278, *280*
three-dimensional electroanatomical
        mapping   111
threshold energy (TE)   45
tiered therapy   8–9
TightRail™   194
TightRail Mini™   194
timing circuit   20
Timothy syndrome   67
tissue Doppler imaging (TDI)   160,
        160, 276–8
torsade de pointes   75
traction tools   191
transcutanous pacing   198–9
   indications   198
   limitations   199
   technical considerations   198–9
transesophageal pacing   199–201
   indications   199–200
   limitations   201
   technical considerations   200–1
transtelephonic monitor (TTM)
        286
transtelephoninc looping   286
transtelephoninc non-looping   286
transvenous leads   13, 44
   air embolism   177–8
   hemothorax   176–7
   miscellaneous access related
        complications   178
   pneumothorax   176
   venous access related
        complications   176
T-wave oversensing   262–3, *263*
Twiddler's syndrome   145. *146*
two-dimensional speckle-tracking
        strain analysis   111

unipolar pacing system   15, *15*, 16
upper limit of vulnerability (ULV)
        126–7

V sensing and refractory (unique to
        devices)   83–4
    following sensed ventricular events
        83–4
vasovagal syncope   43
VDD lead   215
velocity time integral (VTI)   160
venous access related complications
    176
venous thrombosis   184–90
    acute thrombosis   184–5
    chronic venous occlusion   185
    device related failures and
        management   185–6
    battery depletion   186–7
    device malfunctions   187
    lead-related failures   187–90

ventricular electrograms (VEGM)
        template   75
ventricular fibrillation   21
Ventricular Intrinsic Preference
        (VIP)   54
ventricular septal defect (VSD) repair
    39
ventricular synchrony in adult heart
        failure   100–3, 100–1
    alternative strategies for
        resynchronizing failing LV
        102–3
    CRT in restoring failing LV in
        adults   100–2, 100–1
    recommendations for   104
ventricular synchrony in pediatric
        and CHD   103–11

restoring in failing LV   102–5
restoring in failing V   106–9
restoring in failing single ventricle
    109–10
short and midterm outcomes of
    CRT   110–11
ventricular tachycardia (VT)   26
viral myocarditis   39
VV offset   275
VV optimization   276–8

wearable external pacemaker, history
    of   4, 4
Wolff–Parkinson–White syndrome
    283